A Textbook of
Pharmacognosy

A Textbook of
Pharmacognosy

Prof. N.P.S Sengar
M.Pharm, (Ph.D)
STRT Pharmacy, Bhopal.

Ritesh Agrawal
M.Pharm, PGD-PPHC, DPPM

Ashwini Singh
M.Pharm
SIRT Pharmacy, Bhopal.

PharmaMed Press
An imprint of BSP Books Pvt. Ltd.
4-4-309/316, Giriraj Lane,
Sultan Bazar, Hyderabad - 500 095.

A Textbook of Pharmacognosy
by **N. P. S. Sengar, Ritesh Agrawal and Ashwini Singh**

Ninth Reprint 2025

Published by :

PharmaMed Press
An imprint of BSP Books Pvt. Ltd.
4-4-309/316, Giriraj Lane, Sultan Bazar, Hyderabad - 500 095.
Phone: 040-23445688 Fax: 91+40-23445611
E-mail: info@pharmamedpress.com
www.pharmamedpress.com/pharmamedpress.net

Printed at
Repro India Limited.

Price: Rs. 375.00

ISBN: 978-81-8844-981-1 (Papaerback)

Dedicated to

Dr. A.K. Pathak

Head, Department of Pharmacy,
Dean Faculty of Engineering,
Barkatullah University, Bhopal.

Preface

It gives us immense pleasures in bringing out our first book in pharmacognosy for the benefit of the students of B.Pharmacy.

The Chapter on Biogenesis of Phytopharmaceuticals and basic metabolic pathways deals with various metabolic pathways for secondary metabollies. The chapter on Radiotracer techniques, chemical nature of phytoconstituents, screening of drugs covered all necessary and important topics associated with these chapters respectively.

The Aromatic plants, Plant Tissue Culture, Herbs as health food topics also covered in this book.

Various isolation techniques, extraction procedures and anlytical techniques e.g. chromatography, spectral analysis of crude drugs had been extensively covered.

In conclusion, particular thanks are due to Mrs. Parul Sengar for her involvment in proof reading. We are grateful to Er. Sanjeev Agrawal Chairman of SIRT - Pharmacy, Bhopal for his encouragement and continuous support.

We are thankful to Mr. Anil shah and theri staff bringing out this first edition of this book.

Bhopal,
July - 2009.

- Authors

Contents

CHAPTER 1

INTRODUCTION OF PHARMACOGNOSY

1.1 Introduction

Pharmacognosy is branch of science in which we study the medicines derived from natural sources. It is also defined as "the study of the physical, chemical, biochemical and biological properties of drugs, drug substances or potential drugs or drug substances of natural origin as well as the search for new drugs from natural sources". The word." Pharmacognosy" derives from the Greek words pharmakon (drug) and gnosis (knowledge). The contemporary study of pharmacognosy can be divided into the fields of ethnobotany (the study of the use of plants for medicinal purposes), ethnophamarcology (the study of the pharmacological qualities of traditional medicinal substances), phytotherapy (the medicinal use of plant extracts) and phytochemistry (the study of chemicals derived from plants including the identification of new drug candidates derived from plant sources). Mainly pharmacognosy is concerned with crude drugs of vegetable mineral and animals origin; a large number of these crude drugs for e.g. senna from plant origin and kaolin or musk from mineral or animal origin. In brief one might say that pharmacognogy is the scientific study of the structural, physical, chemical and sensory characters of crude drugs of animals , vegetable & mineral origin and include also their history cultivation and collection in other particular relating to the treatment they receive during their passage from the producer to the distributor or pharmacist. Pharmacognosy is concerned mainly with naturally occurring substances having a medicinal action, it is not limited to such substances. Thus surgical dressings prepared from natural fibres disintegrates, filtering and suspending agent, herbicides, allergens, insecticides, toxins etc case is also associated with pharmacognosy.

Pharmacognosy is closely related to botany and plant chemistry. Pharmacognosy, an applied science has played an important role in the development of different branch of sciences. Plant taxonomy, plant genetic, phyto chemistry, zoology, pharmacology, plant tissue culture microbiology , analytical chemistry, genetic engineering etc., and all other developments in other disciplines of science have increased the areas of pharmaconosy. The use of new isolation and analytical techniques and pharmacological testing procedures means that new crude drugs usually find their way into medicine as purified substances rather than in the form of galenical preparations.

Many of the botanical, physical techniques used in pharmacognosy are also applicable to the analysis of other commodities for example (foods, gums, fabrics etc) and are therefore used by public analyst, chemist of quality control, forensic chemists associated with other industries.

CHAPTER 2

BIOGENESIS OF PHYTO-PHARMACEUTICALS AND BASIC METABOLIC PATHWAYS

2.1 Phyto-pharmaceuticals

"Phyto-pharmaceuticals are those pharmaceutical agents derived from plants and other plant related sources".

A higher living plant is considered as a Solar-powered biochemical/biosynthetic factory which manufactures various metabolites from air, water, minerals and sunlight. These *Metabolites* are of two types:

Primary Metabolites	Secondary Metabolites
These are the substances widely distributed in the nature occurring in one form or another in all the organisms. *e.g.* Sugars, Amino acids and fatty acids etc.	These are biosynthetically derived from primary metabolites but are more limited in distribution being restricted to a taxonomic group. *e.g.* Glycosides, Alkaloids, Flavanoids, Volatile oils etc.

Secondary metabolites may represent chemical adaptations or may serve as protective chemicals against microbes, insects and other predators. These metabolites are sometimes considered to be as the waste or secretory products of plant metabolism.

The various biosynthetic reactions occurring in plant cells are enzyme dependent where in enzyme acts as a catalyst of metabolism and is through the control of enzymatic activity that plant metabolism is directed into specific biosynthetic pathways. The enzymatic reactions are reversible and secondary metabolites are synthesized and hydrolysed under the influence of enzymes. The production of secondary metabolites is dependent on the fundamental metabolic cycles of the living tissue. The elucidation of biosynthetic pathways in the plants for production of various plant metabolites have been examined by means of isotopically labelled precursors.

The Biogenesis process of phyto-pharmaceuticals undergone through some metabolic pathways, in which the pharmaceutical products are dissociated in their metabolites form in the presence of enzyme.

2.2 Basic Metabolic Pathways

The Metabolic pathways are also called as Biosynthetic pathways. The major source of carbon is glucose, which is photosynthesized in green plants, and is breakdown and converted to sugar phosphates. This process involved two pathways:

(i) Pentose Phosphate cycle (A direct Pathway)

(ii) Glycolysis (EMI Pathway)

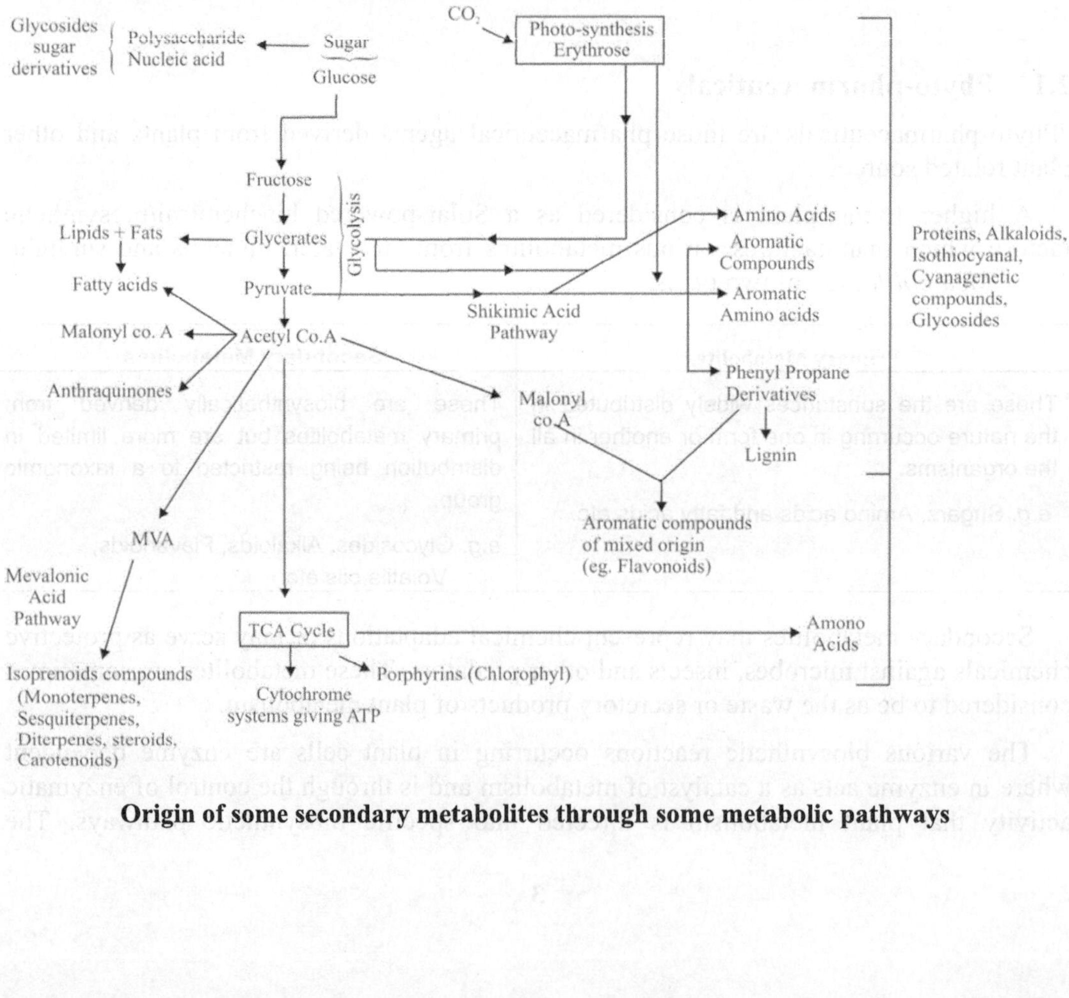

Origin of some secondary metabolites through some metabolic pathways

(a) *Shikimic Acid Pathway*

The shikimic acid is an important intermediate pathway from carbohydrate for the biosynthesis of C_6-C_3 units (Phenyl propane derivatives) *e.g.* Tyrosine and phenylalanine.

1. The shikimic acid serves as an intermediate in the production of tannins, flavones, coumarins and vanillin. It also serves as a precursor of biosynthesis of amino acids.
2. The pathway finds its importance in the genesis of lignin also.

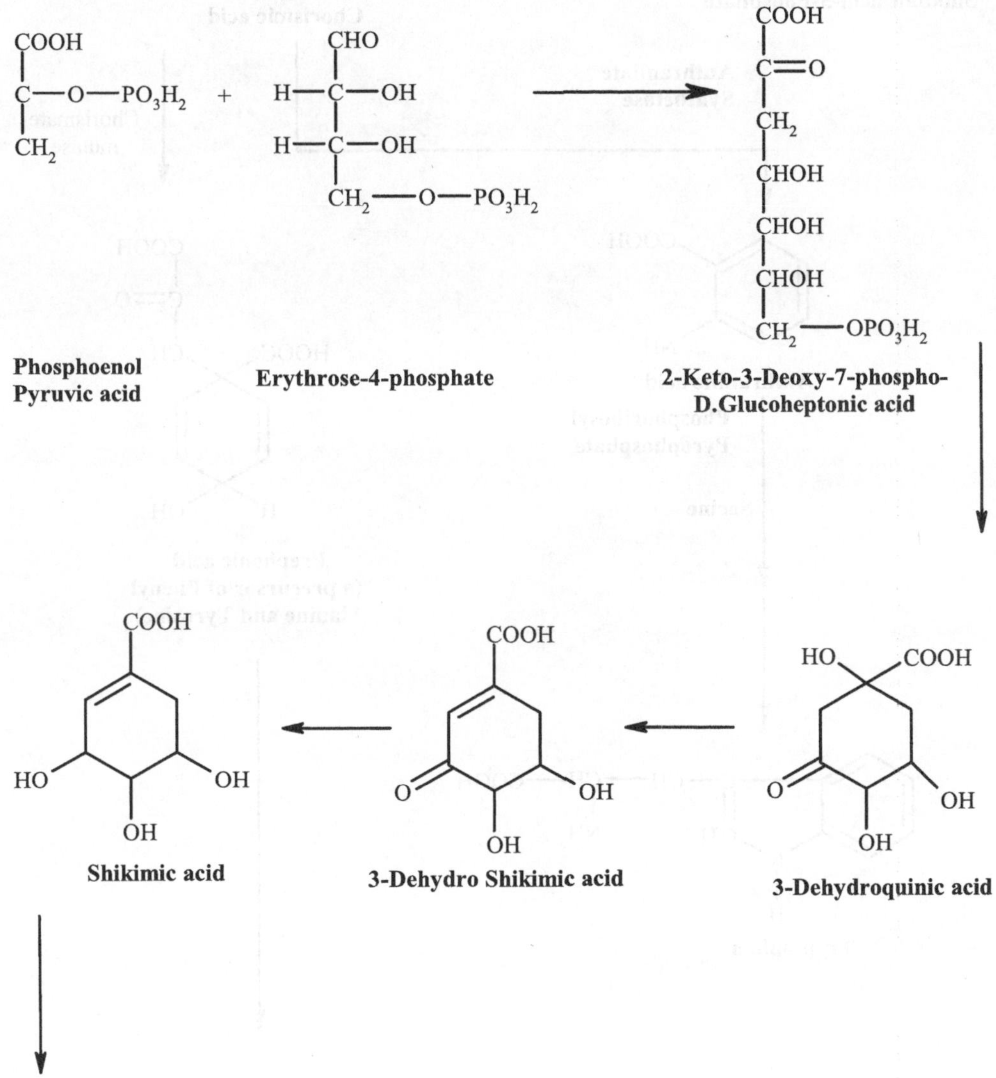

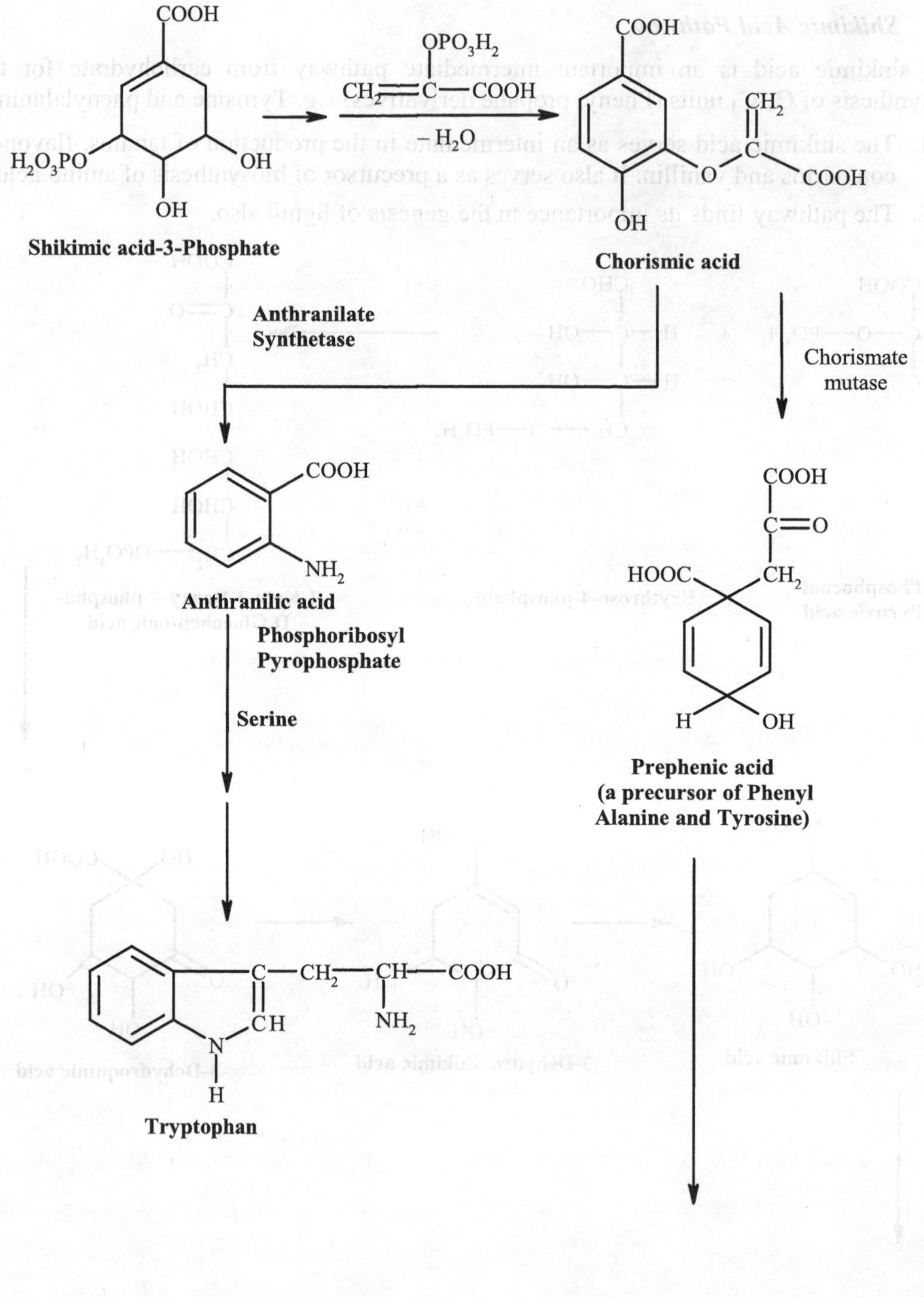
COOH
OPO₃H₂
CH₂=C—COOH
−H₂O
H₂O₃PO
OH
OH
Shikimic acid-3-Phosphate
COOH
CH₂
C
O
COOH
OH
Chorismic acid
Anthranilate
Synthetase
Chorismate
mutase
COOH
NH₂
Anthranilic acid
Phosphoribosyl
Pyrophosphate
Serine
COOH
C=O
HOOC
CH₂
H
OH
Prephenic acid
(a precursor of Phenyl
Alanine and Tyrosine)
C—CH₂—CH—COOH
CH
NH₂
N
H
Tryptophan

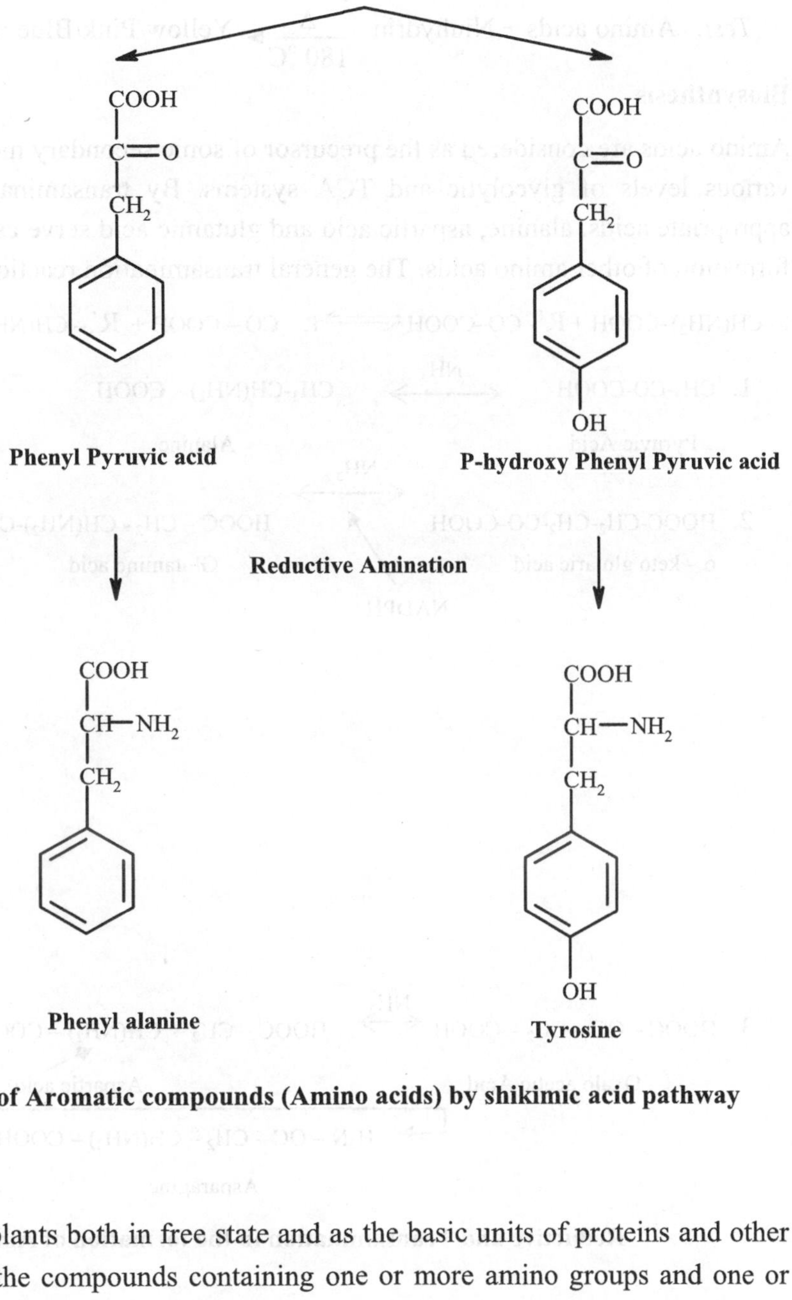

Biosynthesis of Aromatic compounds (Amino acids) by shikimic acid pathway

(b) *Amino Acids*

Amino acids occur in plants both in free state and as the basic units of proteins and other metabolites. They are the compounds containing one or more amino groups and one or more carboxylic acid groups. Most of those present in nature are α-amino acids with an asymmetric carbon atom and general formula R-CH-(NH_2)-COOH. Generally amino acids soluble in water but slightly soluble in alcohol.

Test: Amino acids + Ninhydrin $\xrightarrow[180\,^{\circ}C]{\Delta}$ Yellow/Pink/Blue or violet colour

Biosynthesis

Amino acids are considered as the precursor of some secondary metabolites. They arise at various levels of glycolytic and TCA systems. By transamination reactions with an appropriate acids, alanine, aspartic acid and glutamic acid serve as α-amine donors in the formation of other amino acids. The general transamination reaction may be written as:

$$R\text{–}CH(NH_2)\text{–}COOH + R'\text{–}CO\text{–}COOH \rightleftharpoons R - CO - COOH + R' - CH(NH_2) - COOH$$

1. $CH_3\text{-}CO\text{-}COOH \xleftrightarrow{NH_3} CH_3\text{-}CH(NH_2) - COOH$

   Pyruvic Acid → Alanine

2. $HOOC\text{-}CH_2\text{-}CH_2\text{-}CO\text{-}COOH \xleftrightarrow{NH_3} HOOC - CH_2 - CH(NH_2)\text{-}COOH + NAD$ (NADPH)

   α - keto glutaric acid → Glutamine acid

   $\updownarrow NH_3$

   $H_2N\text{-}OC\text{-}CH_2\text{-}CH_2\text{-}CH(NH_2)\text{-}COOH$

   Glutamine

3. $HOOC - CO - CH_2 - COOH \xleftrightarrow{NH_3} HOOC - CH_2 - CH(NH_2) - COOH$

   Oxalo acetic Acid → Aspartic acid

   $\xrightarrow{NH_3} H_2N - OC - CH_2 - CH(NH_2) - COOH$

   Asparagine

Reductive and Transamination in the formation of Amino acids

(c) Cyanogenetic Compounds

Cyanogenetic compounds are phenyl propanoid derivatives derived from amino acids such as phenyl alanine and Tyrosine (products of shikimic acid pathway).

Biosynthesis

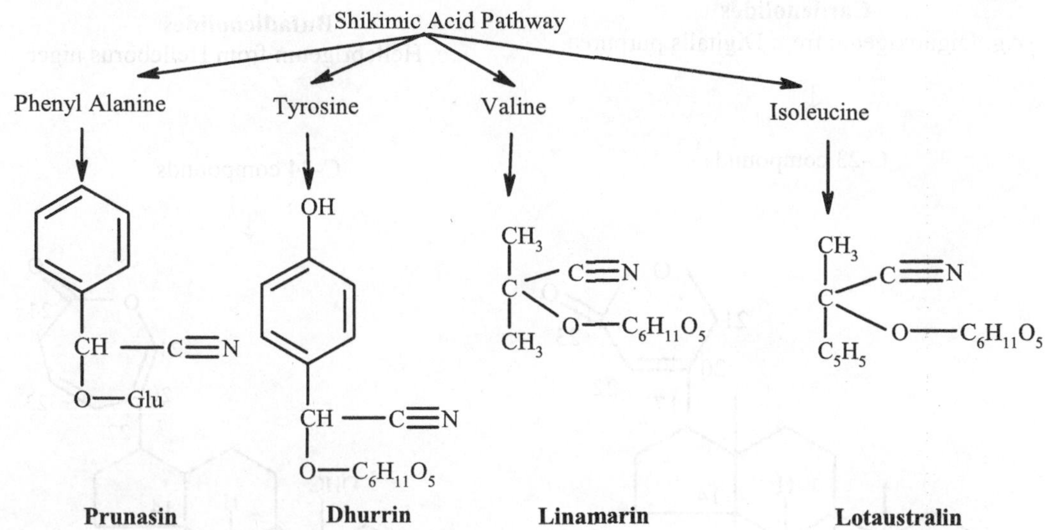

(d) Glycosides (Cardioactive)

The Metabolic processes of glycoside formation essentially consists of two parts. They are:

- The reactions by means of which various types of aglycones are formed.
- Metabolic pathway involving coupling of aglycone with sugar moiety.

Biosynthesis

When the Nucleotide glucoside such as UDP Glucose in the plant cells interact with alcoholic/phenolic group of aglycone, Glycosides are biosynthesized. The principal pathway of glycoside formation involves the transfer of uridylyl group from uridine triphosphate (UTP) to sugar-1 phosphate and the enzymes catalyzing this reaction are called as uridylyl transferases.

$$\text{UTP} + \text{sugar-1 phosphate} \underset{\text{Transferases}}{\overset{\text{Uridylyl}}{\rightleftharpoons}} \text{UDP} - \text{Sugar} + \text{PP}_1$$

$$\text{UDP} + \text{Sugar} + \text{Aglycone} \underset{\text{Transferases}}{\overset{\text{Glycosyl}}{\rightleftharpoons}} \text{Glycoside} + \text{UDP}$$

Furthermore, *cardioactive glycosides*, are used to strengthen a weakened heart and allow it to function more efficiently. Also improves the blood supply to the kidneys.

e.g. Digitalis (Heart drugs), Strophanthus (Arrow poisons)

The therapeutic action by cardioactive glucosides depends on the structure of aglycone and on the type and number of sugar units attached.

Two types of Aglycone are recognized

Cardenolides	**Bufadienolides**
e.g. Digitoxigenin from Digitalis purpurea	*e.g.* Hellebrigenin from Helleborus niger
↓	↓
C-23 compounds	C-24 compounds
↓	↓

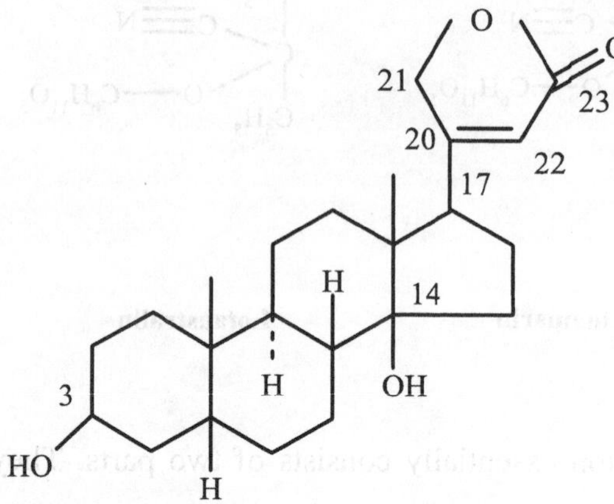

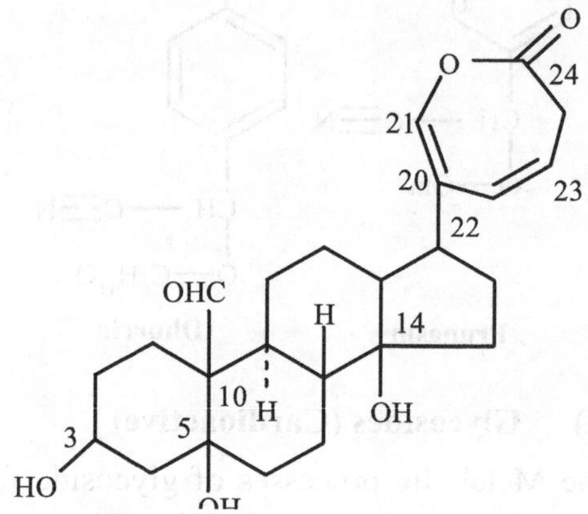

Characteristic Features:

(i) cis-fusion for both A/B and C/D rings

(ii) 3β-and 14 β-Hydroxyl groups with glycoside function at C-3.

(iii) α, β-unsaturated lactone grouping at C-17 β.

(iv) Sugar residues on 3β-hydroxyl group.

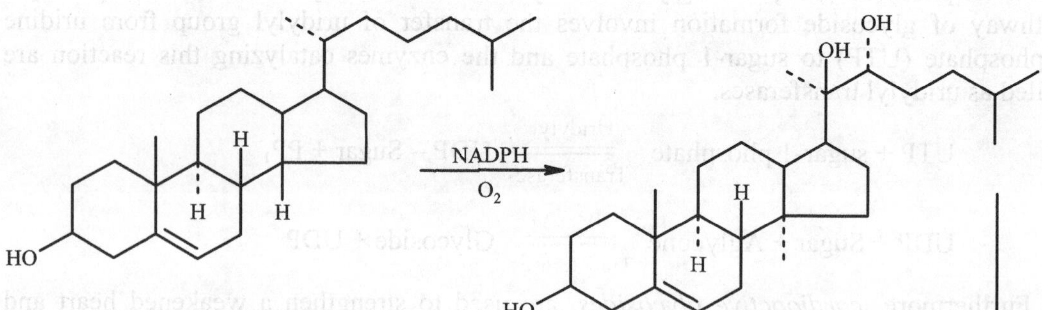

Cholesterol (Stepwise hydroxylation via 22-hydroxy cholesterol)

(Oxidative cleavage between hydroxyls via peroxide)

NADPH O_2

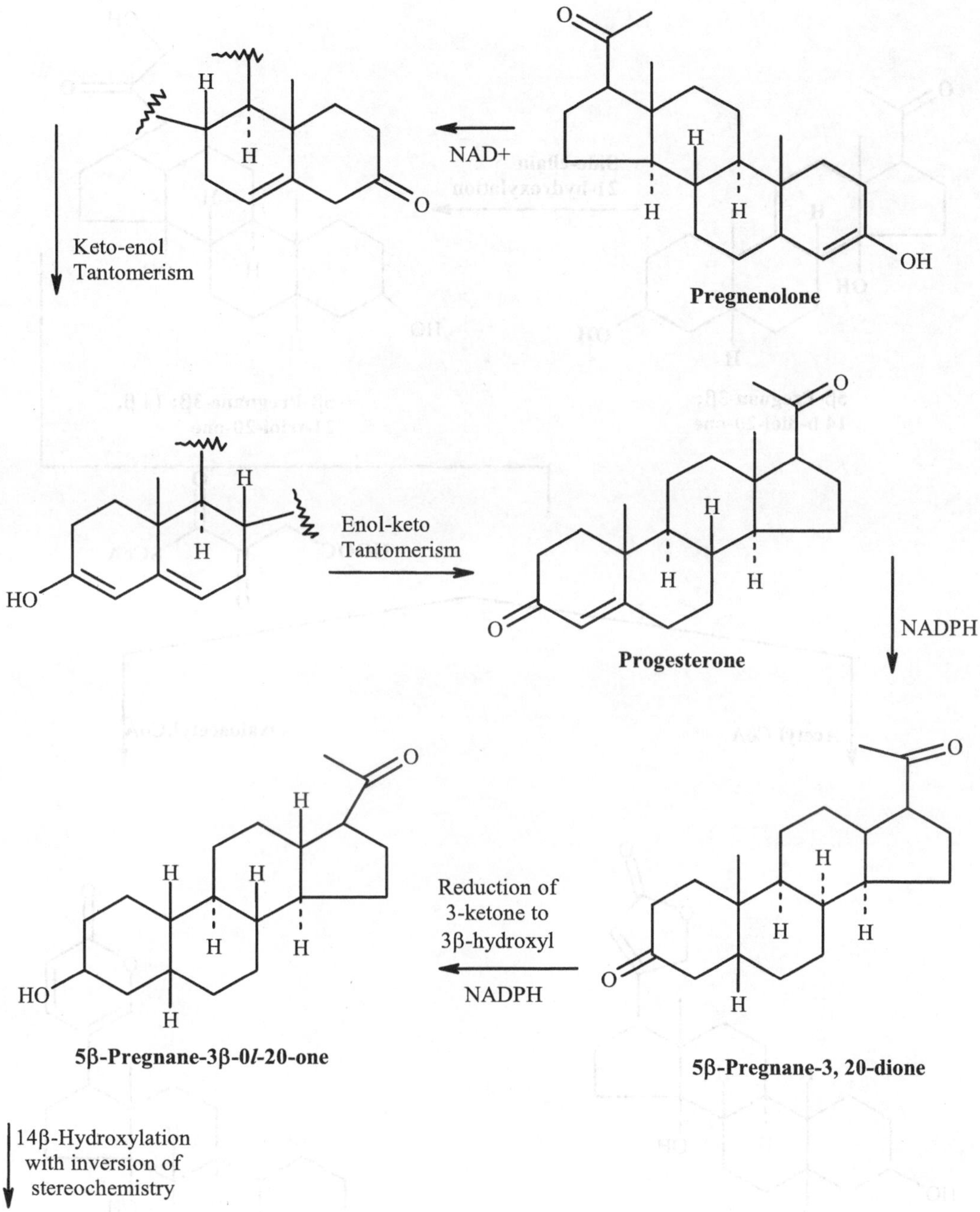
NAD+
Keto-enol Tantomerism
Pregnenolone
Enol-keto Tantomerism
Progesterone
NADPH
Reduction of 3-ketone to 3β-hydroxyl
NADPH
5β-Pregnane-3β-0*l*-20-one
5β-Pregnane-3, 20-dione
14β-Hydroxylation with inversion of stereochemistry

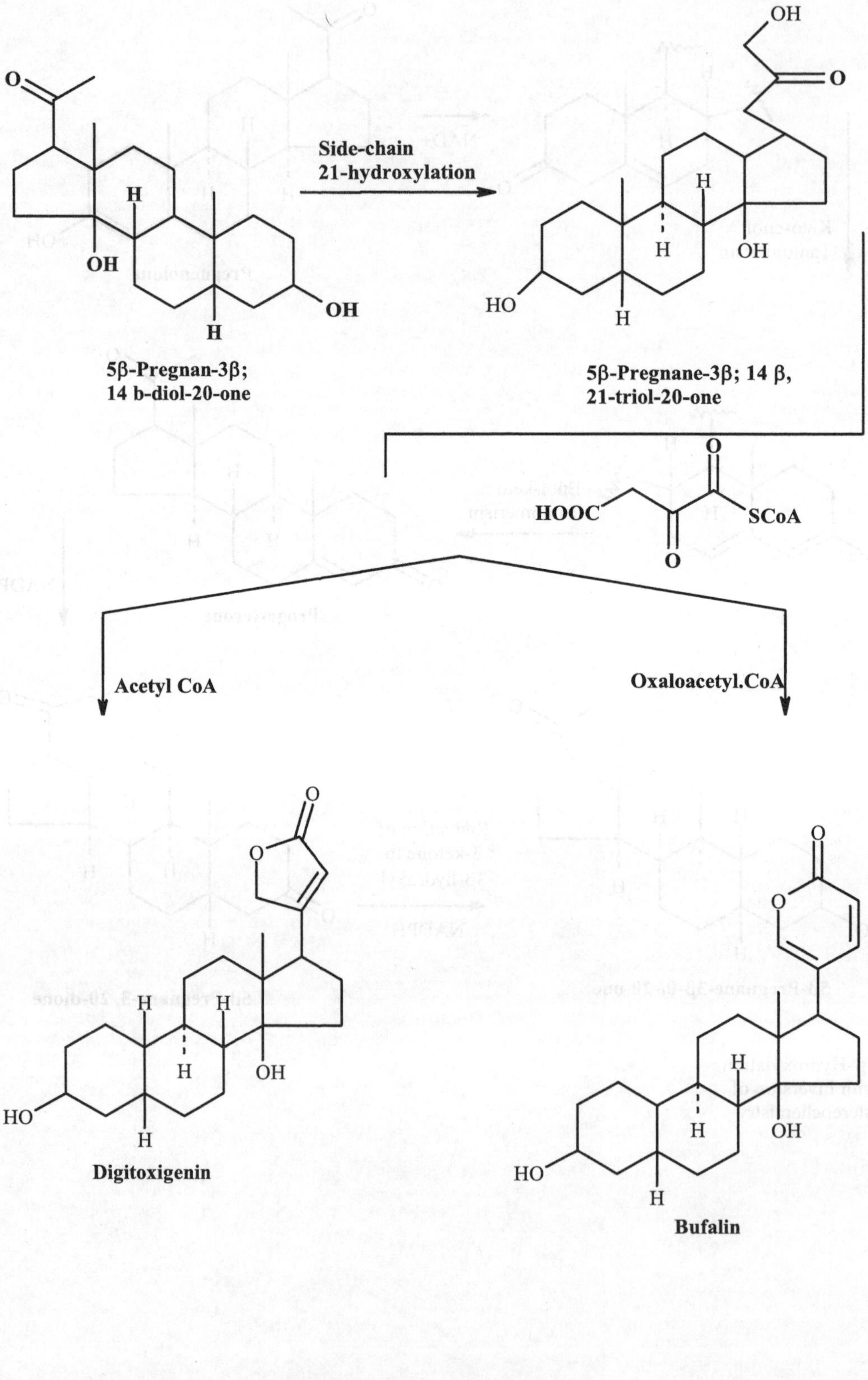
Side-chain
21-hydroxylation
5β-Pregnan-3β;
14 b-diol-20-one
5β-Pregnane-3β; 14 β,
21-triol-20-one
HOOC
SCoA
Acetyl CoA
Oxaloacetyl.CoA
Digitoxigenin
Bufalin

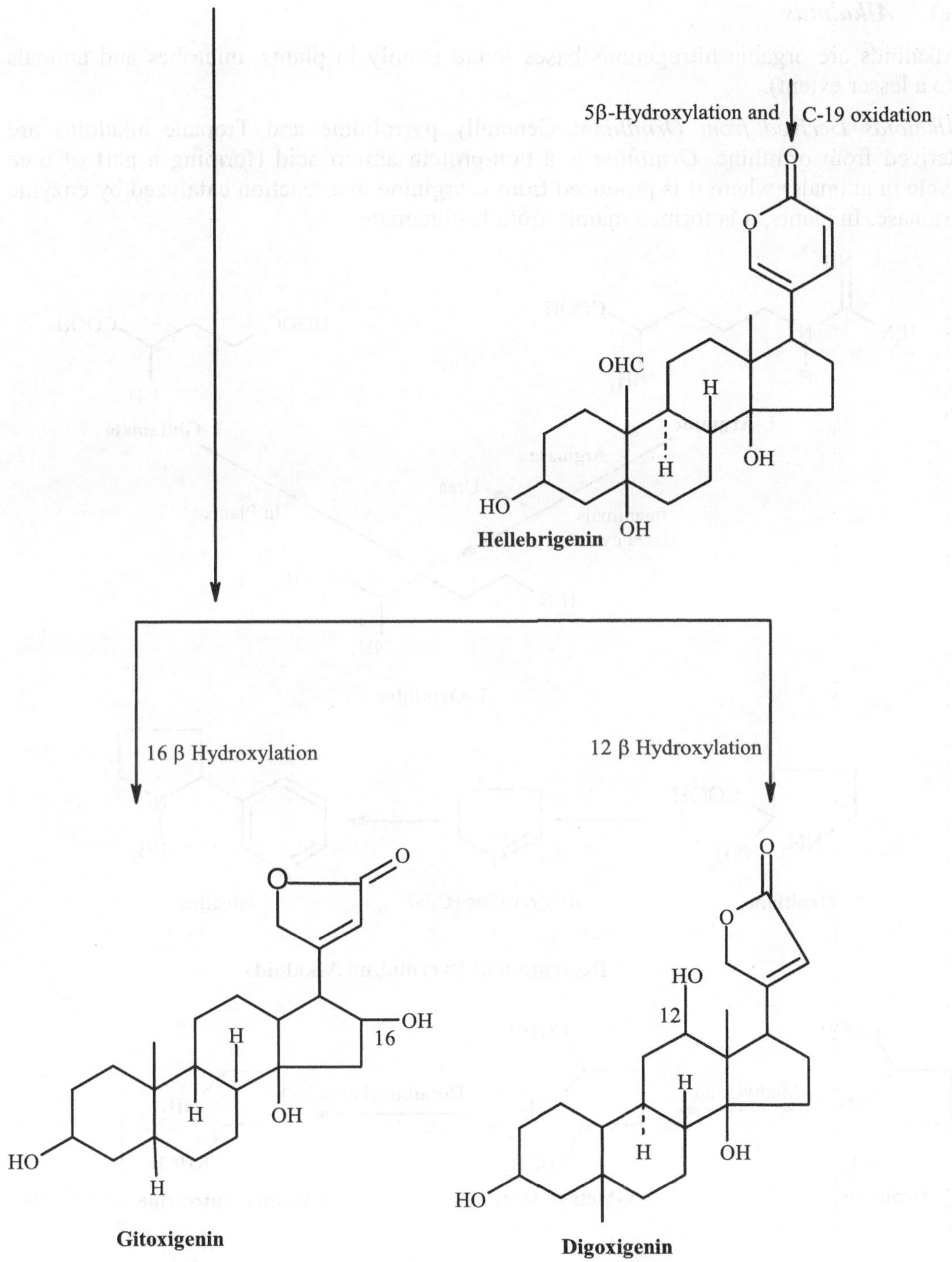
5β-Hydroxylation and C-19 oxidation
OHC
H
H
OH
HO
OH
O
O
Hellebrigenin
16 β Hydroxylation
12 β Hydroxylation
O
O
OH
16
H
H
OH
HO
H
Gitoxigenin
O
O
HO
12
H
H
OH
HO
Digoxigenin

(e) *Alkaloids*

Alkaloids are organic nitrogenous bases found mainly in plants, microbes and animals (to a lesser extent).

*Alkaloids Derived from Ornithin***e:** Generally pyrrolidine and Tropane alkaloids are derived from ornithine. *Ornithine* is a non-protein amino acid (forming a part of urea cycle in animals) where it is produced from L-arginine in a reaction catalyzed by enzyme arginase. In plants, it is formed mainly from L-glutamate.

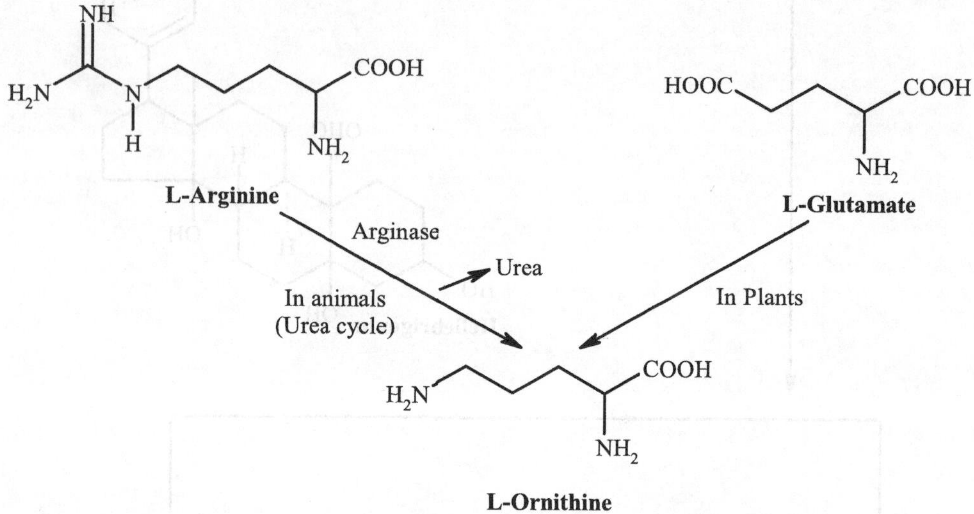

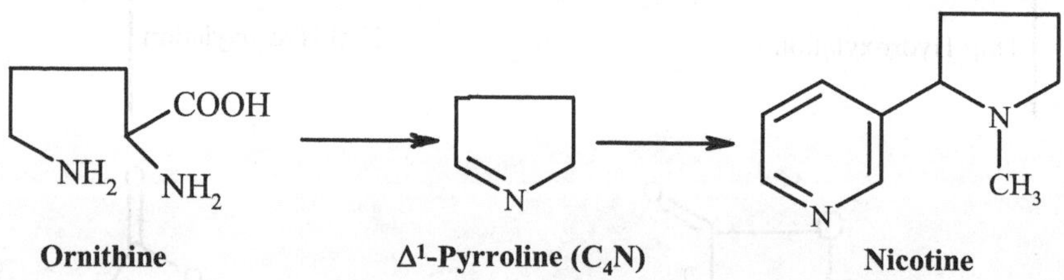

Derivation of Pyrrolidine Alkaloids

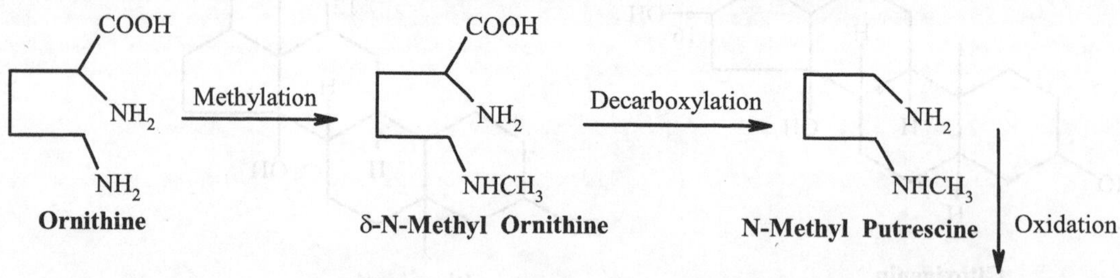

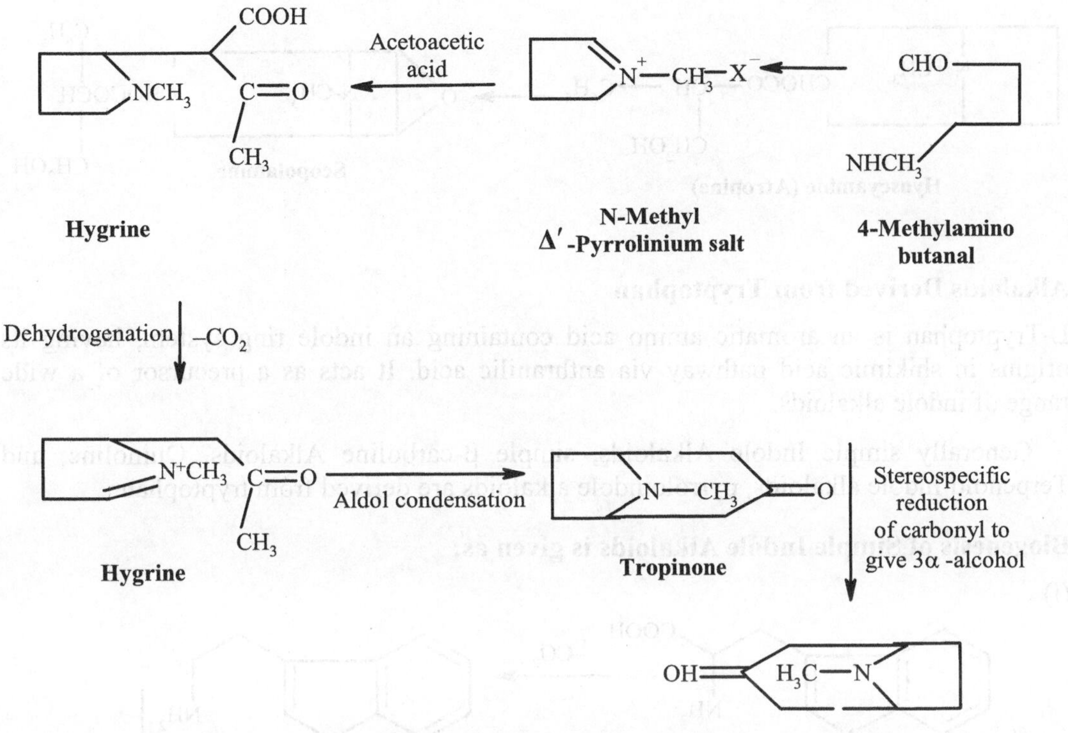

Biogenesis of Tropane Alkaloids

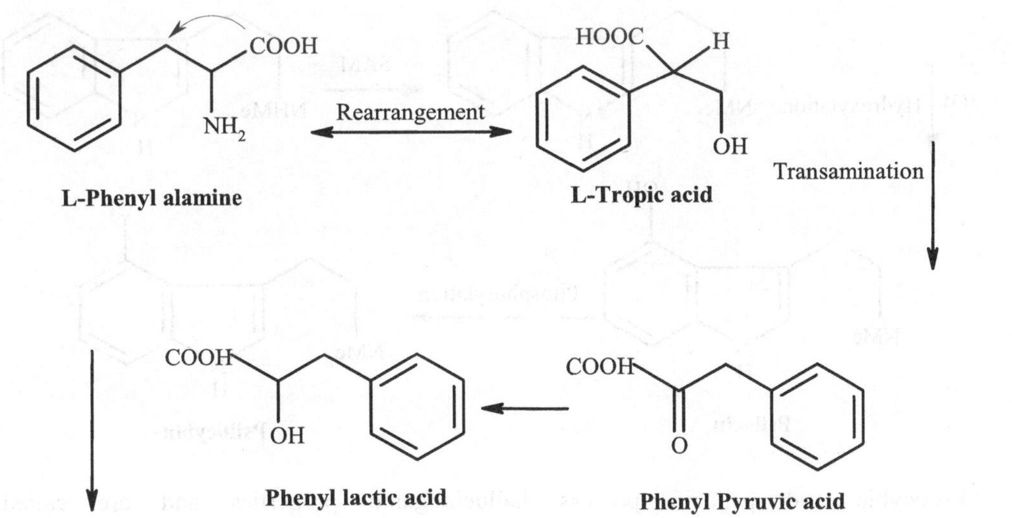

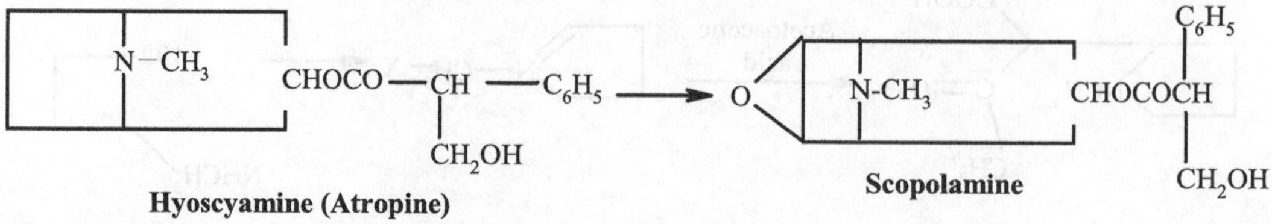

Alkaloids Derived from Tryptophan

L-Tryptophan is an aromatic amino acid containing an indole ring system, having its origins in shikimic acid pathway via anthranilic acid. It acts as a precursor of a wide range of indole alkaloids.

Generally simple Indole Alkaloids, simple β-carboline Alkaloids, Quinoline, and Terpenoid Indole alkaloids, pyrroloindole alkaloids are derived from tryptophan.

Biogenesis of Simple Indole Alkaloids is given as:

(i)

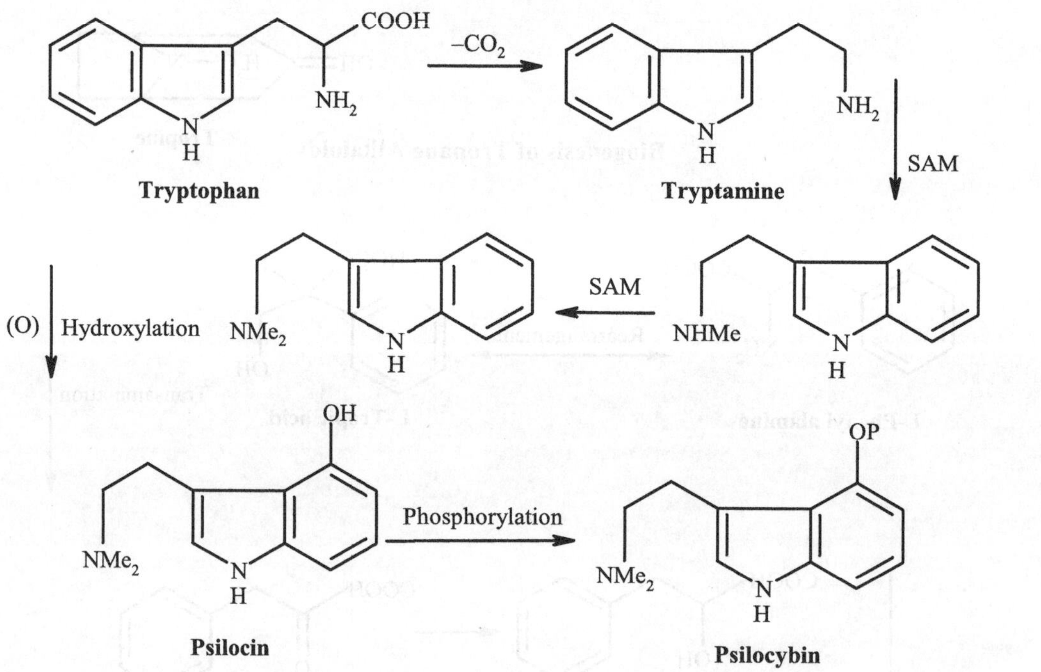

"Psilocybin and psilocin possess hallucinogenic properties and are called as Magic-Mushrooms."

(ii)

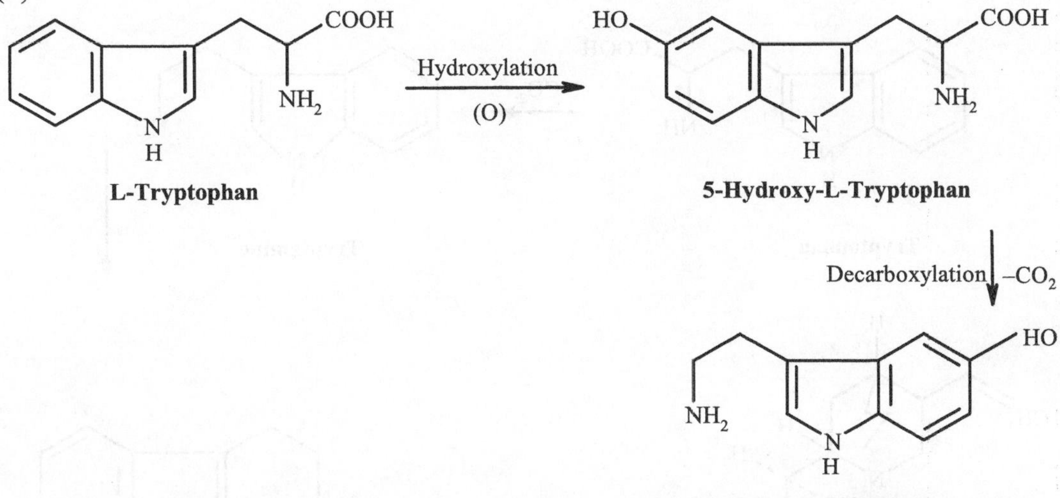

L-Tryptophan → **5-Hydroxy-L-Tryptophan** → **5-Hydroxy Tryptamine (5-HT, Serotonin)**

Serotonin (5-HT) in mammalian tissue acts as a neurotransmitter in the central Nervous system. It stimulates contraction of smooth muscles and is a powerful vasoconstrictor.

Biogenesis of β-Carboline Alkaloids is given as:

(*e.g.* Harmine, Eleagnine)

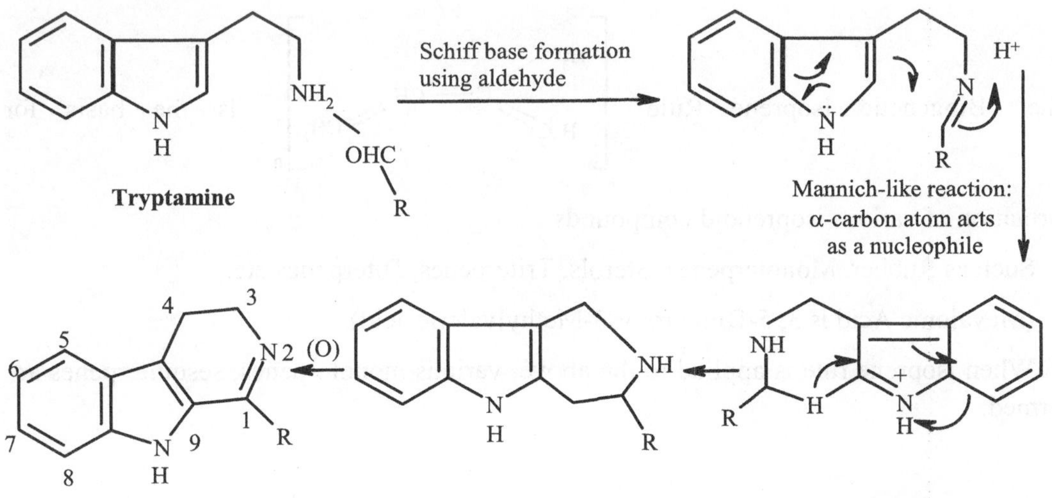

Tryptamine

Tautomerism to restore asomaticity

β-carboline

Biogenesis of Quinoline Alkaloids is given as:

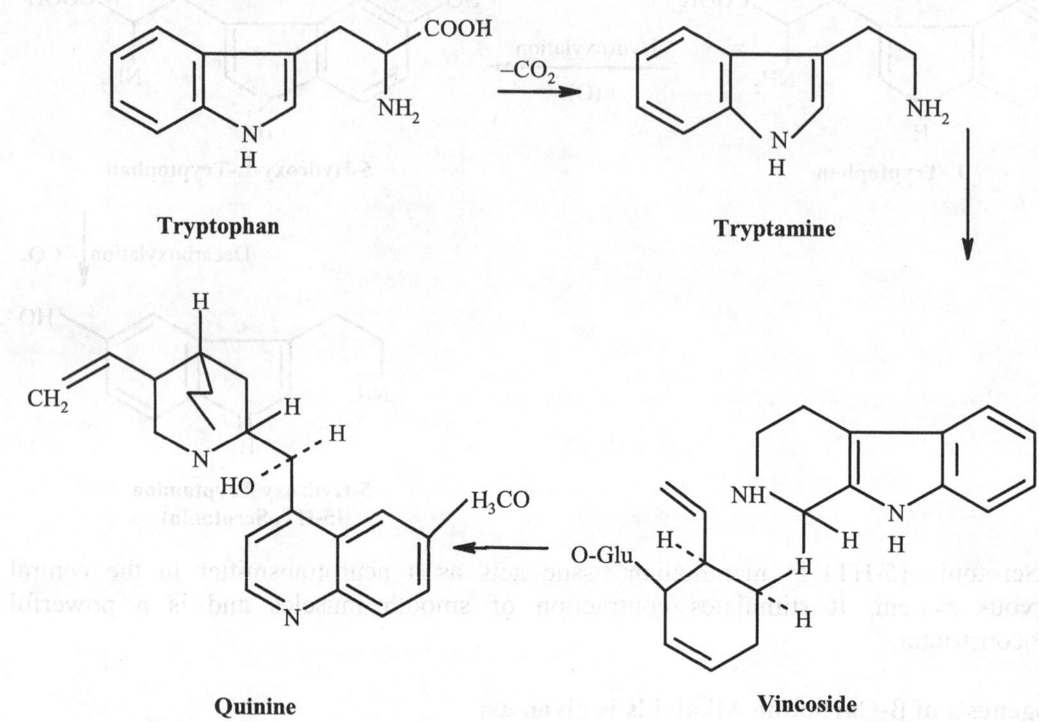

Mevalonic Acid Pathway

The “Biogenetic Isoprene Rule” 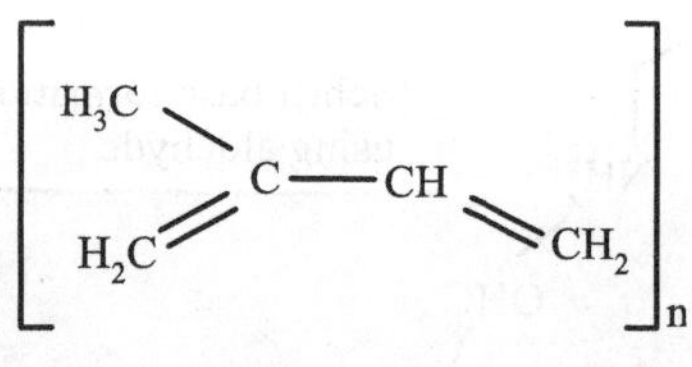 is the basis for formation of various isoprenoid compounds.

Such as Rubber, Monoterpenes, Sterols, Triterpenes, Diterpenes etc.

(Mevalonic Acid is 3, 5-Dihydroxy-3-Methylvaleric acid).

When isoprene rule is applied to the above, various monoterpenes, sesquiterpenes are formed.

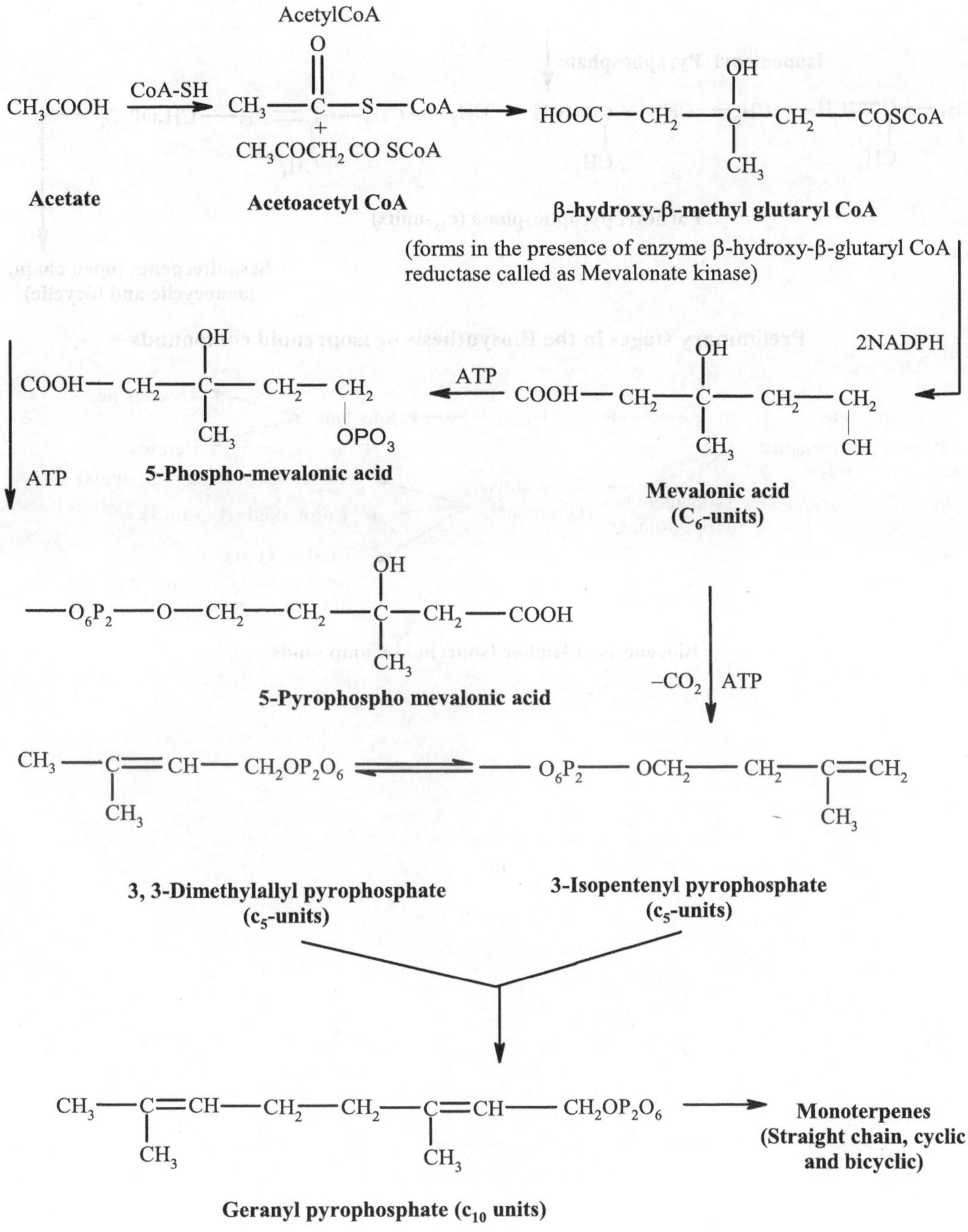
AcetylCoA
CoA-SH
Acetate
Acetoacetyl CoA
β-hydroxy-β-methyl glutaryl CoA
(forms in the presence of enzyme β-hydroxy-β-glutaryl CoA reductase called as Mevalonate kinase)
2NADPH
ATP
Mevalonic acid
(C_6-units)
5-Phospho-mevalonic acid
ATP
5-Pyrophospho mevalonic acid
$-CO_2$ ATP
3, 3-Dimethylallyl pyrophosphate
(c_5-units)
3-Isopentenyl pyrophosphate
(c_5-units)
Geranyl pyrophosphate (c_{10} units)
Monoterpenes
(Straight chain, cyclic and bicyclic)

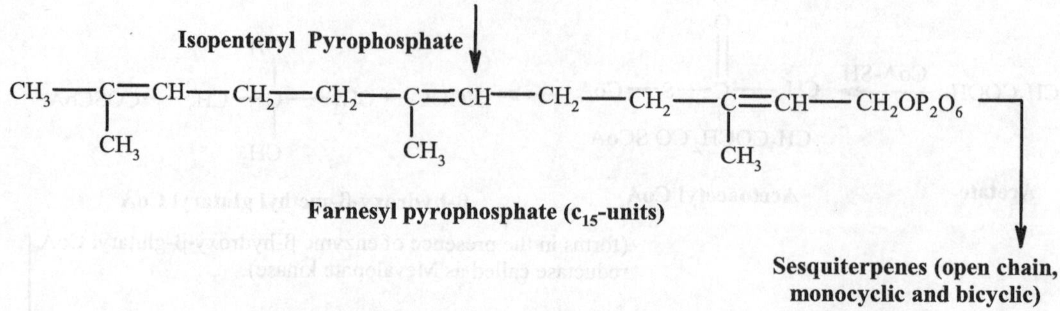

Preliminary stages in the Biosynthesis of Isoprenoid compounds

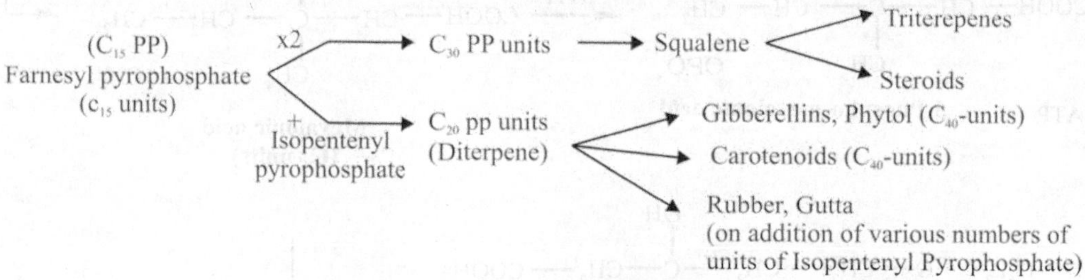

Biogenesis of Higher Isoprenoid Compounds

CHAPTER 3

CHEMICAL NATURE OF PHYTOCONSTITUENTS

3.1 Introduction

The pharmacological actions of crude drugs are determined by the nature of their constituents. The constituents which are synthesized, isolated and purified on a large scale from the nature, are itself used in the preparation of drug and has certain advantages like:

(i) Pharmaceutically it leads to a more suitable and elegant preparation free from undesirable inert constituents.

(ii) Economically it ensures a regular supply at fairly uniform prices.

(iii) Medically it can be guaranteed to provide doses that are more exact.

Importance

The crude drugs and galenicals obtained from plants and animals, with or without purification, are generally employed for medicine. The therapeutically active components obtained from different origins are:

Plant origin	**Animal origin**
↓	↓
Cellulose, Lignin, Suberin, Cutin, Starch, Albumin	Keratin, chitin, Muscle fibre, Connective tissues

(i) Many crude drugs provide natural mixture of medicinal substances which produce a therapeutic action. One component produces desired therapeutic effect whereas the other enhances activity or nullify the side effects of inert materials, extracted crystallized and purified for therapeutic use called as secondary substances.

(ii) The Metabolic processes occurring in plants are of two kinds:

- The Anabolic or building up process where the materials of plant tissues and food reserves including the synthesis of carbohydrates, fats and oils, proteins are formed.
- The Catabolic process consisting of oxidation process arising from plant respiration, hydrolysis of oils and fats, fermentation process where the breakdown of food reservoir takes place, converted into more soluble forms and then utilized by plants for its growth and development.

Various plant drugs chemically consists of a complex but organized mixture of organic and inorganic constituents. Parmaceutically important active constituents are studied under the following categories:

3.2 Alkaloids

The term 'alkaloid' is applied to naturally occurring basic compounds. The term is derived from 'Vegetable alkali' meaning *alkali-like*.

"Alkaloids are a chemically heterogenous group of natural substances comprises of nitrogen containing organic compounds with widely different chemical constituents".

General Chemical Tests

I. Precipitation Reactions

1. *Mayer's Reagent (Mercuric Potassium Iodide solution)*: KI + Mercuric chloride, until precipitation of mercuric iodide redissolves and gives white or pale yellow precipitation except with alkaloid of purine base.
2. *Dragendorff's Reagent (potassium bismuth iodide)*: Adding excess of KI to a solution of bismuth nitrate gives orange or orange red precipitate.
3. *Wagner's Reagent (A solution of Iodine with KI)*: Gives brown or reddish brown precipitate. This test is used in official alkaloidal assay as a test for complete extract of colchicine or emetin.
4. *Hager's Reagent (Saturated solution of picric acid in cold water)*: Gives characteristic crystalline yellow precipitate with many alkaloids. Alkaloid can be identified by its microscopic examination and melting point of its picrate ion formed.

5. Kraut's Reagent (Modified Dragendorff's reagent)

   Bismuth Nitrate + Nitric acid + KI

6. *Marme's Reagent*: A solution of potassium cadmium iodide.

7. *Scheibler's Reagent (Phosphotungstic acid)*: Sodium tungstate + Water + Acidified with HNO_3 acid.

8. *Sonnenschein's Reagent*: (A solution of Phosphomolybdic acid).

9. *Reineckate's Salt Solution Test*: Saturated aqueous solution of Ammonia Reineckate + Hydroxylamine HCl + ethanol + slightly acidified with HCl acid → Pink precipitate.

10. *Gold Chloride Test*: Used for Belladonna Alkaloids.

11. *Picric Acid Test*: Used for Belladonna Alkaloids.

12. *Tannic Acid Test*: A freshly prepared aqueous solution of tannic acid (5% w/v) gives a precipitate soluble in dilute acid or ammonia solution. Used for Belladonna alkaloids.

II Colour Reactions

1. Marqui's Reagent (Conc. H_2SO_4 + 1 drop of 40% CH_3CHO).
2. Selenium dioxide Solution (0.5%)
3. Ammonium Molybdate solution (0.5%)
4. Saturated aqueous solution ammonium vanidate.
5. Solution of Cerric ammonium sulphate (1 gm in 99 gm of 85% phosphoric Acid).
6. Fuming Nitric acid + Alcoholic KOH solution → used for belladonna alkaloids.
7. *Modified Dragendorff's Reagent*: Solution of Bismuth sub nitrate in acetic acid (20%) + 40% of aqueous solution of KI.

III Specific Reagents

1. *Van Urk Reagent*: (used for Ergot Alkaloids).

   Blue or grey green colour. (P. dimethyl amino benzaldehyde in 40% H_2SO_4 and traces of $Fe\ Cl_3$).

2. *Frolides Reagent*: (Sulphomolybdic acid) Morphine gives violet colour.

3. *Vitali Reagent*: Belladonna + Tropane Alkaloids → violet colour. (Fuming HNO_3 acid + Alcoholic KOH solution)

4. *Cerric Ammonium Sulphate acidified with* H_2SO_4 *or* H_3PO_4: Indole Alkaloids such as Nux-Vomica, Ergot, Vinca, Rauwolfia.

5. *Ferric chloride + Perchloric Acid Mixture*: Used for Rauwolfia Alkaloids.

6. Formic Acid (As spraying agent for TLC plates): Cinchona alkaloids, under UV light gives dark and blue fluorescence.
7. *Ferric Chloride Reagent*: In 0.5 N HCl solution for colchicine.
8. *Vanillin Phosphoric Acid*: When sprayed on TLC plates will give colour of steroids. *e.g.* Gluco Alkaloids.
9. Traces of HNO_3: Used for identification of constituents of Nux-vomica seeds.

   Strychnine = Yellow colour
   Brucine = Red colour
10. *Murexide Test*: Used for Purine derivative – caffeine.

    Mixing caffeine + small amount of potassium chlorate ($KClO_3$) + a drop of HCl → evaporating to dryness and exposing the residue to ammonia vapours. A purple colour is produced.
11. Yellow colour by colchicine with mineral acids.
12. Bluish violet to red colour given by Indole alkaloids when treated with H_2SO_4 and P-dimethyl amino benzaldehyde.

Chemical Nature

(i) Alkaloids generally contain one nitrogen atom which may exists as a primary (RNH_2), secondary (R_2NH) and tertiary amine (R_3N).

(ii) As the nitrogen atom contains an unshared pair of electrons, such compounds are basic in nature and possess chemical properties of ammonia.

(iii) The degree of basicity depends on the structure of molecule and presence and location of other functional groups.

(iv) Alkaloids are converted into their salts by aqueous mineral acids.

(v) When the salt of an alkaloid is treated with hydroxide ion, nitrogen gives up a hydrogen ion and free amine is liberated.

(vi) Quarternary ammonium compounds ($R_4N^+X^-$) such as Tubocurarine chloride, have four organic groups covalevetly bonded to nitrogen and the positive charge of this ion is balanced by some negative ion.

(vii) These are basic in reaction.

(viii) Soluble in a number of immiscible organic solvents such as ether, chloroform etc.

(ix) Insoluble in water but salts formed on reaction with acids are usually freely soluble.

(x) Alkaloids are usually classified according to the nature of basic chemical structures from which they are derived. Based on the chemical class they are grouped into:

Group I : Based upon pyridine/piperidine Nucleus

Group II : Based upon Pyrrol/Pyrrolidine Nucleus

Alkaloids in this group include:

Nicotine = From Tobacco

Hygrine = occurs in small quantities in coca leaves.

Group III : Based upon Tropane Nucleus

Group IV : Based upon Quinoline Nucleus

Group V : Based upon Isoquinoline Nucleus

Group VI : Based upon Indole Nucleus

Group VII : Based upon following Nuclei

Glyoxaline → Pyrrolizidine steroid

Quinazoline → Phenanthrene steroid

Group VIII : Substituted Amines

e.g. Colchicine (Colchicum seeds), Ephedrine

Group IX : Purines

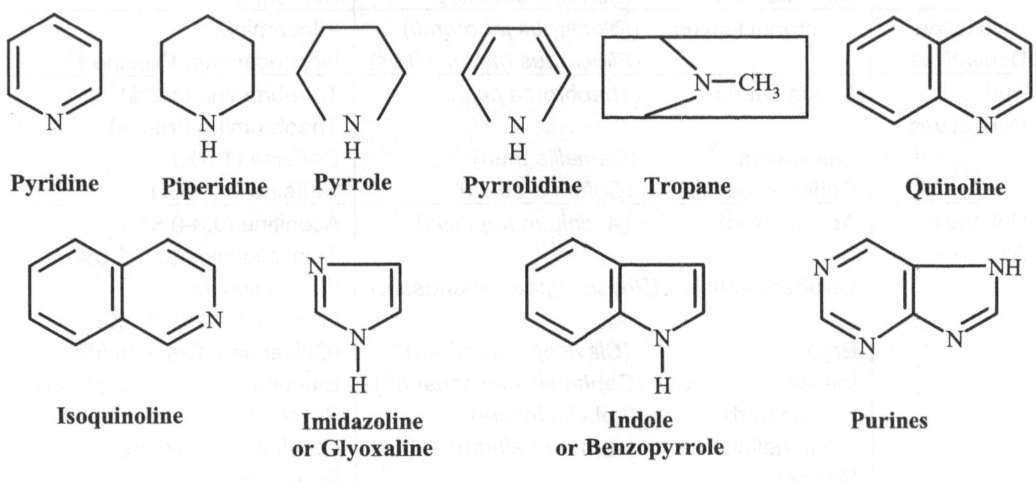

Basic Nucleus of Alkaloids

Drugs Containing Alkaloids

Class of Alkaloids	Name of Crude Drug + Botanical Source	Active Alkaloids
Pyridine derivatives	Areca Nuts (*Areca catechu*) Fenugreek seeds (*Trigonella Foenumgraecum*) Black pepper (*Piper nigrum*)	Arecoline, arecaine Trigonelline, Choline Piperine (5-8%)
Tropane Derivatives	Datura leaves and seeds (*Datura fastuosa*) (*Datura metel*) Henbane leaves and seeds (*Henbane or Myoscyamus niger*) Belladonna leaves and roots (*Atropa belladonna*) Stramonium leaves and seeds (*Datura stramonium*)	Hyoscine (0.2-0.5%) Hyoscyamine (0.05-0.10%) Hyoscine (Traces) Hyoscyamine (0.1-0.7%) Hyoscyamine (0.2-0.5%)
Quinoline Derivatives	Nux vomica seeds (*Strychnos nux-vomica*) Red Cinchona bark (*Cinchona succirubra*)	Strychnine, brucine, total alkaloids 2-3% Quinine, cinchonidine, cinchonine, quinidine, total alkaloids 5-6%.
Iso-quinoline derivatives	Opium (*Papaver somniferum*) Hydrastis rhizome (*Hydrastis Canadensis*) Blood root (*Sanguinaria adensis*) Berberis stem (*Berberis aristata*)	Morphine (7-16%, Narcotine,codeine, thebaine, papaverine Hydrastine (1.5-3.0%) Berberin (3%) Sanguinarine, Protropine Berberine
Glyoxaline Derivatives	Jaborandi leaves (*Pilocarpus jaborandi*) (*Pilocarpus microphyllus*)	Pilocarpine, Isopilocarpine, Pilosine
Purine Derivatives	Cocoa seeds (*Theobroma cacao*) Tea leaves (*Camellia thea*) Coffee seeds (*Coffea arabica*)	Theobromine (1.2%) Theobromine (traces) Caffeine (1.5%) Caffeine (1-1.5%)
Unknown Alkaloids	Aconite Root (*Aconitum napellus*) Calabar beans (*Physostigma venenosum*) Ergot (*Claviceps purpurea*) Ipecacuanha root (*Cephaelis ipecacuanha*) Lobelia herb (*Lobelia inflata*) White hellebore (*veratrum album*) Rhizome	Aconitine (0.3-0.6%) Total alkaloids (0.5-1.5%) Physostigmine, total alkaloids (0.5-1.0) (Gelsemine, Gelsemoidine) Emetine, Cephaeline, Psychotrin Lobeline, Lobelidine, Protoveratrine, Jervine, rubijervine

3.3 Volatile Oils

Synonymns:- (Etheral/Volatile/Essential oils)

(i) The odorous and "Volatile" principles (volatile in the steam) of the plants and animal origin are termed as *Volatile oils.*

(ii) Since volatile oils are responsible for essence/odour of the plant, therefore can be termed as *Essential oils.*

(iii) Due to their "Evaporation" on exposure to air at an ordinary temperature, they are also termed as *Etheral oils.*

Chemical Nature

1. Chemically volatile oils are derived from hydrocarbons (like terpenes) and their oxygenated compounds and are made up of Isoprene units (C_5H_8) and are usually monoterpenes, sesquiterpenes and diterpenes with molecular formulae as $C_{10}H_{16}$, $C_{15}H_{24}$ and $C_{20}H_{32}$ and $C_{20}H_{32}$ respectively.
2. Usually lighter than water and differ from fixed oil in view of that, volatile oil do not leave a permanent grease spot on paper and cannot be saponified by alkalies.
3. Volatile oils have high refractive index and are mostly optically active.
4. Volatile/ essential oils classified according to their main chemical constituents are:-

   (i) Hydrocarbons

   (ii) Alcohols

   (iii) Cineole

   (iv) Aldehydes

   (v) ketones

   (vi) Phenols and Phenolic ether

   (vii) Esters

5. Chemical constituents of volatile oils and spices is divided into two broad categories, based on their methods of preparation by biosynthetic pathways.
   They are:
   - Terpenoid derivatives formed via acetate mevalonic acid pathways.
   - Aromatic compounds formed via shikimic acid – phenyl propanoid pathway.

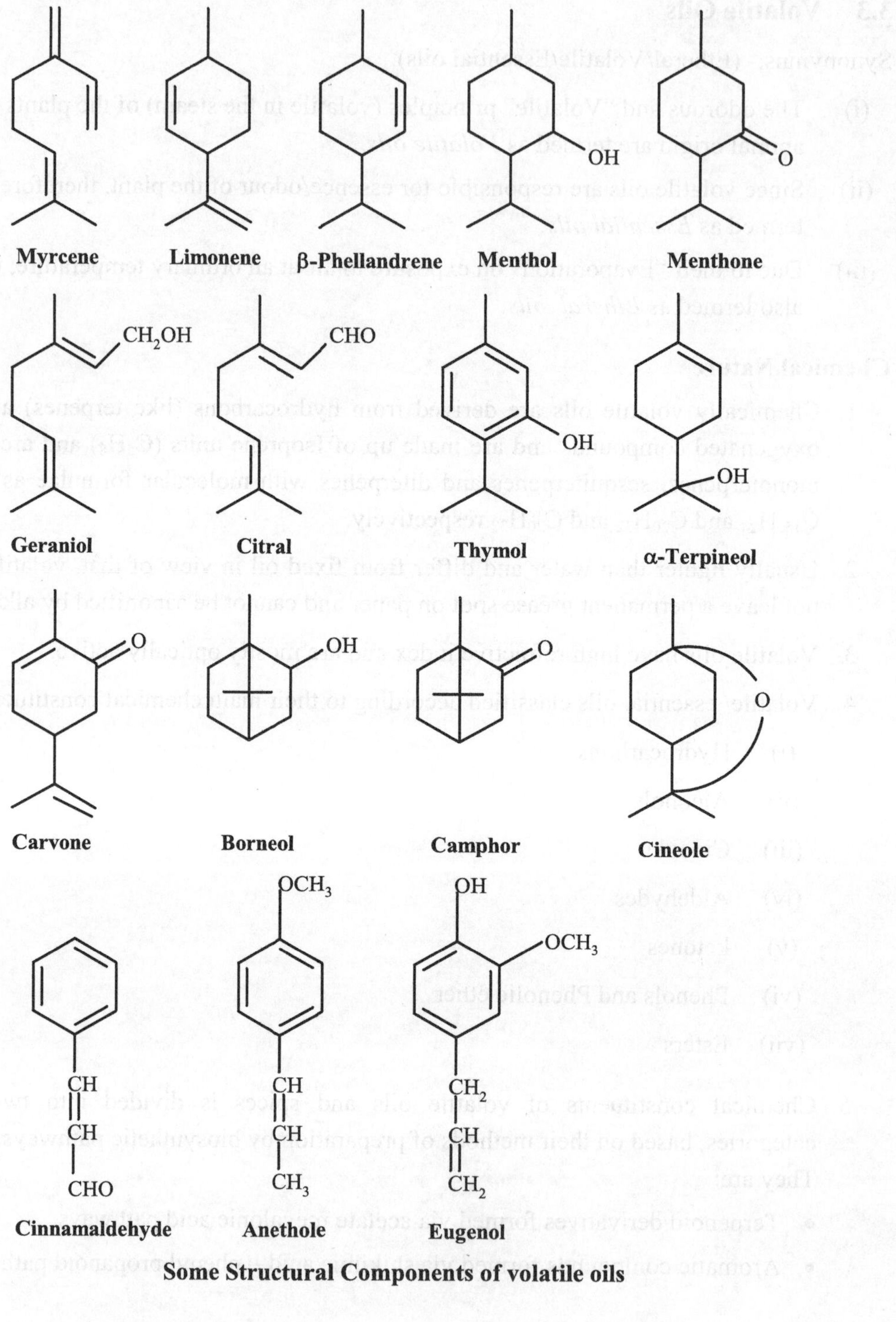

Some Structural Components of volatile oils

Class	Volatile Oil + Botanical Source	Active Constituents
Oils containing Hydrocarbons	Turpentine (*Pinus spp.*) Copaiba (*Species of Copaizera*) Juniper (*Juniperus Communis*)	Terpenes (dand / pinene) sesquiterpenes. Terpenes (pinene), sesquiterpenes (cadcine), terpene alcohols (juniper camphor)
Oils containing Alcohols	Peppermint (*Mentha piperita*) Rosemary (*Rosemarinus officinalis*) Coriander (*Coriandrum satinum*) Sandalwood (*Santalum album*) Rose (*Rosa damascena*) Lavender (*Lavendula vera*)	Alcohols (50-80%, 1-Menthol), esters (5%), aldehydes, ketones Alcohols (Borneol, 10-16%), Esters (Bornnyl acetate, 2-5%) Cineole, ketones (camphor) terpenes Alcohols (d-linalol, 45-70%) Terpenes (20%), sesquiterpene alcohols (α and β santalols, 92-98%). Alcohols 70-75% (geraniol, citronellol), solid hydrocarbons Alcohols (linalol), esters (linalyl acetate), cineole (20-30%)
Oils containing Cineole	Eucalyptus(*species of Eucalyptus*)	Cineole (55%), Hydrocarbones, Terpenes.
Oils containing Aldehydes	Cinnamon (*Cinnamomum zeylanicum*) Lemon grass (*species of Cymbopogan*)	Aldehydes (Cinnamic aldehyde (55-70%), Phenols (Eugenol). Aldehydes 70-85% (citral), alcohols, esters, terpenes.
Oils containing Ketones	Spearmint (*Mentha spicata and Mentha crispa*) Diu (*Peucedanumgraveolens*)	Ketones 91%, carvone 45-60%, alcohols, esters. Ketones (d-carnone, 40-60%)
Oils containing Esters	Wintergreen (*Gaultheria procymbens*) Mustard (*Brassica campestris*)	Esters (methyl salicylate, 99%) Esters (allyl iso-thiocyanate, 92-99%)
Oils containing Phenols and Phenolic esters	Cloves (*Eugenia caryophyllus*) Ajowan (*Carum copticum*)	Phenols (eugenol, 84-95%) alcohols, ketones, esters, phenols (thymol 34-45%) carvacrol, Terpenes.

6. Volatile oils do not become rancid, but on exposure to light and air, they oxidize and resinify.
7. Volatile oils can be distilled from their natural sources, and do not consists of glyceryl esters of fatty acids.
8. As many constituents of volatile oils possess asymmetric carbon atoms, the oil themselves rotate the plane of polarized light.

3.4 Fixed Oils, Fats and Waxes

Waxes: Waxes are present as thin deposits on leaves, stems and fruit, where they have a protective function. Chemically waxes are the esters of higher fatty acids with monohydric alcohol of high molecular weight. The waxes may also contain free acids, free alcohols, high molecular weight ketones and hydrocarbons.

The acids and alcohols used in production of waxes are:

Acid		Alcohol	
Palmitic Acid	$C_{15}H_{31}COOH$	Cetyl Alcohol	$C_{16}H_{33}OH$
Cerotic Acid	$C_{25}H_{51}COOH$	Carnaubyl	$C_{24}H_{49}OH$
Carnaubic Acid	$C_{23}H_{47}COOH$	Ceryl Alcohol	$C_{26}H_{53}OH$
Melisic Acid	$C_{29}H_{59}COOH$	Melissyl Alcohol	$C_{30}H_{61}OH$

Fixed Oils and Fats: "Fixed oils and Fats (*e.g.* Soyabean oil, theobroma oil) consists mainly of triglycerides of fatty acids and a small proportion of sterols."

Fixed Oils – Liquid at room temperature

Fats – Solid at room temperature/semi-solid

Chemical Nature

(i) Chemically they are mixtures of glycerides – esters of glycerol and various acids.

(ii) The glycerides of unsaturated acids are usually liquids (*e.g.* Olein, Linolein) whereas the glycerides of saturated acids are usually solids. (*e.g.* Palmitin, Stearin).

(iii) In the presence of moisture, hydrolysis is possible, giving free acids. This may be brought about by enzyme action or by exposure to air and light.

(iv) Glycerides containing unsaturated acids becomes oxidized and then polymerized to form insoluble resin like substances.

***Fixed Oils of Therapeutic Importance*:**

Almond oil (*Prunus amygdalus*)

Castor oil (*Ricinus communis*)

Olive oil (*Olea europaea*)

Cotton seed oild (*Gossypium spp*)

Soyabean oil (*Glycine hispida*)

Seasame oil (*Seasamum indicum*)

***Fats of Therapeutic Importance*:**

Coconut oil (*Cocos nucifera*)

Hydrocarpus oil (*Hydrocarpus wightiana*)

Theobroma oil (*Theobroma cacao*)

Nutmeg butter (*Myristica fragrans*)

(v) They leave a grease spot when the solvent is allowed to evaporate from a drop of solution placed on paper.

(vi) When the bromine water is added to an unsaturated fixed oils and fats, the colour of bromine disappears rapidly (*e.g.* Linseed oil).

***Acid Value*:** The number of 1 mg of potassium hydroxide required to neutralize the free acid in 1g of the substance is called an Acid value.

***Saponification value*:** The number of 1 mg of potassium hydroxide required to neutralize the fatty acids resulting from the complete hydrolysis of 1g of substance.

Oils and fats are hydrolyzed by boiling with excess aqueous alkali (Alcoholic solution of KOH) and the products obtained are glycerol and alkali salts of acids. These are known as soaps and the process is called as *Saponification*.

***Iodine value*:** The Iodine value of a fixed oil or fat is the weight of iodine absorbed by 100 parts of weight of the substance.

Different values of Pharmaceutically important oils

Name of Oil	Acid Value	Saponification Value	Iodine Value
Almond oil	4.0	187-195	95-100
Arachis oil	2.0	188-193	85-99
Castor oil	4.0	190-195	82-90
Cotton seed oil	0.5	177-187	103-115
Hydrocarpus oil	6.0	198-204	97-103
Linseed oil	5.0	190-198	170-200
Olive oil	2.0	188-195	79-88
Seasame oil	2.0	188-196	103-112
Theobroma oil	3.0	188-196	35-40

3.5 Resins

(i) Resins are solid/semi solid amorphous products of complex chemical nature.

(ii) Resins are usually obtained as an exudate from the plants. (end products of metabolism).

(iii) Resins are produced in plants during normal growth or secreted as a result of an injury/incision to the plant.

(iv) Resins usually occurs in schizogenous/schizosigenous cavities/ducts but yield is usually increased by an injury.

e.g. In case of pinus species.

(v) Resins are generally non-crystallizable, transluscent hard masses and on heating softens and finally melt.

Chemical Nature

Resins are chemically, complex mixture of Resenes (Hydrocarbons), Resin Acids, Resin Alcohols (Resinols) and Resin Phenols (Resinotannols) and Resin esters.

(i) *Resin acids or Resinolic acids*: These acids are of high molecular weight. They combine with alkali and other metallic salts called as Resinates. With aqueous solutions of alkali they form soap like solutions or colloidal suspensions and are used in the preparation of varnishes.

(ii) *Resin Alcohols (Resinols) and Resinotannols*: Resinols and Resinotannols are of high molecular weight and occur free or combined as esters with balsamic acids or resin acids. Resin alcohols are tetracyclic alcohols or pentacyclic alcohols and are usually α and β amyrine derivatives. The Resinotannols because of phenolic (-OH) group give colour reaction with iron salts.

(iii) *Resin Esters*: These esters are of resin alcohol/resinotannol combined with resin acids or balsamic acids.

(iv) *Resenes*: These are complex neutral inert substances and do not show any characteristic chemical properties. These substances are insoluble and do not form salts or esters and are not hydrolysed by alkalis. These are mainly of high molecular weight.

(v) *Glycoresins*: This group consists of glycosidal resins. Glycoresins on hydrolysis yield sugars and complex acids.

e.g. Jalap Resin and Ipomoea resin are glycoresins in convolvulaceae family.

(vi) *Resin Combinations*: Some Resin combinations of pharmaceutical value are:

(a) *Oleo-Resins*: These are homogenous mixture of resins and volatile oils (may be liquid, semi-solid/solid depending upon the amount of volatile oils in mixture).

e.g. Ginger, Capsicum, Malefern

(b) *Oleo-gum Resins*: These are the mixture of volatile oils, gums and resins.

e.g. Myrrh, Asafoetida

(c) *Balsams*: Balsams are very resinous mixture containing various amount of cinnamic acid, benzoic acid or esters of these acids.

e.g. Benzoin (Balsamic Resin), Storax, Balsam of tolu and Balsam of Peru.

(d) *Glycoresins*: These occur in combination with the glycosides.

e.g. Podophyllum, Convolvulaceae family.

3.6 Tannins

Earlier, Tannins was applied to the chemicals that combines with proteins of animal hide to prevent their putrefaction and to convert them into leather. Thus, *Tannins* may be defined as, "The derivatives of polyhydroxy benzoic acid, capable of combining with proteins characterized as non-crystallizable, alcohol and water soluble compounds with an acid reaction and an astringent taste".

They cause precipitation of proteins and alkaloids impart dark blue or green black colour with ferric salts and also cause contraction after applying on smooth muscles.

Chemical Nature

On the basis of chemical nature, tannins can be categorized under as:

1. *Pyrogallol/Depside Tannins*: These tannins give gallic acid as the final production of hydrolysis consists of a glucose molecule in which all the hydroxyl groups are combined with ellagic acid residues. Also called as Non-phloba tannins.

   e.g. Rhubarb, cloves, Logwood, Red Rose petals, Maple, Chestnut

They give following colour reactions:

- Blue colour or precipitate with $FeCl_3$ solution.
- Precipitated by heavy metals.
- Precipitated by gelatin.
- Precipitated by alkaloids, but slowly.
- Do not produce any precipitate with bromine water.
- Yield bulky precipitates with phenazone, especially in the presence of sodium acid phosphate.
- *Metchell's Test*: With iron + ammonium citrate/ iron+sodium tartarate, they give a water soluble iron tannin complex which is insoluble in the solution of ammonium acetate.

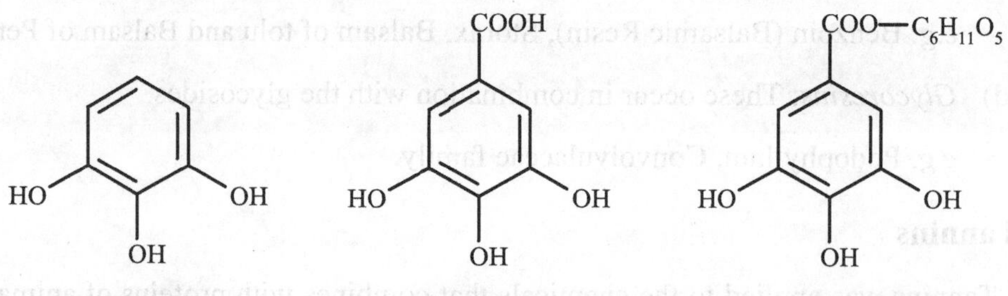

Pyrogallol **Gallic acid** **Glucogallin (Glucose of Gallic acid)**

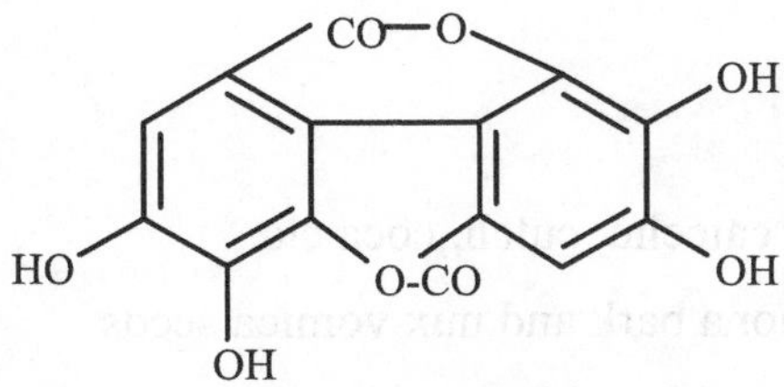

Ellagic acid

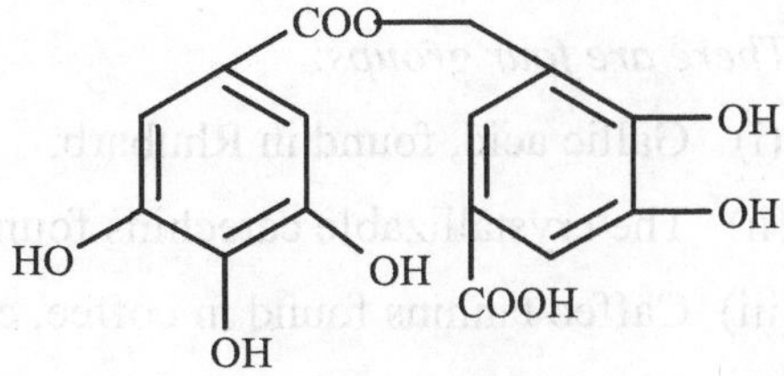

Digallic acid

2. *Ellagic acid Tannins*: These tannins yields ellagic acid on hydrolysis.

   e.g. Oak bark, Pomegranate rind, Pomegranate root bark, Eucalyptus leaves.

3. *Catechol or Phloba Tannins*: These tannins give catechol or paracatechnic acid on alkaline hydrolysis, but with acids or by boiling in air, they are oxidized to red water and alcohol insoluble substances known as *Phlobaphenes.*

   e.g. Cinnamon, Wild cherry bark, Cinchona bark, Oak bark, Acacia bark, Malefern rhizome.

   On dry distillation yields catechol tannins and are related to flavonoids pigments having a polymeric flavan -3 – 0*l* – structure.

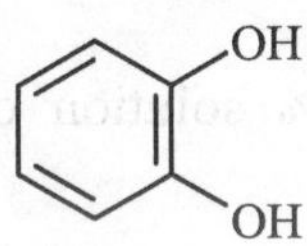

Catechol

   They give following colour Reactions:

   - Green colour with $FeCl_3$ solution.
   - Precipitated by heavy metals.
   - Precipitated by gelatin.
   - Precipitated by alkaloids quite slowly.
   - Phloba tannins produce a leather without a bloom, but the leather produced by depside tannins has a distinct bloom.

4. *Pseudotannins*: These are tannin like substances which respond to most of the chemical tests of true tannins but will not produce a leather. They cannot be hydrolysed. These are the substances of low molecular weight which under certain conditions gives precipitate with gelatin.

There are four groups:

(i) Gallic acid, found in Rhubarb.

(ii) The crystallizable catechins found in catechu, cutch, coca etc.

(iii) Caffeo tannins found in coffee, cinchona bark and nux vomica seeds.

(iv) Ipecacuanha tannins based on ipecacaunhic acid, present in Ipecac root.

Special Test: The presence of phloroglucinol nuclei in the molecule causes the matchstick to stain red when dipped in catechin solution followed by conc. HCl acid and then warmed near a flame.

General Chemical Tests

(i) *Gold-Beater's skin Test*: A piece of Gold-beater's skin (a membrane prepared from the intestine of an ox) + Dilute HCl acid (2% solution) + 1% $FeSO_4$ solution.

↓

Brown/Black colour on the skin denotes the presence of tannins.

(ii) *Phenazone Test*: About 5 ml of an aqueous extract of drug + 0.5 gm sodium acid phosphate + 2% phenazone solution → precipitate of tannins being bulky and coloured oftenly.

(iii) *Gelatin Test*: About 0.5%-1.0% solution of Tannins, precipitate a 1% gelatin solution containing 10% NaCl.

(iv) *Test for chlorogenic acid*: An extract (containing chlorogenic acid) + aqueous ammonia $\xrightarrow{\text{on exposure to air}}$ green colour develops gradually.

3.7 Glycosides

Glycosides are the organic compounds (from plants and animal sources) which on enzymatic or acid hydrolysis give one or more sugar moieties along with non-sugar moiety. The sugar moiety is called *glycone* whereas non-sugar moiety is called *aglycone* or *genin.*

General chemical Tests

(i) *Borntrager's Test*: The drug is powdered, then extracted with ether/immiscible organic solvent
→ filtered ethereal extract is make alkaline either with caustic soda/Ammonia
→ shake it well
→ the aqueous layer shows pink, red or violet colour.

This test is responded by anthraquinone glycosides. Anthranols (reduced forms) show negative test. Anthrones are detected by fluorescence tests.

(ii) *Baljet Test*: Piece of lamina + sodium picrate reagent → Glycoside gives yellow to orange colour.

(iii) *Legal Test*: Glycoside + Pyridine + sodium Nitroprusside solution, made alkaline pink to red colour produced.

(iv) *Keller Killiani Test for Digitoxose*: 1 gm powdered digitalis leaf + 10 ml of 70% alcohol

↓ (i) Boiled for 2-3 minutes
(ii) Filter

5 ml of filtrate + 10 ml of water + 0.5 ml of strong solution of lead acetate

↓ (i) shake it well
(ii) Filter it

Shake the filtrate with 5 ml of chloroform ($CHCl_3$) solution.

↓ (i) Allow to separate
(ii) Pipette off $CHCl_3$
(iii) Removing the solvent in a porcelain dish by gentle evaporation.

Dissolve cooled residue in 3 ml glacial acetic acid with 2 drops of 5% $FeCl_3$ solution.

↓

Carefully transferred this solution to the surface of 2 ml con. H_2SO_4 acid.

↓

A *Reddish Brown* layer is formed at the junction of two liquids and upper layer slowly becomes *Bluish Green*, darkening with standing.

⇓

This confirms the presence of Digitoxose.

(In British Pharmacopoeca, Digitoxose is used as an assay for Digoxin injection and tablets (λmax = 590 nm))

Chemical Nature

(i) Glycosides have an organic radical R in place of hydrogen atom of

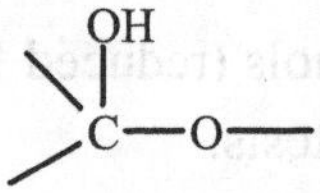 group of sugar ring.

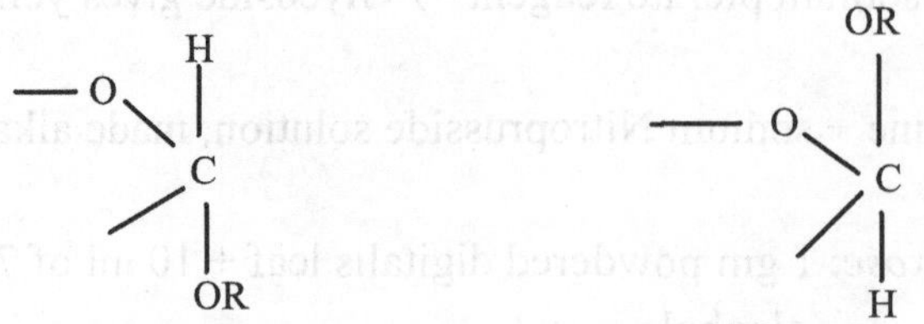

α – Glycoside β – Glycoside

(ii) Glycosides are colourless, except: Flavone glycosides → yellow

Anthracene glycosides → Red/orange

(iii) Glycosides are optically active usually laevorotatory.

(iv) All glycosides contain β-form of sugar except strophanthosides.

(v) Glycosides are usually mixed acetats in which hydroxyl group on the anomeric carbon atom is replaced by a moiety possessing nucleophilic atom.

The sugar hemiacetal reacts with a hydroxyl group of another sugar to form a disaccharide, and further to form a polysaccharide.

- O-Glycosides → The Nucleophilic atom is oxygen present in an alcohol, a phenol or a carboxyl.
- S-Glycosides → Nucleophill atom is sulphur, such as thiol (-SH) group
- N-Glycosides → Nucleosides are formed when the amino group of base reacts with -OH group of ribose /deoxyribose
- C-Glycosides → Nucleophilic atom is carbon in the form of a carbonion

3.8 Carbohydrates

"Carbohydrates are the group of naturally occurring compounds which are either sugars or compounds which produces sugar on hydrolysis."

Sugars are crystalline, water soluble and sweet; whereas non-sugars are amorphons, water insoluble and tasteless substances.

Qualitative chemical Analysis of Monosaccharides:

(i) Depending up on the chemical nature, all carbohydrates will give positive test with Molisch's Reagent → gives purple colour, if treated with alcoholic α-naphthol in the presence of sulphuric acid.

(ii) All carbohydrates reduce Fehling's solution.

(iii) When warmed with an alkali solution, they caramelize to give yellowish brown solutions.

(iv) They all react with phenyl hydrazine to give osazones.

(v) In Pinoff's Test, the fructose gives red colour after boiling it for a very short time.

(vi) In Seliwanoff's test, the fructose gives red colour after boiling for a few minutes but glucose gives colour after a long time.

(vii) Naturally occurring pentoses (ribose, arabinose, xylose etc) when treated with conc. HCl acid → Furfuraldehyde $\xrightarrow{+\text{Aniline}}$ Red colour.

(viii) When treated with a phloroglucinol solution produces red colour.

Qualitative Chemical Analysis of Disaccharides:

(i) It does not reduce Fehling's solution.

(ii) It gives a yellowish, brown colour with alkali.

(iii) It does not form an osazone.

(iv) Disaccharides hydrolyzed to the constituent hexoses by warming with dilute acid (sucrose → Glucose + Fructose)
This, then reduces Fehling's solution if made alkaline.

CHAPTER 4

RADIO-TRACER TECHNIQUES

4.1 Introduction

In *Tracer Technology,* the isotopes may be stable (^{2}H, ^{13}C, ^{15}N, ^{18}O) and the nucleus may be unstable (^{1}H, ^{14}C) of those elements which existed with identical chemical properties but with different atomic weights. These decay with the emission of radiation. To detect these isotopes, they are incorporated into precursors of plant constituents and used in the biogenesis of secondary metabolic pathways.

Radioactive Tracers

(i) The Radioactive carbon and hydrogen are used in biological investigations.

(ii) To study the metabolic pathways of proteins, alkaloids and amino acids with the help of labelled nitrogen atom.

(iii) In biological research, the use of organic compounds with specific labelled carbon atoms led to the synthesis of various inorganic compounds.

(iv) The product synthesized must retain its purity, as the small proportion of a strongly radioactive impurity seriously jeopardizes the results.

(v) Many compounds prepared from natural sources are produced by growing chlorella in an atmosphere containing $^{14}CO_2$.

(vi) The labelling of various Tritium (^{3}H) labelled compounds are effected by:

- By catalytic exchange in an aqueous media.
- By irradiation of organic compounds with Tritium gas.
- By hydrogenation of unsaturated compounds with Tritium gas.

Tritium is a pure β-emitter of low toxicity and its radiation energy is lower than that of ^{14}C.

Radioactive elements used in Biological Research

Isotopes	Toxicity	Half-Life	Energy of Radiation (in Mev)	
			Beta (β)	Gamma (γ)
^{3}H	Low	12.43 years	0.0186	None
^{14}C	Medium (lower group)	5730 years	0.156	None
^{24}Na	Lower group	14.93 hrs	1.39	1.38, 2.758
^{42}K	Lower group	12.4 hrs	3.6, 2.4	1.5
^{35}S	Lower group	87.4 days	0.167	–
^{35}P	Lower group	14.3 days	1.709	None
^{131}I	Medium (upper group)	8.04 days	0.247-0.806	0.080-0.723

4.2 Detection and Assay of Radioactively Labelled Compounds

Liquid Scintillation counter is the instrument used for those radiation which are easily absorbed from ^{3}H and ^{14}C labelled compounds. This instrument depends on the conversion of kinetic energy of a particle into a pulse of light, as a result of its penetrating a suitable luminescent substance.

Liquid scintillation media consists of a solvent in which the excitation occurs and a fluorescent solute emits a light to actuate the photomultiplier.

Other modern instruments measure mixed radiations of ^{3}H and ^{14}C labelled compounds because both a β-emitters and have different radiation energies. These instruments are connected to a suitable ratemeter which records the counts for over a given time.

4.3 Utilization in Biosynthetic Studies

1. For the elucidation of biosynthetic pathways in plants by means of labelled compounds, *Precursor-Product Sequence* is used.

   In this method, a presumed precursor of constituent under investigation, in a labelled form, is fed to the plant and after a suitable time the constituent is isolated, purified and its radio activiy is determined. If specific atoms of the precursor are labelled, it may be possible to degrade the isolated metabolite.

   e.g. Biogenesis of Morphine and Ergot alkaloids is done by using this method only.

2. Another method, *Competitive feeding* is used in determining, which of two possible intermediates is normally used by the plant.

In this method, in the formation of Z from X, two intermediates are used B and B′. Firstly, inactive B and B′ are fed with labelled X to separate groups of plants. If the incorporation of activity into z is inhibited in the plants receiving B, but is unaffected in the group receiving B′, then it is concluded that pathway from X to Z proceeds via B.

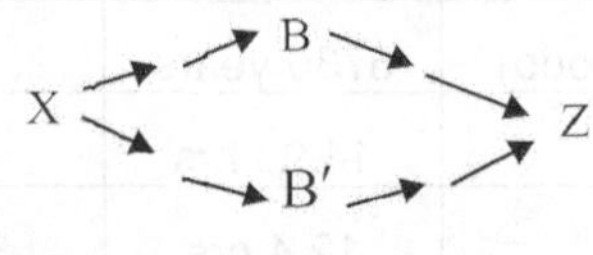

e.g. For the study of rates of demethylation of codeine and unnatural codeine derivatives in papaver orientale, the same plants were used as control and test plant and a mixture of ^{3}H labelled codeine and ^{14}C labelled unnatural codeine derivative was administered to the plant. The metabolites produced were chemically identical due to their characteristic radiations.

3. An *Autoradiography* is a technique used for the location of radioactive tracers isotopes in biological and other material.

   In this method, the specimen is placed in contact with a suitable emulsion. (*e.g.* X-ray sensitive film) and after exposure, the X-ray film is developed. The resulting autoradiograph gives the distribution pattern of radioactive substances in the specimen.

   This method is applied to whole morphological parts (*e.g.* leaves) or to histological sections. The Radioactive compounds on paper and thin layer chromatograms is detected and the relative amounts of radioactivity in different spots is then determined by using density measurements or calibrated films.

4. *Sequential Analysis*: In this method:

   (a) The plants are grown in an atmosphere of $^{14}CO_2$ and analyse at given intervals.

   (b) Then a sequence is obtained in which various related compounds become labelled.

This method is used in elucidation of path of carbon in photosynthesis and also for determining the sequential formation of opium, tobacco and hemlock alkaloids.

e.g. Biosynthetic sequence in Mentha piperita

Piperitone → (–) menthone → (–) menthol

Use of Stable Isotopes

The stable isotopes such as ^{13}C, ^{15}N, ^{18}O and ^{2}H are used as radioactive elements for labelling compounds which are used as intermediates in biosynthetic pathways.

Methods of detection ⇒ Mass spectroscopy (^{15}N and ^{18}O)

NMR Spectroscopy (^{1}H and ^{13}C)

Advantages of Tracer Technique

Following are the advantages of this technique:

(i) Sensitivity of technique is most significant over all other physical and chemical methods.

(ii) The technique can be carried out on living organisms.

(iii) More reliable, easy administration and isolation procedures.

(iv) Gives accurate results (if proper metabolic time and technique is applied)

(v) Wide range of isotopes can be used as per the nature of compound in which label is to be administered.

Thus, a tracer technique is defined as a technique, "which utilizes a labelled compound to find out/trace the different intermediates and various steps in biosynthetic pathway in plants, at a given rate at a given time".

CHAPTER 5

PHYTO-CHEMICAL SCREENING

5.1 Introduction

Medicinal properties of a crude drug usually reside in the secondary metabolites. The plant material subjected to the *PreliminaryPhytochemical Screening* and for detection of various phytoconstituents, must be pure; otherwise test reactions would not be accurate. For this, *purification process* of material is done which consists of sublimation, fractional distillation, crystallization and steam distillation.

The systematic *investigations* of plant material for its phytochemical behaviour involves four different stages:

(i) The availability of raw material and its quality control.

(ii) Extraction, purification and characterization of constituents of pharmaceutical interest in process quality control.

(iii) Investigations of biosynthetic pathways to a particular compound.

(iv) Quantitative evaluation of a crude drug.

The commonly employed technique for separation of an active substance from crude drug is called "Extraction" which involves the use of different solvents. The choice of the plant material for extraction depends on its nature and the components required to be isolated:

1. Fresh plant parts are homogenised, or macerated with a solvent such as alcohol and then used.
2. Dried plant material is directly used for extraction.

Menstruum	:	Solvent/solvent mixture used for extraction
Miscella	:	Solution containing extracted substance
Rinsing	:	Dissolution of extractive substances out of disintegrated cells
Lixivation or Leaching	:	Extraction with water as solvent

These are some common typical terms used in extraction process. Extraction processes for drugs is usually divided into two major groups:

1. Processes which result in the establishment of a concentration equilibrium between solution and solid residue.
2. Processes in which the drug is extracted exhaustively.

Extraction process suddenly stops when the distribution of an extractive substances between miscella and drug residue reaches the value equivalent to K i.e., when the concentration gradient between miscella and residue becomes zero.

$$K = \frac{\text{Concentration of extractive substances in the miscella}}{\text{Concentration of extractive substances in drug residue}}$$

5.2 Procedure for Extraction

During the extraction of phytoactive drugs (Herbal drugs), two processes run parallel with each other in crude drug extracting:

(i) The rinsing of an extractive substances out of disintegrated plant cells. and

(ii) The dissolution of extractive substances out of intact plant cells by diffusion, which requires the following:

   (a) Prior steeping and swelling of the drug plant material in order to increase the permeability of the cells and cell walls.

   (b) Penetration of the solvent into the plant cells and swelling of the cells.

   (c) Dissolution of extractive substances.

   (d) Diffusion of dissolved extractive substances out of the plant cell.

   e.g. The Glycyrrhiza root when extracted with the solvent (0.25% ammonia solution), it penetrates into the roots more rapidly and this process is accelerated by raising the temperature. The steeping and swelling process is strongly influenced by particle size greatly. Upon penetration into the plant material, the solvent becomes enriched with extractive substances and highest content is obtained.

The extract which is obtained is subjected to qualitative tests for various plant constituents namely:

Tannins	:	$FeCl_3$ solution is used
Alkaloids	:	Dragendorff's reagent is used
Glycosides	:	Borhtrager's test is used
Sugars	:	Fehling's and Benedict's solution is used
Saponins	:	Soap forming and Haemolysis activity.

5.3 Evaluation

As far as, the evaluation of a crude drug is concerned, it involves the identity, quality and purity of the material. To protect the extracted material from biochemical reactions or deterioration due to the presence of micro-organisms and their storage, the crude extracted material is subjected to the physical evaluation, Morphological and Microscopical evaluation, chemical evaluation comprising of preliminary phyto-chemical screening including various chemical tests and assays.

General Extraction Scheme of a Drug

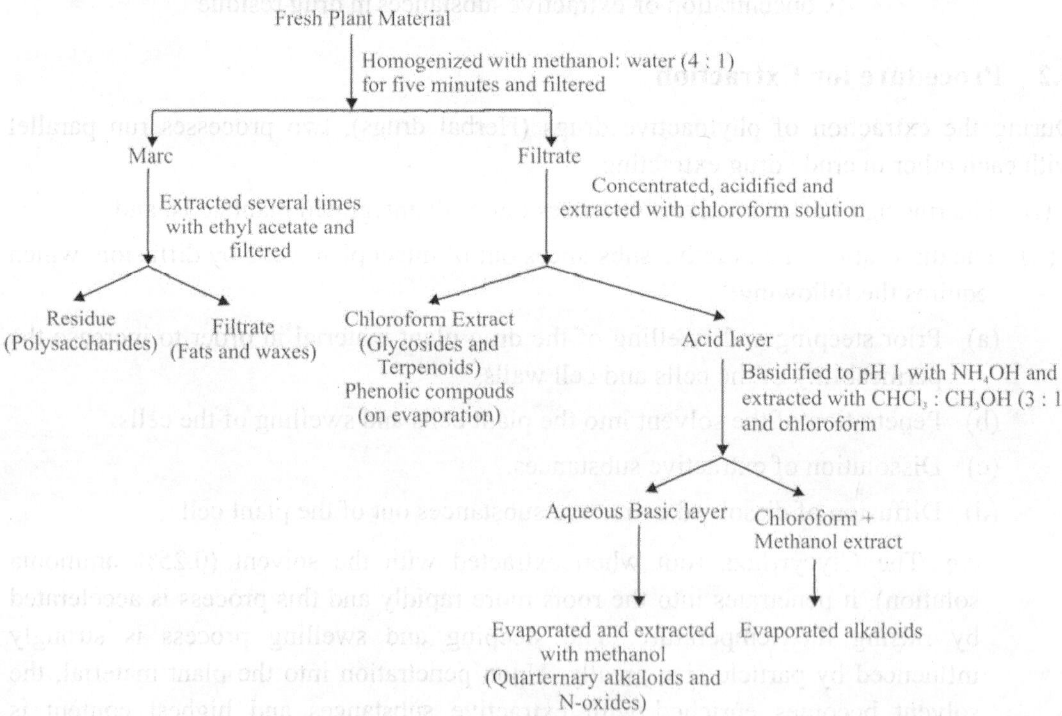

General Protocols for Extraction of phyto constituents and their detection methods through qualitative chemical examination:

1. ***Preparation of De-Tannified Chloroform Extract:***

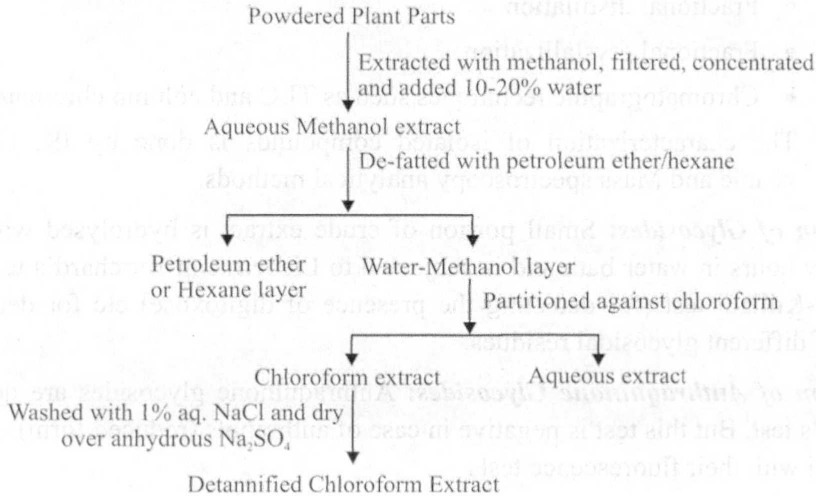

Preparation of Detannified chloroform and Aqueous extract from Methanol extracts

2. ***General Methods of Extraction/Isolation of Glycosides*:** General extraction method is called Stas-Otto Method.

    (i) In this method, Drugs containing glycoside is finely powdered and powder is extracted by continuous hot percolation using soxhlet apparatus with alcohol as a solvent.

    (ii) Drug is extracted during the process and enzymes (present in plant parts) are deactivated due to heating.

    (iii) The thermolabile glycosides should be extracted at temperature below 45 °C temperature.

    (iv) The extract is treated with lead acetate to precipitate tannins and non-glycosidal impurities is eliminated.

    (v) The excess of lead acetate is precipitated as lead sulphide (PbS) by passing H_2S gas through the solution.

    (vi) The extract is then filtered and concentrated to get crude glycosides.

(vii) From the crude extract, glycosides are obtained in pure form by using processes such as:

- Fractional solubility
- Fractional distillation
- Fractional crystallization
- Chromatographic techniques such as TLC and column chromatography.

(viii) The characterization of isolated compounds is done by IR, UV, NMR, visible and Mass spectroscopy analytical methods.

Detection of Glycosides: Small portion of crude extract is hydrolysed with dil-HCl acid for few hours in water bath and is subjected to Liebermann-Burchard's test, Legal's test, Keller-Killiani test (for detecting the presence of digitoxose) etc for detecting the presence of different glycosidal residues.

Detection of Anthraquinone Glycosides: Anthraquinone glycosides are detected by Borntrager's test. But this test is negative in case of anthranols (reduced form). Anthrones are detected with their fluorescence tests.

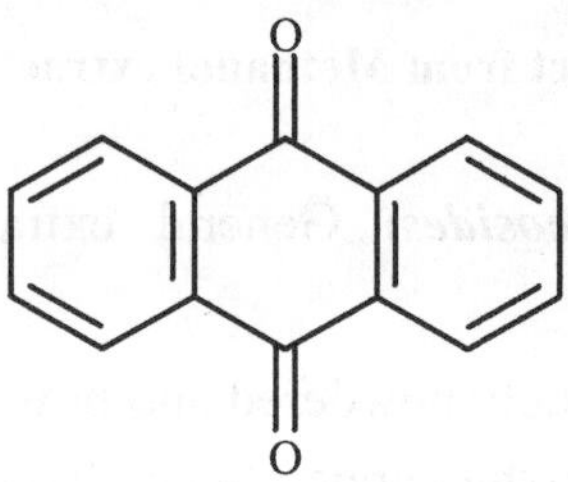

Anthraquinones

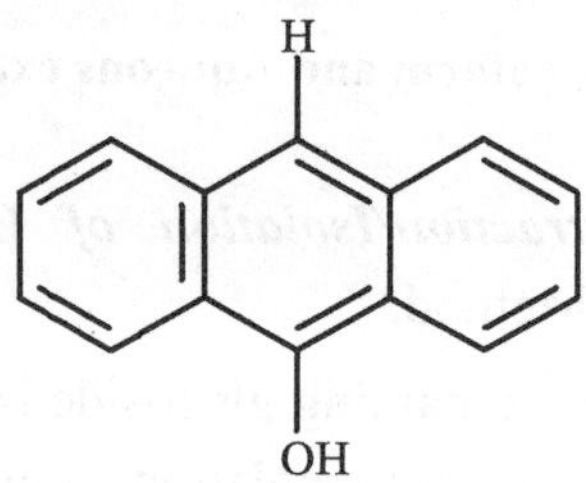

Anthranols

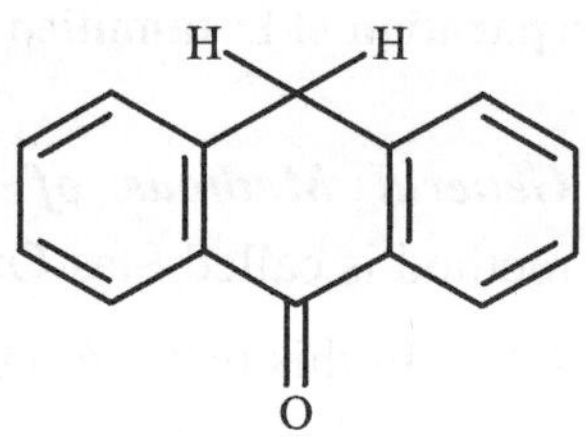

Anthrones

Detection of Flavonoid Glycosides: Flavonoid glycosides dissolve in alkalis, giving yellow solutions which on the addition of acid become colourless.

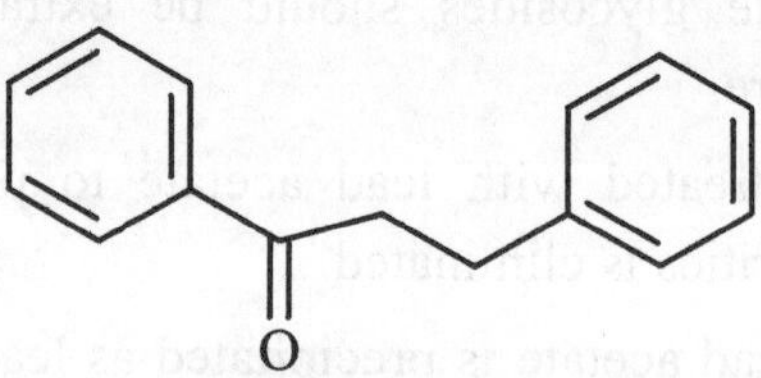

Dihydrochalcone
(Simplest naturally occurring flavonoid)

Detection of Saponins: About 1 ml of alcoholic acid extract and aqueous extract is diluted separately with distilled water to 20 ml and shaken in a graduated cylinder for 15 minutes. One cm layer of foam indicates the presence for saponins.

3. ***Fractionation Method for Extraction of Saponins***:

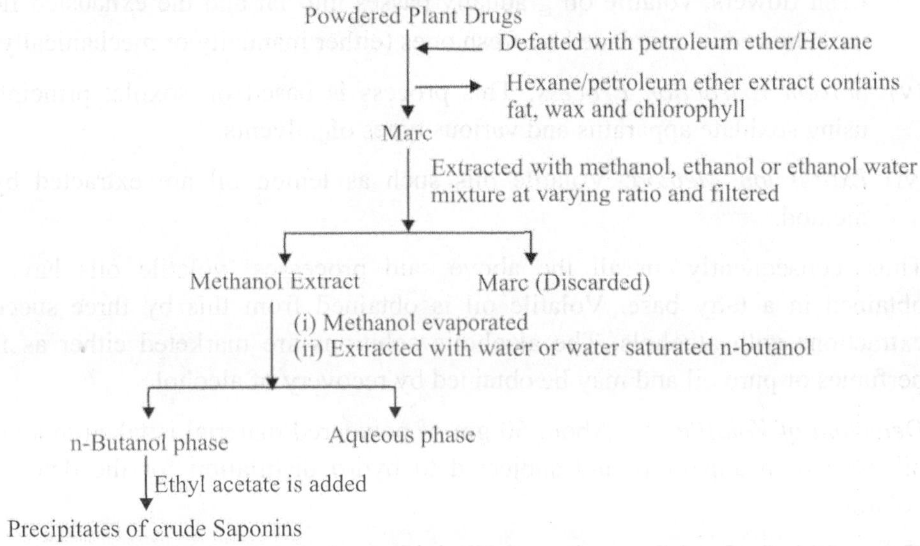

Fractionation Extraction Method for obtaining saponin from crude drugs

4. ***General Methods of Extraction of Volatile Oils***: The methods used generally for extraction of volatile oils are classified and described as follows:

   (i) *Steam Distillation Method*: In this method, the plant is macerated and then steam distilled to obtain the oil.
   e.g. Rose oil (water distillation and water steam distillation method is also used)

   (ii) *Digestion process*: In this method, flowers are gently heated in melted fat until exhausted; after straining out perfume containing fat.

   (iii) *Pneumatic Method*: This method involves the passage of a current of warm air through the flowers. The air, laden with the suspended volatile oil is then passed through a spray of melted fat absorbing the volatile oil.

   (iv) *Mechanical Method*: Under this, two methods are:

Ecuelle: This technique is used for the extraction of citrus oils, where in oil, cells are ruptured mechanically.

Enfluerage: In this method, (similar in principle to pneumatic method), glass plates are covered with a thin layer of fixed oil or fab on which spreading the fresh flowers, volatile oil gradually passes into fat and the exhausted flowers are renewed and replaced by fresh ones (either manually or mechanically).

(v) *Solvent Extraction Process*: This process is based on soxhlet principles by using soxhlate apparatus and various types of solvents.

(vi) *Expression Method*: Volatile oils such as lemon oil are extracted by this method.

Thus, consequently, in all the above said processes, volatile oils have been obtained in a fatty base. Volatile oil is obtained from this by three successive extractions with alcohols. The alcoholic solutions are marketed either as flower perfumes or pure oil and may be obtained by recovery of alcohol.

Detection of Volatile Oil: About 50 gm of powdered material is taken in a volatile oil estimation apparatus and subjected to hydro distillation for the detection of volatile oil.

5. ***General Methods of Extraction of Alkaloids*:**

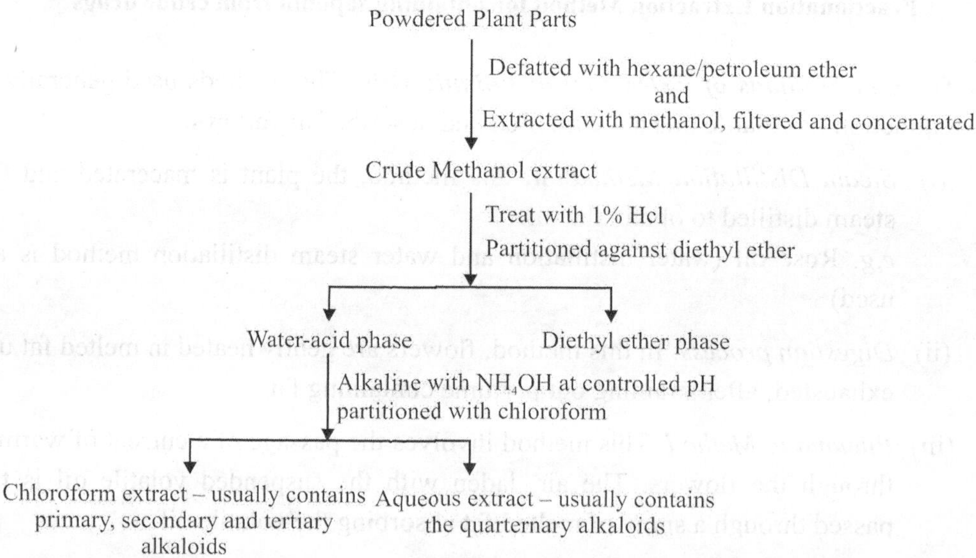

General procedure to obtain an alkaloid extract from the alcoholic crude extract of a plant

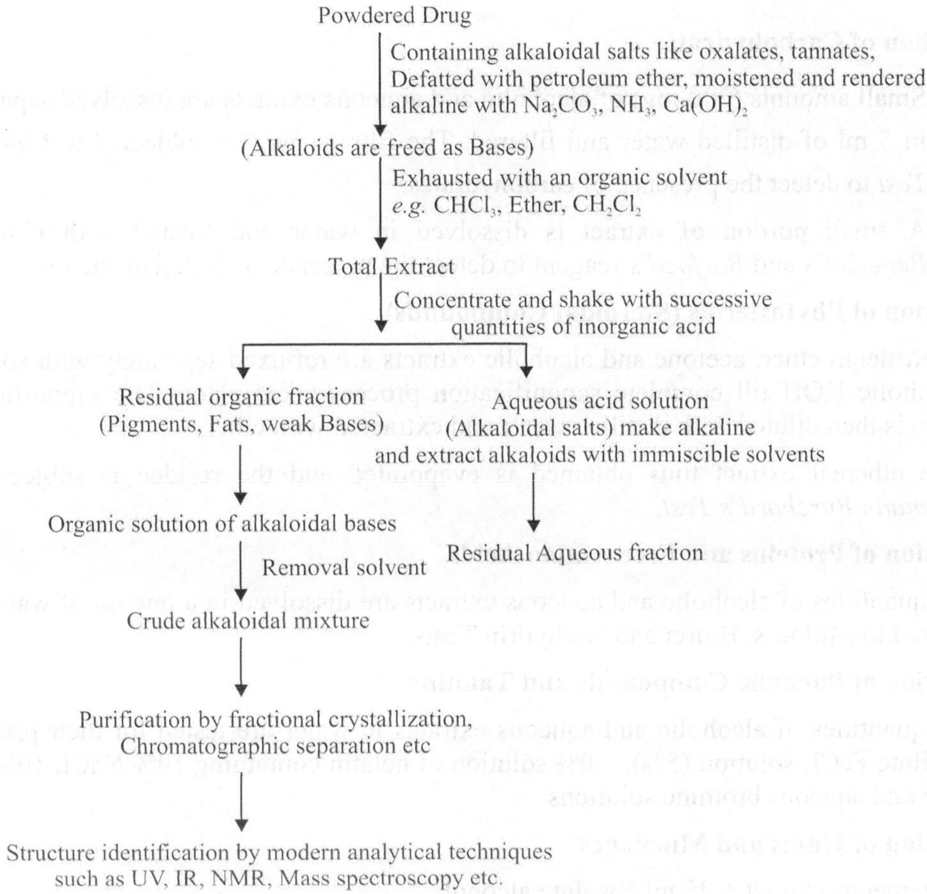

An extraction procedure for alkaloidal crude drugs

Detection of Alkaloids: The small portions of solvent free chloroform alcoholic and water extracts are stirred separately with a few drops of dil. HCl acid and filtered. The filtrate may be tested carefully with various alkaloidal reagents, such as:

Mayer's Reagent. (cream colour precipitate).

Dragendorff's Reagent (Orange Brown precipitate)

Hager's Reagent (Yellow precipitate)

Wagner's Reagent (Reddish Brown precipitate)

Detection of Carbohydrates

(i) Small amounts (200 mg) of alcoholic and aqueous extracts are dissolved separately in 5 ml of distilled water and filtered. The filtrate may be subjected to M*olisch's Test* to detect the presence of carbohydrates.

(ii) A small portion of extract is dissolved in water and treated with *Fehling's Benedict's* and *Barfoed's* reagent to detect the presence of different sugars.

Detection of Phytosterols (Steroidal Compounds)

The petroleum ether, acetone and alcoholic extracts are refluxed separately with solution of alcoholic KOH till complete saponification process takes place. The saponification mixture is then diluted with distilled water and extracted with ether.

The ethereal extract thus obtained is evaporated and the residue is subjected to *Liebermann Burchard's Test.*

Detection of Proteins and Free Amino Acids

Small quantities of alcoholic and aqueous extracts are dissolved in a few ml of water and subjected to Millon's, Biuret and Ninhydrin Tests.

Detection of Phenolic Compounds and Tannins

Small quantities of alcoholic and aqueous extracts in water are tested for their presence with dilute $FeCl_3$ solution (5%), 1.0% solution of gelatin containing 10% NaCl, 10% lead acetate and aqueous bromine solutions.

Detection of Gums and Mucilages

10 ml aqueous extract + 25 ml absolute alcohol

↓ constant stirring

A precipitate is formed which is dried in air and examined for its swelling properties.

CHAPTER 6

MARINE PHARMACOGNOSY

6.1 Introduction

The drugs and medicines used today are obtained synthetically or are natural in origin. Oceans and seas, rich in fauna and flora covers about 70% of earth's surface. The active constituents obtained from marine organisms such as algae, sea weeds are used to cure various human ailments.

e.g. Shark liver oil, cod liver oil, sodium alginate, Agar-agar, Marine fishes, Halibut liver oil, spermaceti, Protamine sulphate, carrageenan, Sea weeds, Polysaccharides agar, alginic acid etc.

Seaweeds, also called as Marine macroalgae are used as crude drugs in treatment of various human diseases. They are:

(i) In treatment of Iodine-deficiency diseases such as Goitre, Hypothyroidism.

(ii) As a source of additional vitamins.

(iii) In treatment of anaemia during pregnanacy.

(iv) In treating various intestinal disorders, used as vermifuges.

(v) Used as hypocholesterolaemic and hypoglycaemic agents. (generally used sea weeds are – *cystoseira barbata, Sargassum confusum* and *Jania rubens*).

(vi) Employed as dressings, ointments and in gynaecology.

(vii) In Hawaii, "Porphyra atropurpurea" is used to dress wounds and burns.

(viii) In Newzealand, "*Durvillea Antarctica*" is used to treat scabies.

Table 6.1 Marine Drugs and their Sources

Name of Drug	Biological source + Family	Chemical constituents	Uses
Chitin	Polysaccharide containing amino and acetyl groups, present in skeletal material of invertebrates, molluscs, annelids, arthropods.	Hard crustacean shell 15-20% chitin. Soft shells of shrimp = 15-30% chitin Mycelia of penicillium = 20% chitin	Used in wound healing preparations; As a sizing agent for rayon, cotton, wool.
Sodium Alginate (Algin) (Alginic acid)	A sodium salt of Alginic acid. Alginic acid is a polyuronic acid composed of reduced mannuronic and glucouronic acids. (Fam : Phaeophyceae) *Macrocystis pyrifera, Laminaria hyperborean, Ascohyllum nodosum.*	Mannuronic acid and Glucouronic acid. It is chemically a polysaccharide	As a suspending and thickening agent. As a binding and disintegrating agent in tablets and lozenges. In food industry, textile industry.
Agar	Dried gelatine substance obtained from *Gelidium amansii* (Fam:Gelidaceae)	Agarose, Agaropectin, (Gel strength of Agar is due to the presence of Agarose which is composed of D-galactose and 3.6% anhydro L-galactose units. 3.5% cellulose + 6% Nitrogen containing substances). (Agar solutions is viscous due to the presence of Agaropectin composed of galactose and uronic acid units, partly esterified with sulphuric acid.	As emulsifying agent. As a bulk laxative, in preparation of jellies and confectionnary items. In preparation of bacteriological culture medium.
Carrageenan (Irishmoss)	A Red Algae obtained from *Chondrus crispus* Fam : *Rhodophyceae* or *Gigartina stellata* Fam : *Gigartinaceae*	On the basis of presence of position of sulphate and presence or absence of anhydrogalactose,carrageenan are of two types: **Kappa (κ)**: D-galactose, 3, 6 anhydrous D-galactose and esters sulphate group → Good gelling agent **Lambda (λ)**: D-galactose and its mono+ disulphate esters → Non-gelling agent i, μ, v Forms of carrageenan	As emulsifying stabilizing gelling agent. In preparation of creams, cosmetic, in food industry in milk products.

Table 6.1 conti…

Name of Drug	Biological soure + Family	Chemical constituents	Uses
Halibut Liver oil	As per BP, a fixed oil obtained from *Hippoglossus vulgaris* Fam : Pleurnectidae	Vitamin A and D. Standard for unsaponifiable matter is not less than 7.0%.	In prevention and cure of rickets in small dose As a vitamin.
Cod-liver Oil	*Gadus morrhu*a and other Spp. Of Gadus Fam: Gadidae	Vitamin A and D. Antirachitic activity is due to vitamin-D_3 (Cholecalciferol) 1g of oil contains not less than 255 g of vitamin-A and 2.125 g of vitamin-D. Oil contains Glyceryl esters of oleic, linoleic, gadoleic, myristic and palmitic acids. 7% eicosapen taenoic acid + decosahexanoic acid 7%.	Used in treatment of rickets and tuber culosis. Used in relief rhematic pains and joint and muscle stiffness.
Shark-liver oil (from Scoliodon, Sphyrna, *carcharias*)	*Hypoprion brevirostris* and *Galeorhinus zyopterus*	one gram of oil should contain not less than 6000 international units of vitamin-A activity. Glycerides of saturated and unsaturated fatty acids.	Shark liver oil Called as Antixero-phthalmic factor, used in deficiency of vitamin-A (but free of vitamin-D). In preparation of shark liver oil emulsion, used in burn and sunburn ointments.

6.2 Shark Liver Oil and Cod Liver Oil

Method of Preparation

The principal and main stages used in the preparation of medicinal oil are:

(i) Refining of crude oil

(ii) Drying

(iii) Winterization

(iv) Deodorization

(v) Standardization for vitamin content.

The livers (shark and cod) free from gall bladder contains about 50% oil, are removed immediately and transferred to steamers in which the oil is released from the tissue. The crude oil is separated and stored.

1. *Refining*: The quality and flavour of various liver oils are improved by refining under air free conditions to avoid oxidation.

   This process is carried out in a continuous, automatic, hermetic refining plant which consists of a battery of mixers linked to centrifuges in the following steps:

   (i) The crude oil is heated to 77 °C–80 °C in a heat exchanger and passed to disc-type mixers.

   (ii) In mixers, reagent is added which removes impurities and causes dissolution.

   (iii) Oil and water are removed in a hermetic separator, without contact with the air.

   (iv) The process is repeated in a second batch as well as third.

2. *Drying*: It is done in vacuum drying tower which evaporates small amount of residual water and discharges a clear, bright and highly refined oil. The plant refines 50-60 tonnes of oil per day.

3. *Winterization*: The oil is cooled to about 0 °C temperature, which causes stearin to separate. The solid is removed by cold filtration and polyunsaturated product is left.

4. *Deodorization*: It is achieved by steaming under vacuum which removes about 0.02% of aldehydic and ketonic impurities, and thus protects the oil from oxidation.

5. *Standardization*: The medicinal oil is standardized for vitamin content by blending. The BP oil should contain not less than 600 units of vitamin A in one gm and not less than 85 units of vitamin D.

Storage: To avoid loss of vitamins, oil should be stored in a well filled airtight containers, protected from light and in a cool place. The addition of small amounts of various antioxidants (such as dodecyl gallate, octyl gallate) is used.

Chemical Tests

1. Dissolve 1.0 ml shark/cod liver oil + 10 ml chloroform + saturated solution of antimony trichloride in chloroform.

↓ Shake it well

A blue colour is developed (Due to vitamin A)

2. 1 gm of shark/cod liver oil + 1 ml chloroform + 0.5 ml sulphuric acid

↓

Light violet colour to purple and finally changes to brown (Due to vitamin A)

6.3 Carrageenan

Carrageenan is generally present in the intercellular matrix and cell wall of algae and contains about 60-80% of dry weight.

Method of Preparation

(i) The dried red sea weed is first cleaned/bleached with cold water by spreading it on the shore to remove salt and other extra matter.

(ii) Then it is extracted with hot water which contains sodium hydroxide or calcium hydroxide solution.

(iii) Then the pH was adjusted to slightly alkaline range (pH = 8-8.2)

(iv) The extract is obtained by filtration and purity of the product is recovered by precipitation with isopropyl alcohol/ethyl alcohol or by drum drying or by freezing.

Chemical Tests

(i) 5% decoction of carrageenan $\xrightarrow{\text{on cooling}}$ a jelly like substance is formed.

(ii) 0.3% solution of carrageenan (cooled) + 1% solution of tannic acid → Gives no precipitate.

(iii) 0.3% solution of carrageenan (cooled) + solution of Iodine → Gives light blue colour.

6.4 Agar

Method of Preparation

The Red Algae is grown on the bamboos spread in the ocean.

1. The algae are taken ashore and dried, beaten or shaken to remove sand and shells.
2. The material is then bleached by watering and exposed to sunlight to remove salt at high altitudes.
3. Then boiled with dilute acidified water (about 1 part of algae with 55/60 parts of water) for 5-6 hours.

4. Then the mucilaginous decoction is filtered through linen cloth and transferred to wooden troughs.
5. On cooling, a jelly is produced which is cut into bars and then passed through the netting under pressure.
6. Narrow strips of agar are prepared and allowed to melt in sun to remove the excess water.

Chemical Tests

(i) Boiled 1.5 gm agar + 100 ml water $\xrightarrow[\text{the room temperature}]{\text{the solution cooled to}}$ A stiff jelly is formed.

(ii) 0.2% solution of agar in water + tannic acid solution → No precipitation is produced.

(iii) When agar is mounted in the solution of ruthenium red and examined under microscope → Mounted particles acquire pink colour.

6.5 Chitin

Method of Preparation

1. The shells of molluscs, annelids, arthropods (contains about 65-70% $CaCO_3$) are pulverized to fine powder and treated to 5% HCl acid for about 24 hours to remove all the calcium and other impurities of shell.
2. The above extract is treated with proteolytic enzymes (pepsin/trypsin).
3. Product, thus obtained in pink colour is bleached by acidified H_2O_2 for 5-6 hours at constant temperature.
4. Then this bleached product is deacetylated at 120 °C temperature with 2 parts of KOH + 1 part of C_2H_5OH + 1 part of ethylene glycol.
5. If the acetyl content is minimum, reaction is stopped.
6. The deacetylated product thus obtained is called *Chitosan*.

Chemical Tests

(i) Chitosan is soaked in Iodine solution + 10% sulphuric acid

↓

A deep violet colour develops

(ii) Chitosan is dissolved in 50% Nitric acid $\xrightarrow[\text{to crystallize}]{\text{Allowed}}$ Sphero crystals of chitosan nitrate obtained.

If the crystals are examined by polarized light, using crossed nicols, a distinct cross is observed.

6.6 Sodium Alginate/Alginic Acid

The algae used for extraction of alginic acid is of brown colour (due to the presence of carotenoid pigment).

Method of Preparation

(i) The sea weeds (red/brown algae) are harvested, dried, milled and macerated with dilute sodium carbonate solution, resulting into a pasty mass.

(ii) This mass is diluted with soft water to separate insoluble matter (Soft water is essential to avoid precipitation of insoluble alginates and to avoid incompatibilities).

(iii) Then, the clear liquor is treated with dilute calcium chloride or dil. sulphuric acid solution for conversion into insoluble alginic acid or its salt, calcium alginate.

(iv) Then it is collected and purified by thorough washing.

(v) The calcium is separated by treating the above with hydrochloric acid and highly swollen pulp of alginic acid is roller pressed and collected.

(vi) It is then neutralized with sodium carbonate to give sodium alginate.

Chemical Tests

(i) 1% solution of sodium alginate in water + dilute sulphuric acid

↓

Heavy gelatinous precipitation

(ii) Aqueous solution of sodium alginate + Calcium chloride solution

↓

Copious precipitation is obtained

6.7 Novel Agents from Marine Sources

These agents are isolated from marine organisms in the form of metabolites and have various medicinal, biomedical, pharmaceutical and agricultural uses. Many of the species also contain numerous toxic compounds derived from marine organisms such as Dinoflagellate, diatoms etc.

The classification and explanation of various Novel agents (from Marine) are discussed in the tabular form:

Table No. 6.2

Name of Novel Agent/Compound	Source	Applications/Actions
1. Cardiovascular substances/Agents		
(i) Eptatretin	Aneural bronchial hearts of Hog fish (*Eptatretus stoutii*)	Potent cardiac stimulant, stimulates action on mammalian myocardium
(ii) D(–)Octopamine	*Octopus macropus*, *Octopus vulgaris*	Adrenergic and cardiovascular response
(iii) Saxitoxin (Str 6.1)	Saxidomus giganteus *Mytilus californianus*	Hypotensive effect
(iv) Anthopleurins	Group of peptides obtained from coelentrates namely *Anthropleura xanthogrammica*	Positive inotropication, produces cardiotonic effect
(v)Spongosine (Methoxy olerivative of adenosine)	*Crypotethia crypta*	Reduces rate and force of contraction of heart
(vi) Eledosin	Posterior salivary glands of cephalopod eledone moschata	Strong hyptensive action as well as acts as vasodilator
2. Antiviral Agents		
(i) ARA-A (Str 6.2)	*Tethya crypta*	Potent and therapeutic antiviral activity
(ii) Eudistomin (str 6.3)	*Eudistoma olivaceum* (Fam : Polycitoridae)	Potent antiviral agent
(iii) Avarol and Avarone	*Disidea avara*	Inhibits immunodeficiency virus and crosses blood-brain barrier. Used in treatment of AIDS
(iv) Patellazole	Ascidian "*Lissoclinum Patella*"	Potent *in vitro* activity against Herpes simplex virus
3. Anti-Parasitic Agents		
(i) α-Kainic acid (str 6.4)	Red alga "*Digenia simplex*"	As a vermifuge As a broad spectrum anthelmintic
(ii) Domoic acid (str 6.5)	Redalga *Chondria armata* and *Alsidium corallinum*	As a potent anthelmintic As a hypotensive agent
(iii) Laminine (str 6.6)	Brown alga, "Lamainariales spp."	As a smooth muscle relaxant and as a potent hypotensive agent.
(iv) Bengamide	Sponges such as Nudi branch and zoanthid	Effect in vitro anthelmintic agent.
(v) Cucumechinoside	Isolated from sea cucumber	Antiprotozoal activity

Table 6.2 conti…

Name of Novel Agent/Compound	Source	Applications/Actions
4. Anticoagulant Agents		
(i) Galactan Sulphuric acid (ii) Carrageenan (iii) Fucoidan	*Iridaea laminariodes* (A Marine algae) *Chondrus crispus*, polyides rotundus. A brown alga, "*Fucus vesiculosus*"	Anticoagulant activity Direct effect on the in vitro inactivation of thrombin Antithrombin effect
5. Anti-Inflammatory and anti spasmodic agents (carrageenan when injected into the synovial fluid of animals, produces an arthritis which can be used to test arthritis specific anti-inflammatory drugs)		
(i) Manoalide (ii)Dendalone-3-Hydroxy Butyrate (iii) Tetradotoxin (iv) Flustramine	*Luffariella varia bilis* *Phyllospongia dendyl* Obtained from liver and ovaries of puffer fishes *Flustra foliaceae*	Have a non-steroidal anti-inflammatory action. It acts by direct inactivation of phospholipase A_2 Used in synthesis of prostaglandins. As an anti-inflammatory agent Strong antispasmodic agent A strong muscle relaxant action.
6. Cytotoxic (Anti-cancer/Anti-tumour) Agents		
(i) Bryostatin (ii) Dolastatin (A group of cyclic and linear peptide) (iii) Asperdiol (iv) Crassin Acetate (v) ARA-C (α-D arakino furanosyl cytosine and cytosine arabinoside) (str 6.7)	Isolated from Bryozoan, *Bugula neritina* Sea hare, "*Dolabella auricularia*." A non-lactonic cembranoid from gorgorian coral *Carribean gorgonian* Carribean sponges such as spongosine and spongouridine	• In treatment of neoplastic Bone-marrow failure. • It triggers activation and differentiation of peripheral • blood cells from lymphocytic leukaemia patients. • Enhances the efficiency of Interleukin-2. • Cell growth activity in vitro As a cytotoxic agent Cytotoxic to Human leukaemic and Hella cells Used in treatment of acute myelogenous leukaemia

Table 6.2 conti…

Name of Novel Agent/Compound	Source	Applications/Actions
7. Antimicrobial/Antibiotic agents		
(i) Cephalosporin-C	Fungus, "*Cephalosporium acremonium*".	Used as an antibiotic drug (Cephalothin sodium is used)
(ii) Istamycins A and B	Produced by fermentation of marine streptomycetes, "Streptomyces tenjimariensis".	Active against Gram(-)ve, and Gram (+) ve bacteria *in vitro*.
(iii) Bromopyrones		Possess antimicrobial activity.
(iv) Fimbrolides	Redalgae, "*Ptilonia australasica*".	Have antimicrobial activity
(v)Tetra bromo Heptane str 6.8	Red algae, "*Delisea fimbriata*". Brown algae, "*Dictyopteris Zonaroides*".	Have antimicrobial activity
8. Prostaglandins		
(i) PGA_2	Soft coral, "*Plexaura Lomomalla*".	Biologically potent substances used as uterine muscle relaxants.
9. Proteins		
(i) Amoebocyte lysate	*Limulus polyphemus*	Detection of Endotoxins (Complex lipopolysaccharides)
(ii) Haemaglutinins (Lectin)	Haemolymph of "*Limulus polyphenus*".	Carbohydrate binding protein
(iii) Sialic acid	Haemolymph of lobster, "*Homarus americanus*".	Binding agent
10.Agrochemical Agents		
(i) Nereistoxin	*Lumbriconeris heteropoda*	As an insecticide (as it is toxic to insects) It affects the nervous system and heart of fish and mammals.
(ii) Capulerpin	Species of caulerpa	Plant growth regulatory activity.

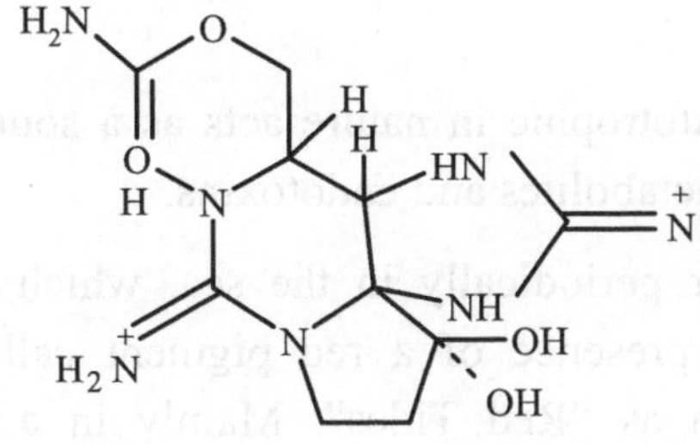

Str 6.1. Saxitoxin

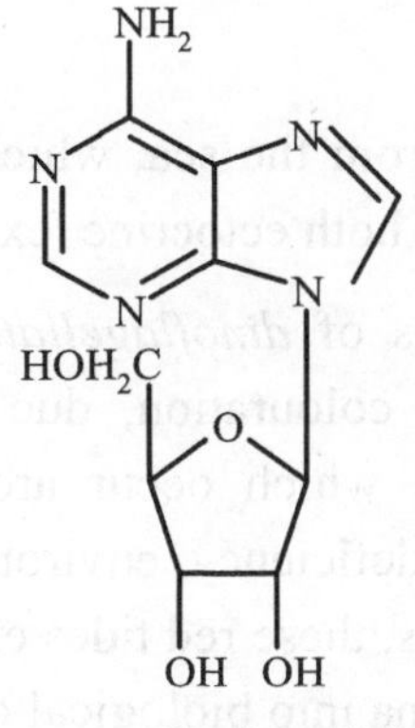

Str 6.2. [ARA-A]

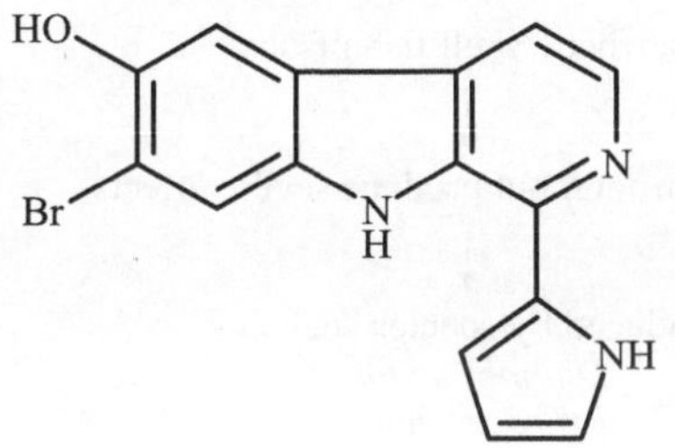

Str.6.3. Eudistomin

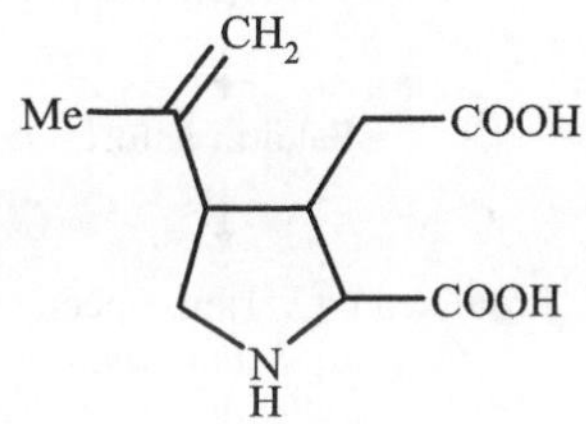

Str 6.4. a-Kainic acid

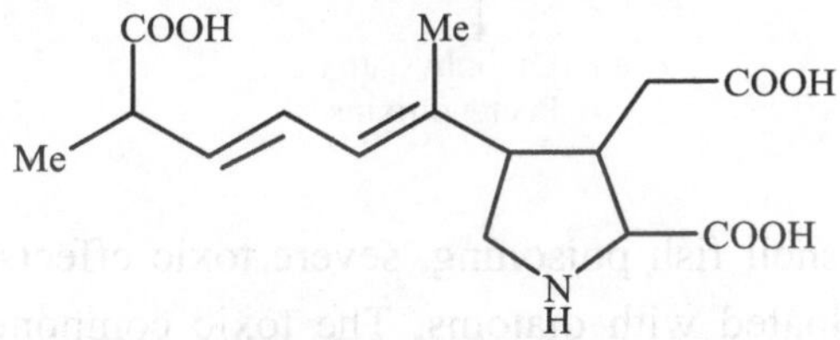

Str 6.5 Domoic acid

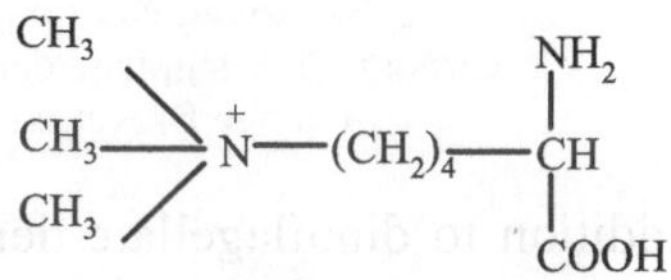

Str 6.6 Laminine

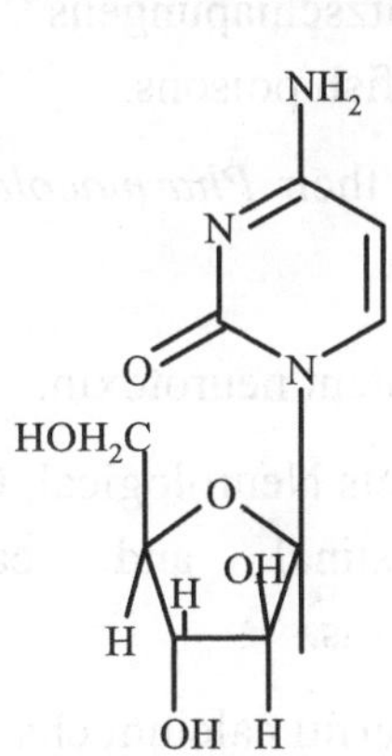

Str 6.7 ARA-C

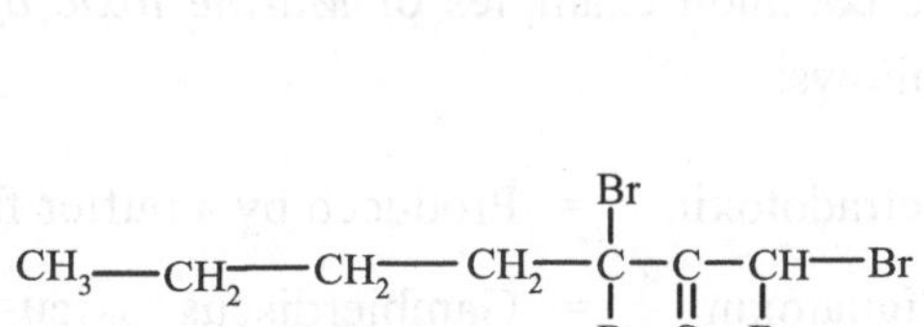

Str 6.8 Tetrabromoheptanone

6.8 Marine Toxins

The micro-organisms from the sea, which are autotrophic in nature acts as a source of toxins. These toxins are both ectocrine /external metabolites and endotoxins.

Large concentrations of *dinoflagellates* occur periodically in the sea, which gives water a brown to red colouration, due to the presence of a red pigment called as *Peridinin*. The blooms which occur are known as "Red Tides". Mainly in adverse conditions like oxygen deficiency, environmental imbalance of nutrients, accumulation of sulphide in surroundings, these red tides exerts drastic effects due to their toxins and turns into a rich flora and fauna into biological desert.

Paralytic shell fish poisons
↓
Fatal in nature
↓
Produced by various species such as:
Alexandrium tamarense
Alexandrium catenellum
Gymnodinium catenatum
Ptychodiscus brevis
↓
e.g. Saxitoxin, Neosaxitoxin, carbomoyl-N-sulphate derivatives of above Brevetoxins

Diarrhetic shell fish pisons
↓
Non-fatal but produce severe effects
↓
Produced by species such as:
Dinophysis fortii
Prorocentrum lima
↓
e.g. Dinophysistoxins, Pectenotoxins

In addition to dinoflagellate derived shell fish poisoning, severe toxic effects results from the ingestion of shell fish contaminated with diatoms. The toxic component was identified as *Domoic acid* produced by diatom "Pseudonitzschiapungens". The poisons produced from this are collectively called as amnesic shell fish poisons.

Some common examples of *Marine toxic agents* with their *Pharmacological effects* are as follows:

1. Tetradotoxin = Produced by a puffer fish = A potent neurotoxin.
2. Ciguatoxin = Gambierdiscus toxicus = Effects Neurological, Gastro-intestinal and cardiovascular systems.
3. Maitotoxin = Gambierdiscus toxicus = Powerful calcium channel activator

4. Lophotoxin (a diterpene Lactone)	= Lophogorgia spp.	= Produces irreversible postsynaptic blockage at neuro muscular junctions.
5. Lyngbyatoxin	= Lyngbya majuscula	= Produces contact dermatitis
6. Debromoaply siatoxin	= Lyngbya majuscula	= Antineoplastic activity
7. Halitoxin	= Haliclona rubens	= A potent neuro muscular blocker
8. Polytoxin	= Palythoa spp.	= Most potent coronary vasoconstrictor

Toxins such as Gonyantoxin and saxitoxin, bind to sodium channels on the outside of excitable membranes and allow an influx of sodium ions in exchange of potassium ions reflux, with the membrane depolarization.

CHAPTER 7

AROMATIC PLANTS AND THEIR UTILIZATION

7.1 Introduction

In India all types of climatic conditions exists varying from temperate in the Himalayas to tropical in South India, dry in central India to humid and wet in Assam and Kerala, thus providing conditions for the growth of aromatic plants.

These plant contains flavouring compounds and have been used in perfumery from the ancient times.

e.g. various aromatic plants grown in India such as Eucalyptus plants grown in Kerala and Tamil Nadu in large scale. Mentha plant is cultivated near Jammu and in Tarai region of Uttar Pradesh. Lemon-grass plant, chenopodium herb etc., are also cultivated in various parts of India.

Aromatic plants contain odorous and volatile principles as active constituents which are known as Volatile oils/Ethereal oils, chemically derived from terpenes and their oxygenated products. They are generally composed of Isoprene (C_5H_8) units. On exposure to air at room temperature, they evaporate easily. *Essential oils* have special aromas and flavour which represent a highly complex class of natural products. Volatile oils are nearly insoluble in water however they dissolve in 1 : 200 parts of water which is sufficient to impart a characteristic smell and taste to water. Their specific gravity is less than 1.

Utilization of Aromatic Plants

The use of aromatic plant products generally exists in:

1. *Industry*: Used in perfumery, soaps, detergents, cosmetics, Agarbattis, Disinfectants, Deodarants, Mosquito repellents, flavouring agents, food, hard and soft drinks, fixatives etc.
2. *Medicine*: Used in Aromatherapy, perfumery products, Tobacco etc.
3. *Agriculture*: Used in Antifeedants, Repellents, Bioinsecticides, Natural Herbicides and as growth boosters.

Use of Essential Oils

Essential oils are used in following industries frequently:

1. *Cosmetic and Toiletries*: Perfumes and sprays, soap and detergents, creams, deodarants, shaving preparations, powder preparations.
2. *Dental Preparations*: Tooth pastes and powders, Mouth washes, Antiseptics.
3. *Medical*: In Pharmaceutical preparations.
4. Food Beverages: Liquor, flavouring agents, preservatives, sauces.
5. Tobacco Industry: Chewing tobacco, cigarettes etc.
6. *Adhesives*: Paste and Glue tapes, cements.
7. Paper and Printing Industry: Carbon paper, Ribbons ink, Labels, wrappers, writing papers.
8. Textile Industry: Finishing deodarants.
9. Petroleum Industry: Oils/Waxes, solvents, Lubricating cream.
10. *Paint Industry*: Paints, Varnishes, Distempers, Dilutants.
11. *Motor Industry*: Polishes, Cleaners and other plastic goods.
12. *Insecticide preparations*: Sprays, Repellants, Disinfectants.

7.2 Aromatherapy

Aromatherapy can be defined,

1. "As the art and science of utilizing naturally extracted aromatic essences from plants to balance and promote the health, body, mind and spirit".
2. "As a holistic approach to medicine, aromatherapy works as both preventative approach and active treatment during acute and chronic stage of illness".
3. "It is a natural, non-invasive treatment system designed to affect the symptom of disease and to balance, regulate, heal and maintain the whole human body".

Aromatherapy uses natural aromatic plant essences in the treatment of a wide range of maladies and as a means of inducing a feeling of well-being. Aromatherapy also provides treatment through the stimulation of the sense of smell using pungent materials.

Hydrosol: It is the water that remains after producing essential oils in steam or water distillation. *e.g.* Rose, Roman Chamomile, Lavender.

Carrier Oils: The essential oils are used after dilution in carrier (or base) oils. These are the vegetable oils mix with the essential oils but do not masks its aroma. *e.g.* Almond oil, Jojopa oils, Soya oils.

7.3 Chemistry of Oils

The chemical compounds in essential oils are broken down into two groups:

1. Oxygen based compounds
2. Hydrocarbons

1. ***Oxygen based Compounds***: These compounds mainly contain oxygen atom such as:

(i) *Phenols*: Stimulates bactericidal and immune boosting activity. Damages liver and skin irritating.

e.g. Eugenol oil (clove), Thymol (Thyme)

(ii) *Alcohols*: Possess antiseptic and antiviral property. Non-toxic and non-irritation to the skin. Less prone to oxidation.

e.g. Linalol (Lavender and Rosewood)

Cetronellol (Geranium Lemon)

(iii) *Esters*: Have fruity aroma

e.g. Neryl acetate (Neroli, lemon), Geranyl acetate (Geranium)

(iv) *Aldehydes*: Possess sedative and anti-inflammatory properties. Oils cause skin-irritation.

e.g. Citral (Lemon-grass, Melissa), Geranial (orange, lemon, eucalyptus) citronellal (citronella)

(v) *Ketones*: Toxic chemicals present in this group causes epileptic seizures, convulsions and mental confusion.

e.g. Fenchone (Fennel), Carvone (Coriander, Peppermint), Menthone (Pepper mint, spearmint)

(vi) *Oxides*: Camphoraceous in nature. Expectorant properties cause convulsant reactions.

e.g. Eucalyptol (Eucalyptus, Rosemary), Piperitonoxide (Peppermint)

2. ***Hydrocarbons***: These contain mainly "Terpenes" which consists of three sub categories:
   1. Monoterpenes
   2. Sesquiterpenes and
   3. Diterpenes

   This stimulates antiseptic and analgesic activity but causes skin irritation.

e.g.	Monoterpenes	=	Limonene (Most citral oils)
			Pinene (pine)
			Campherene (lemongrass)
	Sesquiterpenes	=	Santalol (sandalwood) possess anti-inflammatory properties.
			Chamazulene (Chamomile)

   Diterpenes are very rarely present in essential oils.

7.4 Pharmacological Action

1. The scent (Aroma) of essential oil is conveyed by olfactory nerve to certain areas of brain, which influences emotions and hormonal responses.
2. When used in a bath or massage, the oils are absorbed through the skin and carried out by body fluids to the main body system such as nervous and muscular system for a healing effect.
3. The oil stimulates the healing processes of body by increasing blood flow in the skin.
4. The pungent aromas stimulate the limbic system/emotional centre of brain.

Adverse Reactions

When essential oils applied to the skin, mainly three kinds of adverse reactions are produced.

(i) *Irritation*: Patch test is done.

(ii) *Sensitization*: More complicated than irritation. Once the substance introduced in the skin, it causes permanent changes in the immune system, in a similar manner to vaccination.

(iii) Photosensitization.

Note:

(i) Essential oils (in aromatherapy) are prepared by distillation method using cleavanger apparatus.

(ii) Screening of these oils having aroma is done by skin sensitization testing method using skin patch test.

Applications

Aromatherapy has four areas of applications:

(i) Anaesthesia

(ii) Psycho: These produces effects in changing feeling and mood.

(iii) Holistic: Increases mental and spiritual level.

(iv) Medical: Enhances and maintain a state of homeostasis, nourishes and stimulates skin sensitiveness. Enhances immune system.

(a) *Sandalwood Oil*

Synonyms	:	Oil of sandal wood, East Indian wood oil
Botanical Name	:	*Santalum album Linn*
Family	:	Santalaceae (Samaiaceae)
Part of the Plant	:	Heart wood (By distillation method)

Geographical source

(i) Plants are found in India and Malaysia.

(ii) Santalum species occurring in Australia and islands of Pacific are harvested for their fragrant wood.

(iii) *Santalum spicatum* and *santalum lanceolatum* (Australia),

Santulum elliplicum (Hawaii), *Santalum yasi* (Fiji and Tonga),

Santalum macgregorii (Papua New Guinea),

Santalum austrocaledonicum (Vanuatu and New Caledonia), and *Santalum Insulare* (French Polynesia).

Sandalwood oil has a characteristic sweet and woody odour widely employed in the fragrance industry, particularly in higher priced perfumes.

Habitat

Sandal is a small to medium sized, 8-12 m in height, evergreen semi-parasitic tree found in the dry regions of peninsular India from Vindhya mountains southwards, especially in Mysore and Tamil Nadu.

Description

Indian Standards for Sandalwood oil:

	Characteristics		Requirements
1.	Colour and Appearance	:	Nearly colourless to golden yellow, some what viscid, oily liquid.
2.	Odour	:	Pleasant, sweet, woody and persistent.
3.	Taste	:	Unpleasant.
4.	Solubility	:	Slightly soluble in water and soluble in alcohol and chloroform.
5.	Specific gravity at 30 °C	:	0.962-0.979
6.	Rotation $(\alpha)_D$	:	–15 to –20
7.	Refractive Index at 30 °C	:	1.499-1.506 (not below 1.503)
8.	Esters (calculated as santalyl acetate) percentage by weight	:	20
9.	Free alcohol (calculated as sandal oil) percentage by weight	:	90

Chemical Constituents: The volatile oil is contained in all the elements of wood, medullary rays, cells, wood fibres, vessels and wood parenchyma. The oil contains about 90-97% of sesquiterpene alcohol oils, distinguished for purpose of analysis as "Santalol". This consists of α-santalol (B.P = 300 – 301 °C) and β-Santalol (B.P = 170 – 171 °C)

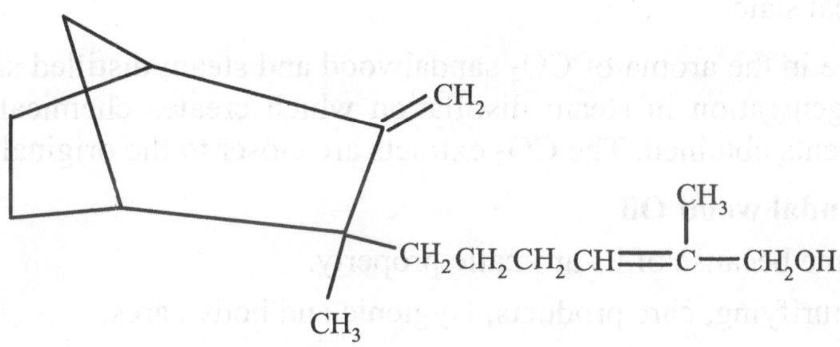

(β-Santalol)

When oil of sandalwood is heated to 150 °C (302 °F) with acetic anhydride, the acetic ester of santalol ($C_{15}H_{25}O\text{-}COCH_3$) is formed.

Isolation of Sandalwood Oil

1. *Cultivation and Collection*: Indian sandal trees of all ages and sizes are liable and more prone to be attacked by *spike disease* and if infected, the disease spread within about three years. Cultivation of sandal in India has had limited success. Cultivation of these plants is undertaken mainly in south India and state of Karnataka.

   Trees more than 25 years of age and above 60 cm girth are selected for collection of oil and are harvested during the post-monsoon period. The plants are uprooted, wood is cut into billets, bark from roots and stems is removed along with little sapwood. The wood is yellowish or pale in colour. It is very much dense, hard heavy and shows darker and higher zones.

2. *Primary Processing*: The wood is cut into small pieces, chipped and then reduced to a powder form, and is then subjected to steam distillation.
3. *Hydro-distillation*: In this method, the powder is allowed to soak in water in a hydrodistiller. A fire from below the vessel then heats the water and carries off the steam which is allowed to cool. The sandalwood oil is then removed from the top of the hydrosol. This hydro-distilling is operated under a moderate pressure, by a controlled temperature in order to avoid thermolabile compounds alteration.
4. *Steam Distillation*: Super heated steam is passed through the powdered wood. The steam helps to release and carry away the essential oils which is locked in the cellular structure of the wood. The steam is then cooled and the result is sandalwood hydrosol and sandalwood essential oil which floats on the hydrosol and is separated, further refined and then filtered.
5. *CO_2 Extraction Method*: The sandalwood CO_2 extraction method is a new technique for extracting essential oils and other constituents from plant materials. It does not use water or steam. But carbon-dioxide (CO_2) is used as a solvent. The CO_2 used under higher pressure expresses both as gaseous and liquid state called as super critical state.

The difference in the aroma of CO_2 sandalwood and steam distilled sandalwood oil is due to the heat generation in steam distillation which creates chemical changes in the aromatic constituents obtained. The CO_2 extracts are closer to the original plant materials.

Utilization of Sandal wood Oil

1. As a perfume because of its aromatic property.
2. Cosmetic purifying, care products, Hygienic and body cares.
3. Antiseptical, Astringent, Diuretic, Calming and soothing.
4. In the preparation of neem cream.
5. Used for medicinal purposes.
6. Natural fragrance widely used for fragrance fixing aromatherapy.
7. Sapwood and sapwood chips are used in preparation of agarbatties.

Pharmaceutical Uses

1. *Heating and Curative Properties*:
   - as a bitter sedative cooling,
   - as a cardiac tonic,
   - used in arresting bleeding,
   - In promoting flow of urine.

2. *Genito-Urinary Disorders*:

   - used in treatment of gonorrhoea,

   - sandal powder is mixed with milk, made into pills to use as a medication,

   - sandal oil is used in treating painful and difficult urination and inflammation of bladder.

3. *Dysentery*:

   About 20 grams of watery emulsion of sandalwood mixed with sugar, honey and rice water to be administered in the treatment of dysentery as well as in curing gastric irritability.

4. *Skin Disorders*:

   An emulsion or a paste of sandalwood is very cooling and is applied in inflammatory itchy and eruptive skin diseases,

   in curing seabies (sandal oil),

   sandal oil mixed with twice its quantity of mustard oil is used for removing pimples.

5. *Prickly Heat*:

   sadalwood paste prevents excessive sweating and heals the inflamed skin,

   dry sandalwood powder mixed with rose water is used in profuse sweating.

6. Sandalwood paste relieves headache and brings down the temperature in minutes.
7. Official medication in Europe against "Gonorrhoea" at the beginning of this century.
8. Used as Pulmonary, Urinary and cutaneous antiseptic.

Commercial Products of Sandalwood Oil

Herbal sandal cleaner (for oily skin types)

Sandal Face wash (normal to oily skins)

Sandal scrubs and Almond scrubs

Note:

1. Sandalwood provides soothing effect for cracked, chopped and irritated skin.
2. Oil of santal is used in the treatment of sub acute and chronic infections of mucus tissues.
3. Sandalwood is best for dry and oily skin and for ache.
4. Oil free sandal seed meal is rich in protein and is used as an animal feed.
5. Must be stored in well-filled closed containers away from light and in cool place.
6. Used for symptomatic treatment of dysurea.

(b) *Mentha Oil*

Synonyms : Peppermint oil

Botanical Source : *Mentha Piperita*

Family : Labiatae

Part of the plant : Fresh flower tops

Geographical source

Mentha species are cultivated in India in U.P. and near Jammu. The world production of Mentha arvensis oil is about 7000 tons of which 3000 tons is produced each in China and India and 1000 tons in the rest of the world mainly in south America. About 4000 tones of *Mentha piperita* oil is produced in United States.

Description

Characteristics		**Requirements**
1. Appearance and colour	:	Almost to pale-greenish yellow liquid
2. Odour	:	Characteristic, pleasant mentha piperita odour
3. Taste	:	Pungent followed by cooling sensation
4. Solubility	:	Soluble in 70% alcohol, ether and chloroform and insoluble in water
5. Specific Gravity	:	0.90-0.91
6. Refractive Index at 20 °C	:	1.479-1.481
7. Optical Rotation	:	(–)24^0 to (–) 26°
8. *l*-Menthol by GLC	:	44% to 50%
9. Ester content (calculated as Menthyl Acetate)	:	4% to 6%
10. Miscibility	:	1 volume with 5 volume (calculated with 70% ethanol at 20 °C)
11. ketone content	:	25% to 30%
12. Mentha Furon by GLC	:	0.7% to 2.5%
13. Availability	:	Throughout the year

Chemical Constituents

As per B.P. and E.P, Pepper mint leaf contains:

- not less than 1.2% of volatile oil
- 4.5% - 10% of esters (Menthyl Acetate)
- not less than 44% of free alcohol (Menthol)
- 15-32% of ketones (Menthone)

There are two main varieties of Mentha:

1. Indian variety (*Mentha arvensis*)
2. Japanese variety (*Mentha Canadensis* variety piperascens) contains 70-90% of menthol.

Menthol is the main constituent in Mentha oil, which contains many constituents in various proportions such as:

l-Menthol, Neo-Menthol, Neo-Iso-Menthol, Iso-Menthol, Menthone, Iso-Menthone, α-pinene, β-pinene, *l*-limonene, *cineole*, Ethylamyl carbinol, Iso-pulegol, Neo-Iso-pulegol, piperitone, β-Hexenol, Furfural and Camphene.

Menthol occurs as colourless, hexagonal usually needle type crystals/fused masses/crystalline powder with a pleasant peppermint type odour.

Melting point of [(–) – Menthol] = 41 °C- 44 °C

Congealing point of [(±) – Menthol] = 27 °C-28 °C

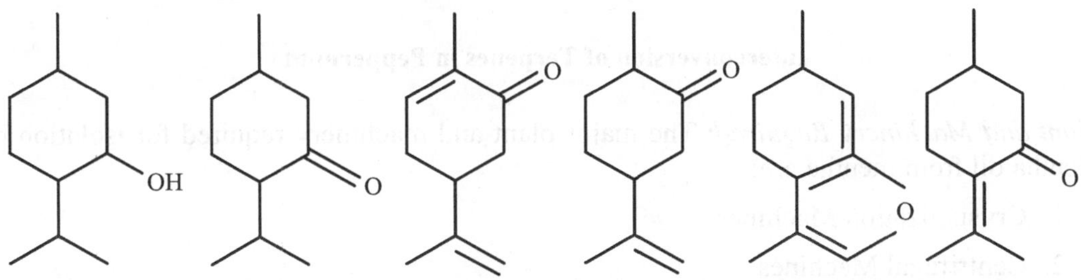

Menthol **Menthone** **Carvone** **Dihydrocarvone** **Mentho-furan** **Pulegon**

Source : ***Mentha piperita*** (Menthol, Menthone)

Source : ***Mentha spicata*** (Carvone, Dihydrocarvone)

Mentha aquatica (Mentho-furan)

Mentha pulegium (Pulegon)

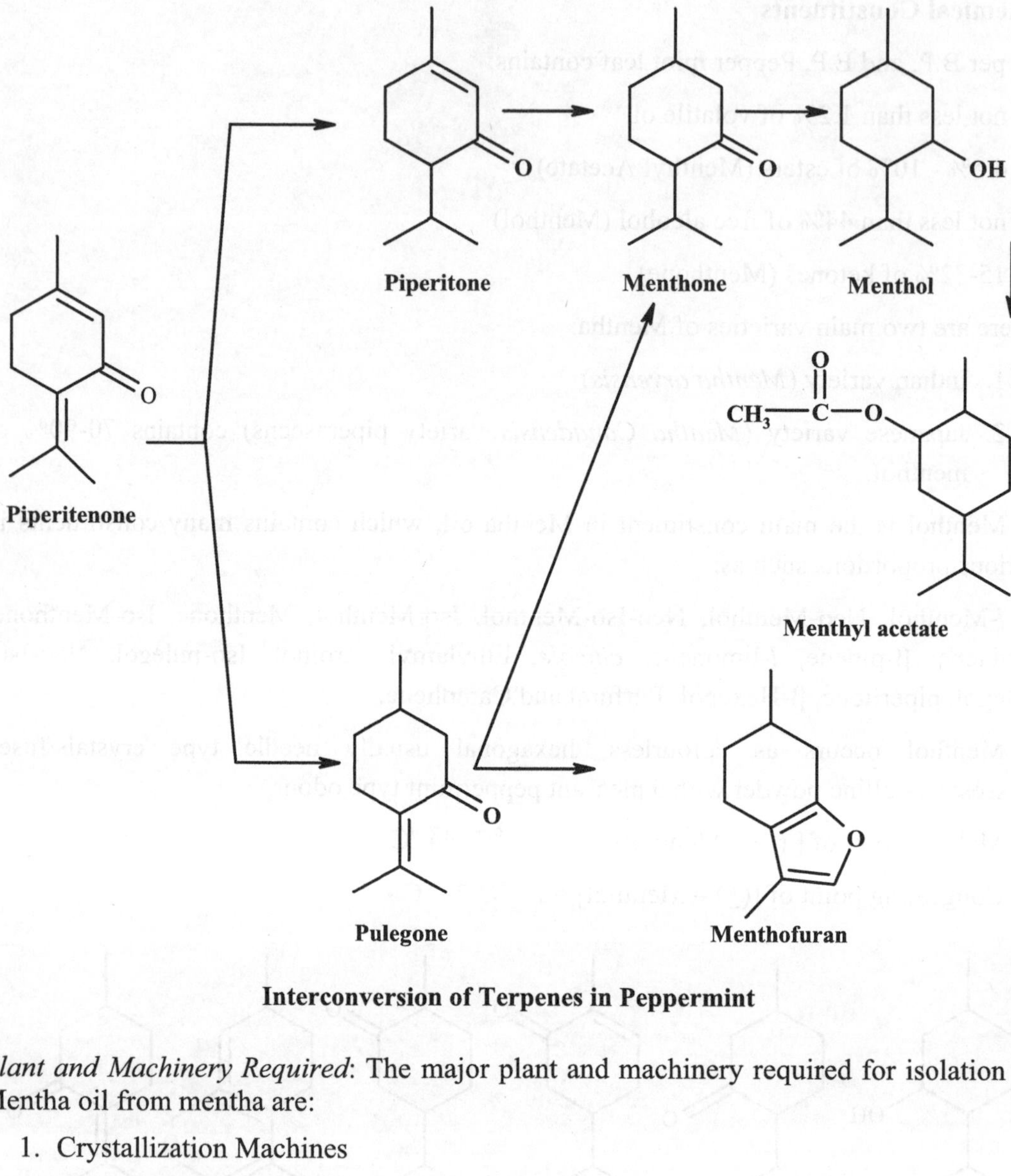

Interconversion of Terpenes in Peppermint

Plant and Machinery Required: The major plant and machinery required for isolation of Mentha oil from mentha are:

1. Crystallization Machines
2. Centrifugal Machines
3. Aluminium containers
4. Filter press and pumps
5. Storage cum melting tank
6. Laboratory instruments.

Cultivation and Collection

For the cultivation of mentha oil, well drained fertile and sandyloam soil. The cultivation is done by vegetative propagation method by using suckers. Stem is generally square and leaves are opposite and decussate, corolla is open and bilabiate, leaves are dorsinentral and have characteristic glandular trichomes which contain volatile oil.

Isolation of Mentha Oil

I *Isolation from Mentha arvensis oil*: L-Menthol, a synthetic menthol is manufactured from "*Mentha arvensis*" oil by slow crystallization, and is produced on technical scale in Europe and USA from m-cresol by alkylation with propene to thymol and hydrogenation to DL-Menthol. The optical isomers are separated and D-isomer is recycled.

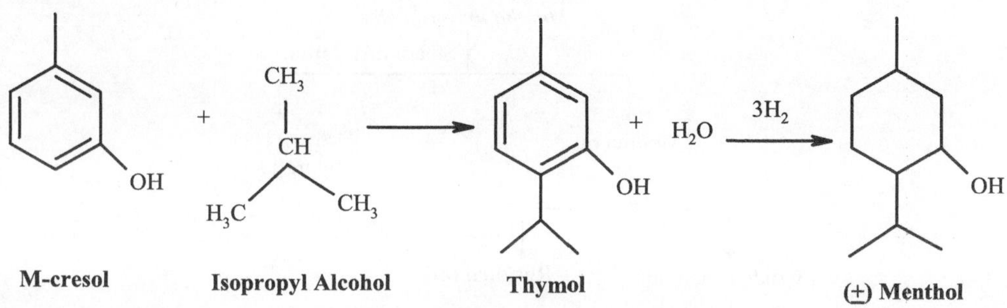

Menthol is a white crystalline chemical product having following properties:

- flavouring agent,
- anti-puritic agent,
- coolant,
- carminative

Menthol Crystals from Mentha Oil

1. In this process, oil is gradually cooled from +15 °C to –40 °C and is then cut and centrifuged.
2. The frozen menthol remains inside the jacket and unfrozen oil is collected at the bottom of centrifugal machine. The dementholised oil is stored.
3. Frozen material is remelted in a tank. The concentration of melted oil is checked and crude mentha oil or menthol powder is added for menthol crystallization at room temperature.
4. This oil is heated to 50 °C and filtered and then poured in small tanks for crystallization.
5. The Mother liquor is slowly cooled from the bottom of container and heated at the top of the container, the crystalline menthol is obtained in 18 to 20 days.

6. After crystallization, the material is taken out and cut into pieces. This process removes oil from crystals and makes them dry.
7. The crystals are subjected to natural drying for 48 hours, sieved and packed. The final product thus obtained is bold sized menthol crystals.

Mentha Oil Distillation

Mentha arvensis after harvesting is distilled by steam distillation and the resulting mentha oil is used for manufacture of menthol. There are two systems of distillation:

1. Centralized system of distillation which consists of a boiler to provide steam and distillation tubs followed by condensers and separators.
2. Decentralized system consists of a still with a false bottom which contains water to produce steam by direct fire. The distillate is condensed and separated.

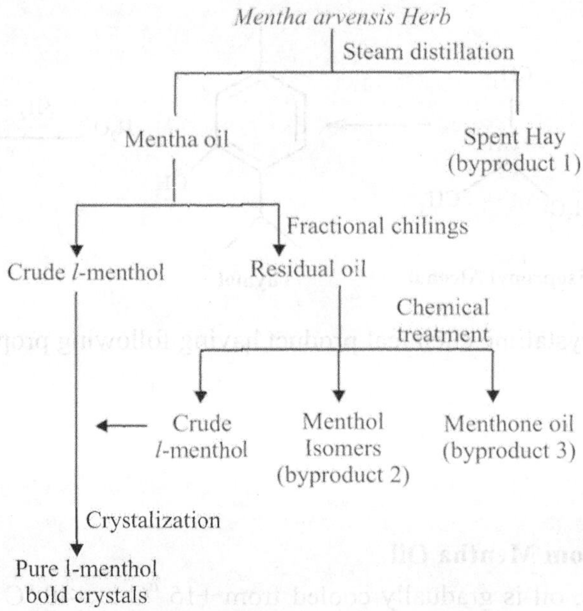

Isolation of Menthol from Mentha oil

Utilization of Mentha Byproducts

Byproduct 1 - *Spent Hay*: Chemical analysis reveals the presence of cellulose and lignin and is used as a supplementing fertilizer for mentha crop and as a fuel of high calorific value.

Byproduct 2 - *Menthol Isomers*: Used in the preparation of peppermint oil blends.

Byproduct 3 - *Menthone oil*: Used for manufacturing of thymol.

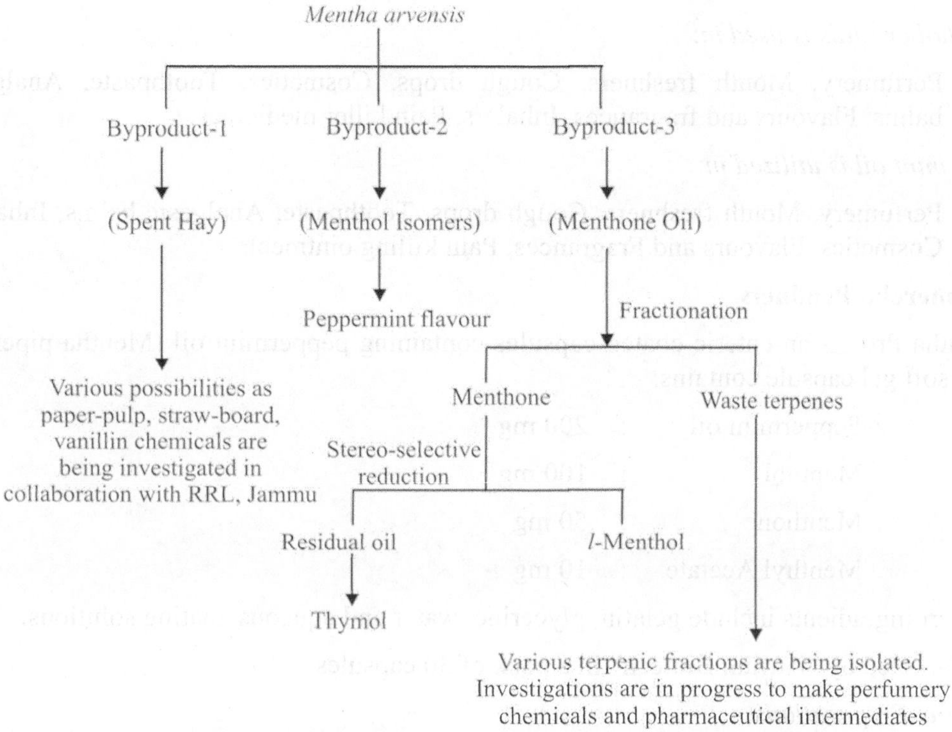

Profitable utilization of Mentha byproducts

II *Conversion of Citronellal from citronella oil*: Java citronella oil contains 30-40% of D-citronellal, which can be isolated from the oil. D-citronellal is converted over an acidic catalyst (active clay) into L-isopulegol, which is then hydrogenated to L-menthol.

III *Conversion of Pulegone from pennyroyal oil*: Pennyroyal oil contains 80-90% L-pulegone, hydrogenated to L-menthone, which is then reduced with sodium in ethanol to L-menthol.

Utilization

Peppermint is used in:

1. Confectionery, Mouth freshners, chocolates, chewing gums, Cough Drops, Analgesic Balm, Inhalers, Tobacco products, Medicated oils, Toothpastes, cosmetics.
2. Peppermint is a powerful diffusible stimulant, carminative, antispasmodic, stomachic.
3. Used to increase the flow of bile from the gall bladder.
4. Perfumery and in pain killer medicines.

Menthol crystals is used in:

1. Perfumery, Mouth freshners, Cough drops, Cosmetics, Toothpaste, Analgesic balms, Flavours and fragrances, Inhalers, Pain killer medicines.

Spearmint oil is utilized in:

1. Perfumery, Mouth freshners, Cough drops, Toothpaste, Analgesic balms, Inhalers, Cosmetics, Flavours and Fragrances, Pain killing ointments.

Commercial Products

"Mentha Pro" is an enteric coated capsules containing peppermint oil (Mentha piperita). Each soft gel capsule contains:

Peppermint oil	:	200 mg
Menthol	:	100 mg
Menthone	:	50 mg
Menthyl Acetate	:	10 mg

Inert ingradients include gelatin, glycerine, water and aqueous coating solutions.

Marketed by "Atrium Biotech" in a pack of 30 capsules.

Various Preparations

1. Aqua *Menthae piperitae*, Peppermint water
2. Oil of Peppermint, Oleum Menthae Piperitae

These various preparations are prepared from the fresh herb by distillation with steam– a greenish-yellow liquid, having a pungent odour and taste. Dose from 1 to 15 minims.

Pharmaceutical Utilization

1. In fevers, with nausea and vomiting, a warm infusion of peppermint is given to produce perspiration (due to diaphoretic property).
2. As a local Anaesthetic (due to presence of menthol)
3. To relieve local pain in the inflamed joints of rheumatism and as a spray in painful inflammation of throat.
4. As an antiseptic to prevent fermentation and promote digestion.
5. Used to cure asthma and chronic bronchitis of the aged persons.
6. To cure irritability state of stomach in cholera in painful diarrhoea and dysentery.
7. In rectal pruritis and in painful papillary growths as the orifice of female urethra, oil of peppermint or menthol is used as a local anaesthetic to relieve itching and pain.

Storage

Mentha oil should be stored in well-filled and air-tight containers protected from light and in cool place. Mentha oil darkens and becomes viscous on storage, as it is a clear and transparent liquid.

(c) *Vetiver Oil*

Synonyms : Khus oil

Botanical source : *Vetiveria zizanioides*

Family : Graminae

Part of the Plant : Root

Geographical source: vetiver is traditionally been utilized as medicinal and aromatic plants in India, Indonesia, Pakistan, Senegal, Srilanka and in Thailand. On commercial level, oil is mainly produced in China, India, Indonesia, Haiti and Reunion Islands.

In India, it is found abundantly in UP, Punjab, Karnataka, Kerala, Rajasthan and Tamil Nadu.

Thailand's vetiver oil is a light golden-yellow brown viscous oil and falls into finest grades of vetiver with high vetiverol content with little or no smokiness. Hence it is considered as Thai's "Liquid Gold".

Properties of Vetiver Oil

Vetiver oil is a light to dark brown, olive or amber coloured viscous oil having a deep smoky, earthy-woody odour with a sweet persistent undertone.

Chemical Constituents

Vetiver oil mainly contains vetiverol, vetivone, Khusimone, khusitone, terpenes (*e.g.* vetiverenes) and sesquiterpenes.

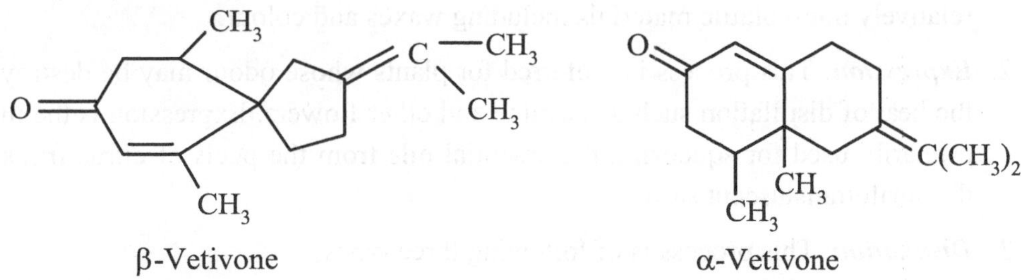

β-Vetivone α-Vetivone

Habitat and Preparation

Vetiver is a tall (2 m in height), tuffed, perennial scented grass with a straight stem, long narrow leaves and a lacework root system that is abundant, complex and extensive. These have rhizome like roots which are dried after washing and distilled immediately or stored for 12-24 months, that enzymatic processes can increase oil yield percentage. The steam distillation produces about 0.3%-1.0% of oil. The oil possess mostly ketonic sesquiterpene having structure of alcohol known as vetiverol, which is fractionated by other chemical methods to produce numerous other compounds such as vetiveryl formate, vetiveryl acetate, vetiveryl propeonale, vetriveryl caprylate, vetiveryl isovalerate and vetiveryl phenylacetate etc.

Vetiver Roots (02 pounds in small pieces) →
- Moistened with little water
- Macerated for 24 hours
- Beated in a marble mortar
- Macerated in alcohol for 8-10 days

↓
- Strained with pressure and filtered through filter paper in a fort-night

Vetiveryl Acetate ← Acetylated ← Vetiverol (Main Alcohol)

***Isolation of Vetiver Oil*:** There are mainly three production methods to obtain essential oils. They are:

1. Extraction
2. Expression
3. Distillation

1. ***Extraction*:** Extraction uses volatile solvents such as hexane and alcohol to wash out the aroma components from the plant material. The process also captures relatively non-volatile materials including waxes and colour.
2. ***Expression***: This process is preferred for plants whose odour may be destroyed by the heat of distillation such as jasmine and other flowers. Expression is the method primarily used for squeezing the essential oils from the peels of citrus fruits from the small transluscent sacs.
3. ***Distillation***: This process is of following three types:
   - (i) Water distillation
   - (ii) Water and steam distillation
   - (iii) Direct steam distillation

(i) ***Water Distillation***: Water + Drug $\xrightarrow{\text{Heated with agitation}}$ Boiled → Condensation takes place

(ii) ***Water and Steam Distillation***:
freshly cut green plant material placed over a layer of water in the base of still,
water is then boiled in a steam coil and jacket,
steam produced in the boiling vessel remains saturated and at low pressure.

(iii) ***Direct Steam Distillation***:

Most widely practised system. Vetiver roots are cut, chopped and dried and are packed on well-spaced supporting grids in stills or cylindrical tanks.

Live steam is injected through perforated coils in the base of the still at about 3 bar pressure. (necessary for vetiver oil rich in c-15 sesquiterpenoids and boiling points within 200 °C or above range temperature),

The super-heated steam forces the oil from the roots and carries away the volatile oil in a vapourous state from the top of the still to a water-cooled condenser,

In the condenser, the steam is cooled and droplets of water and oil are form on the sides,

Now they are collected in a "Florentine flask" where the oil being insoluble in the water floats on the top and is drawn off.

The above isolation process can be summarized as below:

Step I	=	Preparation → Vetiver roots are dried and chopped.
Step II	=	Loading → Roots are loaded into the still on grids
Step III	=	Distillation → Steam distilled for 16-24 hours at 3 bar atmospheric pressure
Step IV	=	Condensation → Steam and oil mixture cooled
Step V	=	Separation → Oil is separated from distillation water
Step VI	=	Maturation → 01 month for "still note" to disperse.

Utilization

Vetiver Oil is mainly utilized as:

- used as a fixative in fine perfumery,
- as a fragrance ingredient in soaps, cosmetics and perfumes,
- used to flavour sharbat and as food preservatives for asparagus

In Aromatic Plants

- Bulk of sweetly scented roots are used for cooling purposes,
- used to prepare refreshing drinking water in hilly regions of Karnataka,
- dried roots are used to give fragrance to linen clothes.

In Herbal Drinks

Vetiver root drink - A Thai traditional beverage
(Nam Ya Faek)

Preparation

Handful vetiver roots and leaves + 04 glasses of water (in equal proportion)

↓ Boiled until the liquid is concentrated to a quarter of glass.

Prepared Herbal Drink.

In Pesticides

- Used as insect repellents/insecticides,
- used to repel moths, flies and cockroaches,
- as an anti-fungal agent.,
- noot katone, a sesquiterpene present in vetiver oil, repels and even kill termites.

Pharmaceutical utilization

1. Produces sedating and strengthening effect on central nervous system.
2. Used in treatment of depression, nervous tension, debility and insomnia.
3. As an aphrodisiac agent.
4. It stimulates the circulatory system and makes a useful massage oil for elderly or debilitated people with poor circulation.
5. It stimulates production of RBCs.
6. Best suited for deep massage of muscular aches, pains, sprains, stiffness, rheumatism and arthritis.
7. In skin care to balance the secretion of sebum.
8. Used as a tonic for women suffering from post-menstruation syndrome.
9. Vetiver oil is also used in aromatherapy.
10. In traditional medicine, it is used as diaphoretic, antiseptic, antispasmodic, rubefacient, sedative, stimulant, tonic and vermifuge.

(d) *Eucalyptus Oil*

Synonyms : Eucalyptus, Dinkum oil

Botanical source : *Eucalyptus globulus, Eucalyptus australiana, Eucalyptus viminalis, Eucalyptus smithii*

Family : Myrtaceae

Part of the plant : Leaf

Geographical source	:	Eucalyptus species are natives of Australia and Tasmania. Now it is cultivated in France, Spain, Portugal, Brazil, Zaire, India and USA. Eucalyptus globulus is a large tree attaining a height of 90-100 metres or more in India, it grows in Annamalai, Nilgiri Hills in South India. Eucalyptus requires plenty of water and is grown to dry marshy lands.

Description

Appearance and colour	:	Colourless or pale yellow liquid
Taste	:	Pungent and camphorous followed by cool sensation
Odour	:	Aromatic and Camphoraceous
Solubility	:	Soluble in 90% alcohol, fixed oils, fats and in paraffin. But insoluble in water
Weight per ml	:	0.897-0.916 gm
Refractive Index	:	1.457-1.469
Optical Rotation $(\alpha)_D$	:	0° to $+10^{\circ}$

Chemical Constituents

Eucalyptus oil contains volatile oil, resins, tannic acids, dihydroflavonol, p-coumaric acid, cinnamic acid, eucalyptic acid, aromadendrin-7-methyl ether.

Eucalyptus oil chiefly contains cineole (about 80%) called as eucalyptol. Also contains pinene, camphene, and traces of phellandrene, citronellal, and geranyl acetate.

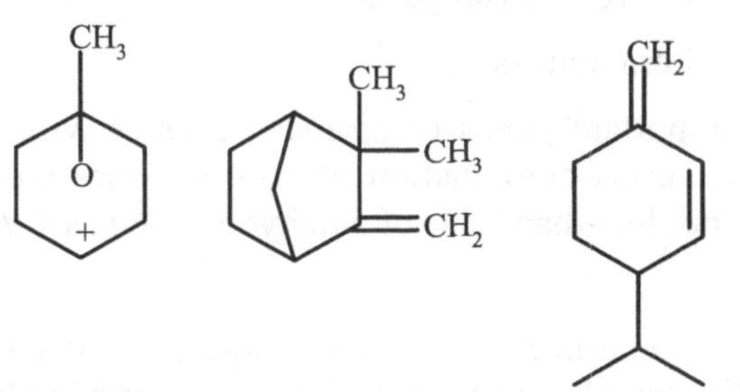

Cineole **Camphene** **Phellandrene**

Isolation of Eucalyptus Oil: Eucalyptus oil is mainly produced in Nilgiris:

(i) Leaves are firstly cut and collected. (about 1000 kg of leaves per hectare).

(ii) Leaves are dried in shade for about 3 days and is then subjected to steam distillation.

(iii) Distillation unit consists of false perforate made from copper.

(iv) During the process, each and every time 350 kg leaves are used with sufficient quantity of water. Then steam under pressure is passed through it.

(v) The distillation process is completed in 06 hours and oil thus produced is collected in the receiver.

(vi) The crude oil is rectified by treating it with NaOH, and is then filtered and filled in suitable containers.

Utilization

1. Used as disinfectant, counter-irritant, diuretic, flavouring agent, expectorant, and as a diaphoretic agent.
2. Used to relief cough, chronic bronchitis in the form of inhalations.
3. Used as an ingredient of several ointments and liniments.
4. Used to increase apetite and digestion.
5. Eucalyptus oil + Olive oil = used as a rubefacient for rheumatic disorders.
6. Used also as a mosquito repellant.

(e) *Lemon-Grass Oil*

Synonyms	:	East India Lemon-Grass oil, Indian Melissa oil
Botanical source	:	*Cymbopogon Flexuousus* *Cymbopogon citrates* *Cymbopogon pendulus*
Family	:	Graminae, Poaceae
Part of the Plant	:	Leaves, Aerial parts
Trade Name	:	Lemongrass

Cymbopogon is an important genus of aromatic grasses with about 140 species and many varieties having a varied combination of both terpenes and non-terpene phenolic constituents. It contains not less than 75% of aldehyde called as *Citral.*

Geographical Source

grown widely throughout India in Kerala, Tamil Nadu, Karnataka and Maharashtra, also occurs in west Africa, Guatemala and East Africa, also found in Cochin, Travancore, and Tinnevelly in India.

West Indian lemon grass oil (Cymboxogon citratus) is collected from plants grown in Gujarat, Maharashtra and Punjab.

Habitat: A Perennial aromatic grass

Description

Indian requirements for oil of lemon grass are:

	Characteristics		Requirements
1.	Colour and Appearance	:	Dark yellow to light brown
2.	Odour	:	Resembling to lemon like
3.	Taste	:	Similar to lemon oil
4.	Solubility	:	03 volumes of ethyl alcohol (70% by volume) occasionally with slight turbidity.
5.	Relative density (27 °C)	:	0.886-0.906
6.	Optical Rotation	:	–3° to +1°
7.	Refractive Index	:	1.4774 to 1.4834
8.	Citral content	:	75 (% by minimum volume)
9.	Storage	:	Well closed containers in cool place and away from light.

Chemical Constituents

lemon grass oil chiefly contains citral, (75-85%) in addition to methyl heptenone, decyl aldehyde, geraniol, dipentene, Linalool, limonene, methyl heptenol, nerol and citronellal,

β-ionone from which vitamin is synthesized is made from citral.

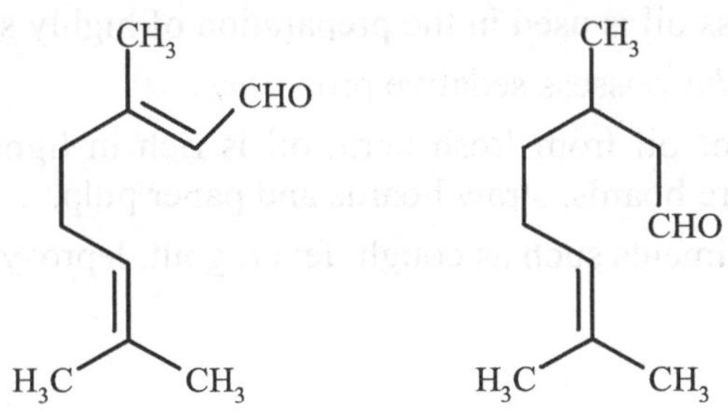

Citral **Citronellal**

Isolation of Lemon Grass Oil

1. ***Harvesting Techniques***: The first harvest of lemongrass is obtained in 4-6 months after planting and subsequent harvests are obtained at an interval of 3-4 months, depending upon the fertility of soil, temperature and humidity.

In North Indian plains, two harvests are obtained during the first year and three harvests during the subsequent years. While in Tropical areas, 4-5 harvests are obtained in subsequent years. The crop is kept in the field for 5-6 years, pulled up and rotated with other crops. Harvesting is done by sickle by cutting the leaves 10-15 cm above the ground level. The grass should be allowed to wilt for 12-24 hours before distillation.

2. ***Distillation***: The distillation of lemon-grass oil is carried out by Hydro-distillation or in directly fired distillation stills which are operated by a boiler. Steam distillation gives better yield of oil and higher citral content as compared to hydro distillation. (To save energy and fuel, the grass is chopped before charging it into stills)

   The distillation is completed within 2½ - 3 hours. The oil content is variable ranging from 0.3%-0.8%. Distillation studies over a period of 2½ hours shows that about 24-33% of oil is distilled out in first hour, 13-21% in second hour and about 3-5% in the last half an hour.

Utilization of Lemon-Grass Oil

1. As a flavouring agent and in perfumery.
2. Vitamin-A synthesized from β-ionone is prepared from citral.
3. Citral is converted into nerol and lonones which are perfumery materials.
4. Used in soaps, detergents, Cosmetics and is suitable as fumigent against flies and mosquitoes.
5. Lemongrass is a good crop for checking soil erosion on hilly areas.
6. Infusion of grass is sometimes used as a refreshing beverage. (called as Hirva cha or green tea)
7. In Java, lemongrass oil is used in the preparation of highly spiced sharbat.
8. *Cymbopogon nardus* possess sedative properties.
9. After distillation of oil from fresh herb, oil is rich in lignocellulosic material for manufacturing fibre boards, straw boards and paper pulp.
10. Used in Human ailments such as cough, fever, gout, leprosy and stomach disorders.

CHAPTER 8

PLANT TISSUE CULTURE

8.1 Introduction

Tissue culture is an experimental technique through which a mass of cells (callus) is produced from an explant tissue.

Utilization of Callus: The Callus produced during the process is used for:

regenerating plantlets,

extraction of 1°/2° metabolites,

manipulation of 1°/2° metabolites, for increasing the production through genetic engineering.

Under aseptic conditions, plant tissue culture is utilized for:

protoplast culture

cell culture

tissue culture

organ culture

Cell culture : Growth of any cell (Microbe, Plant or Animal cell)

Tissue culture : Cultivation of a plant/mammalian cell which normally forms a multicellular tissue.

Salient Characteristics of Tissue Culture

1. The culture of cells/tissues is carried out in a sterile medium under controlled conditions.
2. Clones generated through tissue culture are identical in terms of size, developmental stage and rate of metabolic activities.

3. The rate of tissue multiplication is rapid within a small area.
4. Clones are capable of performing the transformative activity to produce 1° and 2° metabolites in tissue culture medium.

Historical Development of Plant Tissue Culture

The important achievements in the development of plant tissue culture technology and production of secondary metabolites are given as under:

Table 8.1 Brief History of Plant cell Culture Technology

Year	Researchers	Work carried out
1902	Gottlieb Haberlandt (Germany)	Culturing of single cells isolated from plant tissues in a simple nutrient media
1904	Haning	Embryo culture
1922	Robbins and Kotte	Efficiency of vitamins as growth promoters
1934	White	Establishment of actively growing tomato roots
1937	White	Discovery of importance of vitamin-B for the growth
1937	Went and Thimann	Role of ouxin in plant tissue culture
1939	White, Gautheret	Establishment of callus culture
1941	Van Overback	Culture of plant embryo
1950	Street	Role of vitamins in plant growth
1954	Muir, Haberlandt	Establishment of cell suspension culture
1955	Welmore & Sorokin	Established the role of auxins and vitamins as growth regulators
1957	West & Kika	Achievement of callus production
1959	Tulecke	Developed submerged suspensions
1960	Berg,amm	Single cell cloning
1960	Cocking	Isolation of protoplast
1962	Murashigae and Skoog	Medium for the growth of callus

Table 8.1 contd...

Year	Researchers	Work carried out
1964	Morel	Micro propagation
1970	Cocking	Protoplast fusion
1972	Carson et.al	Production of first somatic hybrid
1976	Bajaj et.al	Regenerated plants from cryo-preserved plant tissues
1977	Murashigae	Proposed artificial seed production
1977	Street	Cultivation of single cell
1978	Melchers, Holder & Sacristan	Production of somatic embryo
1983	Bartan et.al	Demonstrated gene transfer into the protoplast by using plasmid vectors
1983	Chilton	Transformed tobacco plamts
1994	Calgene (USA)	Production of Novel transformed plant

Table 8.2 Milestones for Production of Secondary Metabolites from Plant Cell Cultures

Year	Milestones achieved	Researchers
1934	Plant tissue culture obtained	Gautheret
1939	Discovery of auxin	Gautheret
1942	Secondary metabolite produced in callus culture (diosgenin)	Gautheret
1954	Cell suspension culture	Muir
1955	Production of secondary metabolites in cell cultures	Mothes & Kala
1959	Large scale cultivation of plant cells	Tulecke & Nickell
1967	Yields of phytopharmaceuticals equal to intact plant	Kaul & Staba
1977	Cultivation of tobacco cells in 20000 litres bioreactor	Noguchi et.al
1979	Immobilization of plant cella by sodium alginate	Bordelins
1981	Use of hollow fibre reactor for secondary metabolite production	Shuler
1983	First plant tissue culture process commercialized	Curtin
1995	Taxol produced from plant cell culture on commercial scale	Phyton Newsletter

Nutritional Requirements of Plant Cell Culture

Tissue culture technique requires a controlled and an aseptic environment to proceed with the establishment of callus in the nutrient media. The nature of the explant and composition of nutrient medium generally determines the successful establishment and growth of plant cells *in vitro.*

- Media containing nutrients of plant origin that are chemically not precisely characterized are called complex or highly enriched media.
- Media containing exclusively chemically defined compounds are called synthetic or regular media.

An ideal nutrient medium for plant tissue culture contain five classes of ingredients:

1. ***Inorganic Components***: Cultured plant tissues require a continuous supply of certain inorganic chemicals. Basic media are solutions of inorganic salts in different concentrations, called as macro and micro nutrients.

Inorganic Components

Macro-Nutrients	**Micro-Nutrients**
(in m mol/*l*) ↓ N, P, K, Ca, Mg, S (Concentration >30 ppm)	(in μmol/*l*) Iodide, Boric Acid, Salts of B, Mn, Zn, Cu, Mo, Cl, Ni, Al etc. (Necessary as cofactor, *e.g.* Ni used for urease synthesis)

2. ***Organic Components***

   Amino acids: These are added for substitution of nitrogen supply. *e.g.* Threonine, Glycine, and valine reduces ammonium utilization by inactivating glutamase synthetase located in chloroplasts and cytoplasm.

   Vitamins(μ *mol/l*):

   (i) Thiamine(vitamin-B_1) is the only essential vitamin, added as thiamine hydrochloride in amounts ranging from 0.1-10 mg/*l*.

   (ii) But Nicotinic acid (Niacin) and Pyridoxin (vitamin – B_6) may stimulate the growth.

   (iii) p-aminobenzoic acid (PABA), Ascorbic acid (vitamin-C), Tocopherol (vitamin-E), Biotin (Vitamin-H), Cyanocobalamin (Vitamin-B_{12}), Folic acid, Riboflavin (vitamin-B_2) and calcium pentothenate.

   Complex extracts: Required for increasing the growth rate of cells in bio-mass e.g. Coconut milk (liquid endosperm), Yeast extract, Malt extract, Protein hydrolyzates, Tomato juice, Potato extract.

3. ***Carbon Source***: Carbon source is added in the form of carbohydrates. Sucrose or glucose is used as a concentration of 20-30 g/*l* (2-4%). Myoinositol is also used.

   Plant Cell cultures utilizing galactose) are (*Daucus Carota, Pentunia hybrida*) or lactose (*Caffea arobica, Datura innoxia, Daucus carota, Medicago sativa*:

   Various carbon sources used in plant tissue culture media:

   Commonly used: Glucose, Sucrose, Glycerol, Pentoses, Uronic acid,

   Scarcely used: Lactose, Galactose, Non-refined carbohydrates, Molasses, Potato starch, Grain starch.

4. ***Plant Growth Regulators***: "Plant growth regulators are organic compounds, which affect the morphological structure or physiological process of plants in low concentrations." Phytohormones or plant hormones are naturally occurring growth regulation, which in low concentrations control the physiological process in plants. The main five naturally occurring plant harmones are:

   Auxins, Ethylene, Abscisic acid, cytokinins and Gibberellins. Some new natural growth substances with regulatory roles in tissue cultures have been discovered. *They are*: Polyamines, Jasmonates, Brassinosteroids, Oligosaccharins, Sterols, Phosphoinositosides, Salicylic acid.

5. ***Water***: Demineralized and double distilled water is used.

   Note: Agar as a gelling agent is required for growth when the surface is solid.

Table 8.3 Composition of Murashige and Skoog Medium

Compound	Concentration in medium mg/*l*	Amount of stock solution	Stock volume (in m*l*)
NH_4NO_3	1650	8.25 g	400
KNO_3	1900	9.50 g	400
$MgSO_4.7H_2O$	370	1.85 g	400
KH_2PO_4	170	0.85 g	400
KI	0.83	4.18 mg	400
$MnSO_4.4H_2O$	22.30	111.50 mg	400

Table 8.3 contd...

Compound	Concentration in medium mg/l	Amount of stock solution	Stock volume (in ml)
$ZnSO_4.\ 7H_2O$	8.6	43.00 mg	400
Myo-inositol	100	0.50 g	400
$CaCl_2.\ 2H_2O$	440	2.20 g	400
$FeSO_4.\ 7H_2O$	27.8	139.25 mg	100
Na_2 EDTA. $2H_2O$	37.3	186.25 mg	100
$CuSO_4.\ 5H_2O$	0.025	12.5 mg	100
$Na_2MoO_4.\ 2H_2O$	0.25	12.5 mg	10
$CoCl_2.\ 6H_2O$	0.025	12.5 mg	100
Nicotinic acid	0.50	25.0 mg	10
Pyridoxine .HCl	0.50	25.0 mg	10
Thiamine .HCl	0.10	5.0 mg	10
Glycine	2.0	100 mg	10
Sucrose	30g/l	-	-

Surface Sterilization of Explants

An explant is a detached portion of the plant body which is used in tissue culture to produce callus tissues. The commonly used surface sterilizing agents are:

Sodium hypochlorite (1-2%), Bromine water (1-2%), Hydrogen Peroxide (10-12%), Mercuric Chloride (0.1-1.0%) and silver nitrate (1%).

The aerial portions of plant such as bud, stem and leaf are sterilized by submerging for 2-3 minutes in 70% ethanol followed by 2-3 rinses in sterile distilled water.

The seeds are treated with 70% ethanol for about 2 minutes, washed with sterile distilled water and treated with surface sterilizing agent for a specific period, once again rinsed with sterile distilled water and kept for germination under aseptic conditions.

Establishment of Cultures: Two types of cultures are established:

1. Agar gel culture
2. Suspension culture
   a. Batch suspension cultures
   b. Semi continuous cultures
   c. Continuous cultures

1. ***Agar gel Culture*:** The surface sterilized plant material is aseptically transferred on solidified nutrient medium in flasks or culture tubes and allowed to incubate at 26-28 °C in dark. After 3-4 weeks, the callus should be about 5 times, the size of the explant. The callus develops from the tissue not in contact with and not immersed in the solidified culture medium. The well developed callus is cut into small pieces with a sterile knife, and transferred into proliferation media to induce the proliferation of callus. In this media, the callus tissues multiplies more rapidly.

2. ***Suspension Culture*:** This culture contains homogenous individual plant cells in its liquid medium.

   - *Batch suspension cultures*: In this technique, the cells multiply in a liquid medium which is being continuously agitated to break up any cell aggregates.

   - *Semi-continuous cultures*: Here, an open system is designed for the periodic removal of culture and addition of a fresh medium, by which means the growth of the culture is continuously maintained.

     Continuous cultures: This open system has two forms:

     (a) Chemostat system

     (b) Turbostat system

The main feature is that, cell proliferation takes place under constant conditions.

Growth Profile and Maintenance of Plant Cell Culture

Growth of cell and callus suspension culture is monitored and maintained by increase in fresh or dry weight or increase in cell number. For cell suspension cultures increase in packed cell volume. Packed cell volume pcv) is also a good indicator of growth.

Cell Culture Growth Profile

(i) *Lag-phase*: From subculture into the fresh medium, the cell regains the ability of division and the tissue shows slow growth.

(ii) *Exponential phase*: This stage involves rapid cell division.

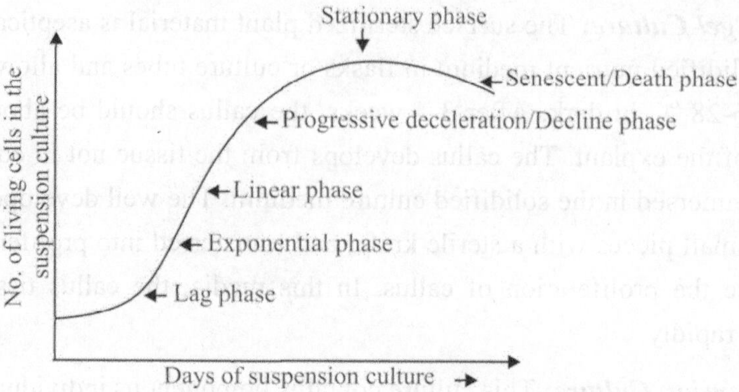

Growth curve of single cell culture

(iii) *Linear Phase*: Growth is in linear pattern with respect to time.

(iv) *Progressive decelaration phase*: The rate of cell division declines with the aging of the culture.

(v) *Stationary phase*: The rate of production of cells is equal to the rate of their death.

(vi) *Senescent Phase*: The cells are dying in this phase.

Callus Culture Growth Profile

(i) *Lag Phase*: Cells undergo cell division and tissue resumes its growth.

(ii) *Exponential phase*: This phase have vigorous growth with rapid cell division. The tissues consume nutrients from the medium.

(iii) *Decline Phase*: Elements from medium deplete which leads to a decline in the growth of callus tissue.

(iv) *Stationary phase*: From this stage, no growth is evident.

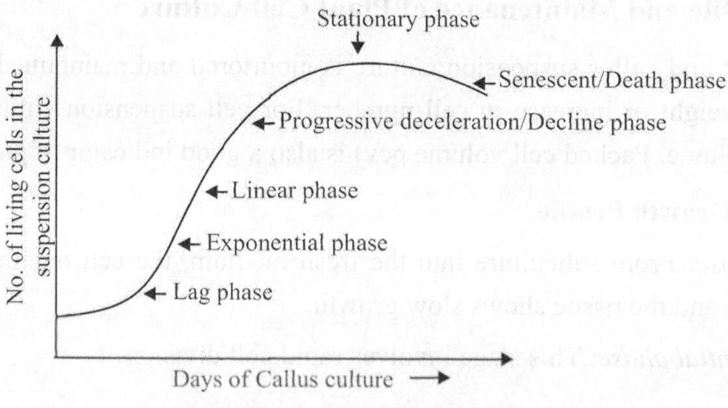

Growth curve of callus culture

Growth Determination

Several techniques are used for measuring culture growth:

1. *Fresh and Dry Weight Measurements*:

$$\text{Growth Index (GI)} = \frac{\text{Final Weight of Callus or Cells}}{\text{Initial Weight of Callus or Cells}}$$

2. *Increase in cell number*: A haemocytometer is used for determining cell numbers in a fine suspension culture. An ideal macerating fluid for callus or cell aggregates from suspension cultures consists of equal volumes of 10% chromic acid and 10% nitric acid.
3. *Packed cell volume (pcv)*: Expressed as a percentage of total volume in tube and useful for suspension cultures.
4. *Molecular Protein and DNA*:
5. *Mitotic Index*: It is an estimate of number of cells of population in mitosis stages.

$$\text{Mitotic Index} = \frac{\text{Number of Nuclei in mitosis}}{\text{Total number of nuclei stored}} \times 100$$

6. Medium component calibration
7. Conductivity of medium
8. *Cellular protein*: The total α protein and Growth/amount of cells and is estimated by Bardford's reagent.

Types of Culture

Plant tissue culture, covers all type of aseptic plant culture and is distinguished into various types of cultures under organogenic differentiation.

1. *Seed Culture*: Culture of seeds *in vitro* to generate seedlings/plants.
2. *Organ Culture*: Culture of isolated plant organs. Some types of organ culture can be distinguished as follows:
   - *Meristem-tip-culture*: Meristem is the mass of undifferentiated parenchyma cells found at the extreme tip of the shoot and root systems. They have the potency for regenerate into plant leaves.
   - *Shoot-tip culture*: This method is used with both monocot and dicot species. Actively growing shoot-tip is surface sterilized and is placed on a defined culture medium under sterile conditions.
   - *Microspore and Anther Culture (Pollen culture)*: Microspore culture utilizes a true haploid cell system with gametophytic chromosome number and develops directly into embryos within 15 days.

In another culture, dissected grains + liquid beaker suspension is filtered through a millipore nylon filter which contains only microspores, which is centrifuged at 1000 rpm for 5 minutes.

3. *Embryo culture*: Culture or excised mature/immature embryo from seeds.
4. *Callus culture*: Culture of a differentiated tissue from explant is allowed to differentiate, *in vitro* and so called callus tissue is produced.
5. *Suspension culture*: The liquid suspension culture consists of mixtures of cell aggregates, cell clusters and single cells.
6. *Protoplast culture*: Culture of plant protoplasts i.e., cells devoid of their cell walls.
7. *Plant cell culture*: Culture of isolated cells or very small aggregates remaining dispersed in liquid medium.
8. *Flower organ and fruit organ culture*

Major Advantages of Plant Tissue Culture

1. Useful natural compounds can be produced under controlled environmental conditions, independent of soil conditions and changes in climatic conditions.
2. Used in studying biogenesis of secondary metabolites.
3. Technique used for synthesis of medicinal compounds which are too difficult to synthesize chemically.
4. Absolutely uniform biomass is managed under regulated and reproducible conditions.
5. Possible to attempt biotransformation (steroidal) reactions in plant cell cultures.
6. Cells of any plant (topical/temperate) is multiplied to yield specific metabolites.
7. Cultured cells could be maintained free from any microbial contamination and insect attack.
8. It can create a large number of clones from a single seed/explant.
9. For species that have long generation time (*e.g.* Taxol), low levels of seed production or seeds that do not readily germinate, rapid propagation is possible.
10. Easy to select desirable traits directly from culture set up (*in vitro*).
11. It allows for the internal exchange of sterilized plant materials.
12. Eliminates plant diseases through careful stock selection and sterile techniques.
13. Enables the cold storage of large numbers of viable plants in a small space.

Limitations

1. It is costly (as aseptic conditions is to be maintained) technique.
2. It requires highly skilled personnel.
3. Ability to grow off the plantlets will limit the production.

4. Care and handling of plantlets is required prior to their transfer into the containers.
5. Maintenance of disease and insect free stock plants is done with a low titer of bacterial and fungal contamination.

Applications of Plant Tissue Culture in Pharmacy

1. To study respiration and metabolism: During study, callus tissue homogenates and its cellular fraction provide means of separating normal and diseased growth.

   For e.g. Enzymatic differences in tissue of crown gall and normal origins exists even after growth in culture. A reduction in respiratory levels in crown gall tissue culture has also been noted.

2. *Studies of plant diseases and their elimination:* During the study the gall tissue was found to be more growth substance active than normal tissue *in vitro*. Callus tissues infected with TMV and other viruses have been examined to clarify virus infection and multiplication.

3. *To study polarity and organ function*: Isolated tissues are useful for conducting studies related to polarity and organ function. Three major types of proliferation are developed in isolated tissues.

   (i) Proliferation of unorganized parenchyma

   (ii) Proliferation of specialized cambial layer

   (iii) Proliferation of organized growing points.

   These may develop in fresh plants or in established cultures.

4. *The production of Haploids*: The haploid plants are characterized by having only a single set of chromosomes in their cells. For production of haploid; ovule or pollen grain culture is established in the medium. These haploid plants are employed in improving the field and agricultural crops. Pollen incompatibility can be removed by mentor pollen technology.

5. *Single cell culture of higher plant cells*: Single cell clones of tissue from marigold crown gall tissue have shown constant differences in growth rate, texture and colour. Some clones with varied media developed shoots/roots in culture.

   Single cell clones may be further evaluated for additional chemical, morphological, genetical and pathological similarities and differences.

6. *Procurement of commercial products*: Commercial products like cardiac glycosides, morphine alkaloids, essential oil and original rubber is produced by exploiting tissue culture. Cardiac glycosides are found only in morphologically differentiated cell cultures with concentrations of only 1mg/*l* suspension. Even

morphine and codeine are present in about 1.5 mg/gm dry weight in the cell cultures of papaver species.

7. *Germplasm storage*: Generally a large number of individual tissues are stored in a limited area. This type of storage is called as Germplasm storage. The germplasm in the growing stage is used for storage of tissues.
8. *Embryo rescue*: When normal fertilization fails, the fertilized egg on immature, embryo is removed from the immature fruits and cultured in the tissue culture medium to generate hybrids. This process of embryo culture is referred as embryo rescue and is used for embryo culture, ovule culture and ovary culture.
9. *Somaclonal modification*: The formation of variant clones from the cultured callus tissues is called somaclonal variation. The somaclonal variables can be desirable and undesirable. Desirable variants are useful in crop improvements. A variety of somaclonal variants have been raised from plants like sugarcane, maize, rice and other cereals.
10. *Production of artificial seeds*: An artificial seed (a synthetic seed) is made up of a somatic embryo surrounded by the nutrient medium and is protected by a thin synthetic membrane. They are identical and contain only somatic embryos of known strain. The seeds are encapsulated in a synthetic membrane made up of a polyoxyethylene, sodium alginate or polyacrylamide gel.
11. *Clonal propagation and Micro propagation*:

    Clonal propagation involves propagation through the techniques of cell, tissue and organ culture.

    Advantages

    - Rapid multiplication of superior clones.
    - Maintenance of genetic uniformity
    - Multiplication of sexually derived sterile hybrids.

    In this technique shoot tips/auxillary buds are utilized for propagation on culture media.

    Micro propagation technique is used both at research level and commercial level. It can be employed for the mass production of plants including nursery stock species, ornamental vegetables and field crops. This method produces selected genotypes in large number.

    Micro propagation is conducted into four main stages:

    (i) Selection and sterilization of elite plants.

    (ii) Establishment of auxillary buds and culture.

(iii) Multiplication in culture.

(iv) Rooting of *in vitro* plants and transfers to compost.

12. *Mutant selection*: The selection of mutant cells is usually performed by addition of toxic substances to cells followed by isolation of resistant cells.
13. *Endosperm culture*: Endosperm is triploid in its chromosomal constitution. It supplies nutrition to developing embryo. Triploid plants are useful for production of seedless fruits of banana, watermelon etc. Triploids are generally obtained by crossing colchicines-induced tetraploids with diploid followed by rescue of triploid embryos.
14. *Nucellus culture*: In citrus plant, adventative embryos develop from nuclear cells is utilized for micro propagation. It is grown on Whites medium supplemented with case in hydrolysate to obtain callus which may give rise to pseudobulbils differentiating into embryoids.
15. In production of high-yielding, herbicide, salt-resistant and insect resistant crops.
16. In micro propagation of medicinal and aromatic plants.
17. Used in production and analysis of secondary metabolites.
18. Used in production of phyto pharmaceuticals, food flavours, colours from plant cell cultures.

CHAPTER 9

HERBS AS HEALTH FOODS

9.1 Herbs

Depending on the perspective, the word "herb" has different meanings:

1. In commercial terms: Herb generally refers to plants used for culinary purposes.
2. In Horticultural terms: Herb refers to "herbaceous", which describes the appearance of the plant.
2. In Taxonomic terms: Herb refers to above ground/aerial parts, such as leaf, flower and stem.
4. In terms of Herbal Medicine: Herb refers to plants used in various forms/preparations, valued for their therapeutic benefits.

Herbal Medicine: "It is an approach to healing which uses plant or plant-derived preparations to treat, prevent or cure various health conditions and ailments."

Philosophy

(i) Modern medicine drugs contain a single active ingredient.

(ii) Combinations of plants are used, each having different compounds as well as individual properties.

(iii) Single plant medicines are considered by herbalists to be polypharmacy.

(iv) Single plant may contain hundreds of different chemical compounds.

(v) Modern medicine drug produced by development of a synthetic chemical ingredient or by identifying and extracting a specific active compound from a plant and then producing it synthetically to obtain a pure form of the entity which has the desired pharmacological effect.

(vi) In herbal medicine, it is accepted that, even if a specific compound is identified and its action understood, it is the effect of other supporting or modifying compounds present in the whole plant which complement the therapeutic action and minimizes side effects and adverse reactions in herbal medicines.

(vii) The chemical compounds in each one will be different, which is the strength of herbal medicine.

WHO guidelines for Herbal Medicines

1. Finished, labelled medicinal products that contain as active ingredients – aerial or underground parts of plants, or other plant material, or combinations thereof, whether in the crude state or as plant preparations.
2. Plant material includes juices, gums, fatty oils, essential oils and any other substance of this nature.
3. Herbal medicines may contain excipients in addition to active ingredients.
4. Medicines containing plant material combined with chemically defined active substances including chemically defined, isolated constituents of plants, are not considered to be herbal medicines.
5. The main objectives are:
   (i) Provisions for recommended general test methods.
   (ii) General limits for contaminants for herbal drugs.

Utilization of Herbal Remedies

A 'Herbal Remedy' is that in which main therapeutic activity depends upon the plant or fungal metabolites which it contains.

Some of the herbal preparations/formulations with their therapeutic effects and applications are listed below:-

Herbal Preparations	Ingredients (Herbs) present	Applications/ Uses	Therapeutic effects
Thyme and lungwort syrup	Liquorice (*Glycyrrhiza glabra*) Thyme (*Thymus vulgaris*) Lungwort (*Pulmonaria officinalis*) Anise seeds (*Pimpinella anisum*) Honey	Used in chesty coughs	Thyme, a useful antiseptic for respiratory system. Lungwort leaves, for chest infections.
Wild cherry and Hyssop syrup	Wild cherry bark (*Prunus serotina*) Hyssop (*Hyssopus officinalis*) Honey	Used in irritant coughs	Wild cherry, a mild sedative and good for suppressing irritable coughs. Hyssop a traditional remedy for stubborn coughs.
Boneset and elderflower tea	Boneset (*Eupatorium perfoliatum*) Elderflower (*sambucus nigra*) Peppermint (*Mentha piperita*) Yarrow, water	Common colds	Boneset, used for bone-shaking fevers. Elderflower, is added to combat catarrh
Elecampane and Vervain mixture	Elecampane root (*Inula helenium*) Pleurisy root (*Asclepias tuberose*) Vervain (*Verbena officinalis*) Liquorice root (*Glycyrrhiza glabra*) Boneset (*Eupatorium perfoliatum*) Water	Used in bad cold as flu	Elecampane, an excellent tonic expectonant and restorative. Vervain encourages sweating to help reduce fevers and aids the digestion.
Catmint and Vervain Tea	Catmint (*Nepeta cataria*) Vervain (*Verbena offcinalis*) Boneset (*Eupatorium perfoliatum*) Water	Fevers	A cooling mixture used when the fever is at the hot and sticky stage. Catmint, a sedative herb encourages sweating. Vervain, a good digestive stimulant.

Table conti...

Herbal Preparations	Ingredients (Herbs) present	Applications/ Uses	Therapeutic effects
Sage and Rosemary Gargle	Sage leaves (*Salvia officinalis purpurea*) Rosemary leaves (*Rosemarinus officinalis*) Lady's mantle leaves (*Alchemilla vulgaris*) Water	Sore throats and laryngitis	Rosemary and sage are aromatic, antiseptic and rich in potent healing oils. Lady's Mantle an astringent is used to reduce inflammation.
Cleavers and sage tincture	Cleavers tincture (*Galium apparine*) Sage tincture(*Salvia officinalis*) Echinacea tincture (*Echinacea angustifolia*) Golden seal tincture (*Hydrastis Canadensis*)	Tonsillitis	Cleavers, a cleansing and healing agent for lymphatic system. Sage, an antiseptic and immune stimulant which helps to combat tonsillitis.
Myrrh and rosemary mouthwash	Myrrh tincture (*Commiphora molmol*) Rosemary (*Rosemarinus officinalis*) Water	Mouth ulcers	Myrrh, an extremely antimicrobial agen is a less pleasant herbs. Rosemary infusion is added to help disguise the flavour.
Sandalwood and pine inhalant	Sandalwood oil (*Santalum album*) Pine oil (*Pinus sylvestris*) Lavender oil (*Lavendula angustifolia*) Peppermint oil (*Menta piperita*) Balsam (*Styrax benzoin*)	Catarrh (Excess passing of mucus through nasal passage)	Steam inhalants are one of the most effective ways of treating upper respiratory tract problems. These oils are astringent, antiseptic and have soothing agent.
Magnolia and Elderflower tincture	Magnolia flower tincture (*Magnolia liliflora*) Elderflower tincture (*Sambucus nigra*) Ground ivy tincture (*Glechoma hederacea*) Echinacea tincture (*Echinacea angustifolia*) Bayberry tincture (*Myrica cerifera*) Ginger tincture (*Zingiber officinalis*) Peppermint tincture (*Mentha piperita*)	Sinusitis	Magnolia, an anti-inflammatory agent for the mucous membranes. Elderflower, a traditional remedy for catarrh and phlegm.

Table contd...

Herbal Preparations	Ingredients (Herbs) present	Applications/ Uses	Therapeutic effects
Mullein and pasque flower ear drops	Pasque flower tincture (*Anemone vulgaris*) Infused Mullein oil (*Verbascum thapsus*) Golden seal tincture (*Hydrastis Canadensis*)	Earache	Pasque flower, a good sedative and analgesic seems to have a specific affinity with the ears. Mullein is a herb with soothing properties that helps repair damaged tissues.
Goldent rod and Gingko mixture	Golden rod tincture (*Solidago virgaurea*) Gingko tincture (*Gingko biloba*) Ribwort plantain tincture (*Plantago lanceolata*) St.John's wort tincture (*Hypericum perforatum*) Pasque flower tincture (*Anemone vulgaris*)	Chronic ear infection (otitis media region)	Golden rod is a good anticatarrhal helpful in ear conditions. Gingko and pasque flower have an affinity with ear problems helping to focus healing mixtures on the ear.
Marigold compress	Marigold petals (Calendula officinalis) Water	Styes (an inflammation of glands present at the base of eyelashes)	Marigold, an astringent and antiseptic, and an excellent remedy for local skin infections and inflammations.
Eyebright and marigold eye bath	Eyebright (*Euphrasia officinalis*) Marigold petals (*Calendula officinalis*) Water	Conjunctivitis and Blepharitis (inflammation of eye lid)	Eyebright is a herb used to treat eye infections.
Ju hua and wood betony tea	Ju hua (*Chinese chrysanthemum flowers*) (*Chrysanthemum morifolium*) Wood betony (*Stachys betonica*) Gotu kola (*Centella asiatica*) Peppermint (*Mentha piperita*) Water.	Used in tired eyes and eye strain	In Chinese medicine, eyes are associated with liver and herbs such as Ju Hua and wood betony clean and stimulate that organ, thus helping to revive the eyes.
Heartsease and red clover tea	Heartsease (*viola tricolour*) Red clover flowers (*Trifolium pratense*) Stinging nettle (*Urtica dioica*) Burdock (*Arctium lappa*) Fumitory (*Fumaria officinalis*) Skullcap(*Scutellaria lateriflora*) Water	Used in eczema	Heartsease is a good cleansing and anti-inflammatory herb, which acts as a gentle circulatory stimulant. Red clover helps to clear toxins from the system and has a diuretic action.

Table contd…

Herbal Preparations	Ingredients (Herbs) present	Applications/ Uses	Therapeutic effects
Figwort Tea	Burdock root (*Arctium lappa*) Yellow dock root (*Rumex crispus*) Figwork (*Scrophularia nodosa*) Red clover flowers (*Trifolium pratense*) Water	Psoriasis	Figwort and red clover functions as cleansing and anti inflammatory herbs
Agrimony and chamomile tea	Agrimony (*Agrimonia eupatoria*) Chamomile flowers (*Matricaria recutita*) Stinging nettles (*Urtica dioica*) Heartsease (*Viola tricolor*)	Urticaria (hives) (Red rashes and itchy lumps present on the skin)	Preparation is a soothing infusion in which agrimony calms the gut irritations and chamomile has anti-allergic properties.
Marigold and tea tree ointment	Infused marigold oil (*Calendula officinalis*) Tea tree oil (*Melaleuca alternifolia*) Bees wax (*Anhydrous lanolin*)	Ringworm and athlete's foot	Marigold and tea tree oil possess antifungal property. Combining the two oils for use as a lotion is a convenient alternative.
Slippery elm poultice	Powdered slippery elm (*Ulmus fulva*) Eucalyptus oil (*Eucalyptus globulus*) Water	Boils and carbuncles (Cluster of boils)	Slippery elm is effective in drawing the core from boils. Eucalyptus oil is added as an antiseptic.
Lavender and Yarrow facial	Tea Tree oil (*Melaleuca alternifolia*) Rosewater (*Rosa damasiena*) Distilled witch hazel (*Hamamelis virginiana*) Lavender flowers (*Lavandula angustifolia*) Yarrow flowers (*Achillea millefolium*) Elder flowers (*sambucus nigra*)	Used in Ache	Steam is used to open the pores and then a lotion is applied to cleanse the skin. The antiseptic and anti inflammatory herbs added to the steam helps to combat the symptoms of ache.
Rosemary and Nettle shampoo	Rosemary leaves (*Rosemarinus officinalis*) Stinging nettle root (*Urtica dioica*) Tea tree oil (*Melaleuca alternifolia*) Soft soap (*Methylated alcohol*)	Dandruff	Rosemary is a stimulating warming herb for traditional hair rinse, helping to keep hair shiny and healthy. Stinging Nettle root is used as a hair conditioner.
Tea tree and lavender oil	Tea tree oil (*Melaleuca alternifolia*) Lavender oil (*Lavendula angustifolia*) Sweet almond oil	Cold sores	These have specific antiviral properties and used topically to treat infections caused by Herpes simplex virus.

Table contd…

Herbal Preparations	Ingredients (Herbs) present	Applications/ Uses	Therapeutic effects
Thuja and tea tree lotion	Thuja tincture (*thuja accidentalis*) Tea tree oil (*Melalucea alternifolia*)	Warts and verrucae (*viral infections*)	Thuja, a traditional remedy for treating warts. Tea tree has powerful antiseptic and antifungal properties.
Elderflower and dandelion tincture	Elderflower tincture (*Sambucus nigra*) Dandelion root tincture (*Taraxacum officinale*) Vervain tincture (*Verbena officinalis*) White horehound tincture (*Marrubium vulgare*) Siberian Ginseng tincture (*Elentherococcus senticosue*)	Hayfever and allergic rhinitis	Elderflower, strengthens the mucous membranes and Dandelion cleanse the liver to fight with allergens and reduce symoptoms.
Sundew and Hyssop mixture	Sundew fluid extract (*Drosera rotundifolia*) Hyssop tincture (*Hyssopus officinalis*) Elecampane tincture (*Inula helenium*) Thyme tincture (*Thymus vulgaris*) Chamomile tincture (*Matricaria recutita*) Liquorice fluid extract (*Glycyrrhiza glabra*)	Used to cure asthma of allergic character	Sundew, an antispasmodic and relaxing expectorant is the most effective herb used for allergic asthma.
Marigold and Agrimony tea	Echinacea root (*Echinacea angustifolia*) Marigold petals (*Calendula officinalis*) Agrimony leaves (*Agrimonia eupatoria*)	Candidiasis	Marigold is good antifungal agent used internally/externally. Agrimony helps to soothe the gut irritation caused by allergens and heals mucous membranes.
Marshmallow and Lemon balm tea	Marshmallow root (*Althaea officinalis*) Fenugreek seeds (*Trigonella foenum graecum*) Dang shen (*Codonopsis pilosula*) Fresh lemon balm leaves (*Melissa officinalis*) Agrimony (*Agrimonia eupatoria*)	Food intolerance	Marshmallow protects and coats the gut and sooth it. Lemon balm is a carminative and used for digestive upsets.

Table contd...

Herbal Preparations	Ingredients (Herbs) present	Applications/ Uses	Therapeutic effects
Wild yam and Chamomile mixture	Wild yam root tincture (*Dioscorea villosa*) Chamamile flower tincture (*Matricaria recutita*) Bistort tincture (*Polygonum bistorta*) Hop tincture (*Humulus lupulus*) Liquorice fluid extract	Irritable bowel syndrome	Wild yam, an effective antispasmodic agent relaxes the gut and relieves over activity. Hops and chamomile act as relaxants while bitterness of hops helps restore normal digestion.
Liquorice and Dandelion decoction	Dandelion root (*Taraxaccum officinale*) Yellow dock root (*Rumex crispus*) Dried anise seeds (*Pimpinella anisum*) Dried liquorice root Water	Used in constipation	Dandelion is a good liver tonic. Yellow dock has a gentle laxative action. Chronic constipation is improves by bitter herbs which stimulates the liver and increases production of digestive enzymes.
Fennel and Chamomile tea	Fennel seeds (*Foeniculum officinalis*) Chamomile flowers (*Matricaria recutita*) Peppermint (*Mentha piperita*) Water	Flatulence	The calming and anti-inflammatory actions of fennel and chamomile provides a soothing mixture for relief of wind.
Tormentil and Marshmallow decoction	Tormentil root (*Potentilla erecta*) Marshmallow root (*Altaea officinalis*) Cinnamon bark (Cinnamomum zeylanicum) Arrow root	Diarrhoea	This mixture of herbs and arrow root is soothing and nutritious. Tormentil root rich in tannins is highly astringent which helps to reduce inflammation. Marshmallow is a soothing agent.
Pilewort ointment	Pilewort leaves (*Ranunculus ficaria*) Sunflower oil Bees wax Anhydrous lanolin	Haemorrhoids	Pilewort is a very astringent plant and is extremely helpful for haemorrhoids.
Fennel and Lemon balm tea	Fennel seeds (*Foeniculum officinalis*) Lemon balm leaves (*Melissa officinalis*) Cinnamon bark (*Cinnamomum zeylanicum*) Water	Indeigestion and heart burn	Both these herbs calms the stomach. Lemon balm also relaxes the nerves if stress or anxiety is arised.

Table contd…

Herbal Preparations	Ingredients (Herbs) present	Applications/ Uses	Therapeutic effects
Meadow - sweet tea	Meadowsweet (*Filipendula ulmaria*) Water	Gastritis	Meadowsweet is a cooling and soothing herb which eases inflammation and helps to reduce acidic secretions in the stomach.
Ginger capsules	Powdered ginger (*zingiber officinalis*) Size oo gelatine capsules	Nausea and vomiting	Ginger is excellent for nausea and vomiting and is safe and effective even in pregnancy.
Ginger and Cinnamon tea	Ginger root (*Zingiber officinalis*) Gui Zhi (*Cinnamon twigs*) (*Cinnamomum cassia*) Angelica root (*Angelica archangelica*)	Poor circulation and chilblains	These herbs (Cinnamon and ginger) stimulates the circulation. Gui Zhi herb produces heat to the peripheries.
Hawthorn and chrysanthemu m tea	Hawthorn flowering tops (*Crataegus oxyacantha*) Ju Hua (*Chrysanthemum morifolium*) Linden flowers (*Tilia europaea*) Yarrow (*Achillea millefolium*)	Used to lower high blood pressure	Hawthorn improves coronary circulation making the heart more efficient. Chrysanthenum flowers relaxes the heart and improves blood flow.
Stinging nettle and melilot tea	Stinging nettle (*Urtica dioica*) Dried melilot (*Melilotus officinalis*) Shepherd's purse (*Capsella bursa pastoris*) Buckwheat (*Fagopyrum esculentum*) Horsetail juice (*Equisetum arvense*) Water	Varicose veins	Herbs rich in silica, such as stinging nettle and horsetail helps to strengthen the vein walls. Shepherd's purse and buck whea contains flavonoids.
Apricot iron tonic	Fresh apricots Stinging nettle juice (*Urtica dioica*) Dandelion root tincture (*Taraxacum officinale*) Red wine Honey or sugar + water	Used in Iron-deficient anaemia	Apricots are rich in iron and provides a good base for this tonic. Stinging nettles and dandelion are added to provide extra nutrients and to stimulate the liver.

Table contd...

Herbal Preparations	Ingredients (Herbs) present	Applications/ Uses	Therapeutic effects
Wood betony tea	Wood betony (*Stachys betonica*) Chamomile (*Matricaria recutita*) Skull cap (*Scutellaria lateriflora*) Water	Tension headaches	Wood betony herb is a potent pain killer and relaxant.
Lavender and Pine inhalation	Lavender oil (*Lavandula angustifolia*) Pine oil (*Pinus sylvestris*) Eucalyptus oil (*Eucalyptus globulus*) Thyme oil (*Thymus vulgaris*)	Simus headache	Lavender + pine contains potent essential oils which reduces inflammation and infection.
Feverfew and valerian tincture	Feverfew tincture (*Tanacetum parthenium*) Valerian tincture (*Valeriana officinalis*) Lavender tincture (*Lavandula angustifolia*)	Migraines	Feverfew fresh leaves is highly effective for treating migraine attacks.
Skullcap and Passion flower mixture	Skullcap tincture (*Scutellaria laterifolia*) Passionflower tincture (*Passiflora incarnata*) Lemon balm tincture (*Melissa officinalis*) Pasque flower tincture (*Anemone vulgaris*)	Anxiety and tension	Soothing herbal nervines, encourages relaxation and reduces tensions. Skull cap is a restorative and relaxant. Passionflower has an effective sedative action.
Lemon balm and Oat mixture	Oat tincture (*Avena sativa*) St.John's wort tincture (*Hypericum perforatum*) Vervain tincture (*Verbena officinalis*) Lemon balm tincture (*Melissa officinalis*) Liquorice tincture	Depression	Oats are good antidepressant and restorative for nervous system. Lemon balm oil is a CNS relaxant. St.John's wort is an antidepressant.
Nightcap and Passion flower tea	Californian poppy (*Eschscholzia californica*) Passion flower (*Passiflora incarnata*) Wood betony (*Stachys betonica*) Lavender flowers (*Lavandula angustifolia*)	Used to cure Insomnia	Californian poppy is a sedative remedy and is far less powerful then opium poppy. It gives a gentle and soothing effect.

Table contd...

Herbal Preparations	Ingredients (Herbs) present	Applications/ Uses	Therapeutic effects
Lavender and thyme rub	Lavender oil (*Lavandula angustifolia*) Thyme oil (*Thymus vulgaris*) Juniper oil (*Juniperus communis*) Pine oil (*Pinus sylvestris*) Eucalyptus oil (*Eucalyptus globulus*) St John's wort oil (*Hypericum perforatum*)	Used to cure Backache and sciatica	Lavender oil is a mild analgesic and relieves many types of back ache. Thyme is an antispasmodic which relaxes over-tense muscles. Both combined with warming oils to soothe aches and pains.
Bogbean and Meadowsweet tea	Bogbean leaves (*Menyanthes trifoliata*) Meadowsweet (*Filipendula ulmaria*) Yarrow (*Achillea millefolium*) Liquorice fluid extract Water	Rheumatism	Bogbean and Meadowsweet are anti-inflammatory in action and also used as digestive stimulants. Thus, it clears the build-up toxins associated with muscle and joint disorders.
Celery and Heather tea	Celery seed (*Apium graveolems*) Heather flowers (*Calluria vulgaris*) Yarrow (*Achillea millefolium*)	Used to treat gout	Celery seed and heather flowers are effective diuretics, and clears excess uric acid from the system.
St.John's wort and Celery mixture	St. John's wort tincture (*Hypericum perforatum*) Celery seed (*Apium graceolens*) Bogbean (*Menyanthes trifoliate*) Angelica root (*Angelica archangelica*) Yellow dock (*Rumex crispus*) Liquorice tincture (*Glycyrrhiza glabra*)	Osteoarthritis	This combination of tinctures helps to cleanse the system, stimulate the circulation and digestion and reduces inflammation
Saw palmetto and Siberian ginseng mixture	Saw Palmetto tincture (*Serenoa repens*) Siberian ginseng tincture (*Elentherococus senticosus*) Echinacea tincture (*Echinacea angustifolia*)	Used in prostate disorder	Saw palmetto is used as a sexual tonic and is effective in treating prostate problems both for inflammation and enlargement.

Table contd…

Herbal Preparations	Ingredients (Herbs) present	Applications/ Uses	Therapeutic effects
Buchu and Couchgrass tea	Buchu leaves (*Barosma betulina*) Couchgrass rhizome (*Agropyron sepens*) Dried corn silk (*Zea mays*)	Urethritis	Buchu bush has antiseptic and diuretic properties and it gently stimulates kidneys. Couch grass rhizomes provide mucilages to soothe and heal the affected area.
He Shou Wu and Cinnamon wine	He Shou Wu (*Polygonum multiflorum*) Cinnamon bark (*Cinnamomum zeylanicum*) Dried liquorice root (*Glycyrrhiza glabra*)	Generally used in infertility of males	He Shou Wu is used as a reproductive energy tonic by Chinese and is used to increase the sperm count.
Lady's mantle and Shepherd's purse tea	Lady's mantle (*Alchemilla vulgaris*) Shepherd's purse (*Capsella bursa pastoris*) Raspberry leaves (*Rubus idaeus*) Marigold petals (*Calendula officinalis*) Mugwort leaves (*Artemisia vulgaris*)	Used in heavey periods of females	Lady's Mantle acts as a good astringent and helps to regulate menstrial imbalances. Shepherd's purse is used to reduce excessive bleeding.
Dang Gui and Paeony decoction	Dang gui (*Chinese angelica*) (*Angelica sinensis*) Bai Shao (*White paeony root*) (*Paeonia lactiflora*) Chen Pi (*Tangerine peel*) *Citrus reticulata*) Dried liquorice root Fresh ginger root Vervain and peppermint	Used in pre-menstrual syndrome (PMS) (A hormonal imbalanced condison)	These herbs are given to relieve the energy blocks related to PMS
Black haw tincture	Black haw bark tincture (*Viburnum prunifolium*) St. John's wort tincture (*Hypericum perforatum*) Pasque flower tincture (*Anemone vulgaris*)	Used to control periodic pain	Black haw, a relaxing herb acts on uterus. St. John's wort and pasque flower has antispasmodic properties.

Table contd…

Herbal Preparations	Ingredients (Herbs) present	Applications/ Uses	Therapeutic effects
He Shou Wu and Vervain mix	He Shou Wu tincture (*Polygonum multiflorum*) Vervain tincture (*Verbena officinalis*) Sage tincture (*Salvia officinalis*) Wild yam root tincture (*Dioscorea villosa*) Lavender tincture (*Lavandula angustifolia*) Liquorice tincture (*Glycyrrhiza glabra*)	In curing Menopause	He Shou Wu acts on kidneys. Vervain, a good liver tonic provides sedation to emotions. Sage and wild yam helps to cure menopausal problems.
Marigold and Tea tree pessaries	Cocoa butter Marigold oil (*Calendula officinalis*) Tea-tree oil (*Melaleuca alternifolia*) Thyme oil (*Thymus vulgaris*)	Used for vaginal infections	Marigold is a useful antifungal agent. Tea-tree is most effective herbal antiseptics.
Simple tinctures	Ginger tincture (*Zingiber officinalis*) Chamomile tincture (*Matricaria recutita*) Chen Pi tincture (*Citrus reticulata*) Black horehound tincture (*Ballota nigra*) Peppermint tincture (*Mentha piperita*) Lemon balm tincture (*Melissa officinalis*)	Used in morning sickness	Placing a few drops of tincture on the tongue is the best way to take remedies when feeling nanseous.
Cornsilk and Dandelion tea	Dandelion leaves (*Taraxacum officinale*) Cornsilk (*Zea mays*) Couchgrass rhizome (Agryopyron repens) Water	In curing fluid retention (oedema) during pregnance period.	Dandelion leaves are rich in potassium. Cornsilk is used for its soothig property in the urinary tract.
Marshmallow and Corn silk mixture	Marshmallow tincture (*Althaea officinalis*) Bearberry tincture (*Arctostaphylos spp.*) Corn silk tincture (*Zea mays*) Couch grass tincture (*Agropyron repens*) Yarrow tincture (*Achillea millefolium*)	Used in urinary tract infections such as cystitis (inflammation of bladder)	Marshmallow is rich in mucilage to ease inflamed membranes. Yarrow acts as astringent and heals the infections.

CHAPTER 10

CONCEPT OF STEREOISOMERISMS

10.1 Stereoisomerisms

Stereochemistry of a molecule i.e., a relative spatial arrangement of atoms, or 3-D structure of molecule plays a major role in the pharmacological properties. Stereochemistry alone is responsible for difference in degree of pharmacologic activity between isomers.

Thus, "When isomerism is caused by different arrangements of atoms or groups in space, the phenomenon is called *Stereoisomerism"*. The stereoisomers have the same structural formulas but differ in atoms arrangement in space.

Types of Stereoisomers

Stereoisomers

- Conformational Isomers
  - Rotation about single bonds
  - Amine Inversion
- Configurational Isomers
  - Cis-trans Isomers
  - Isomers that contain asymmetric centres

Basically Stereoisomers are of following types:

1. *Optical isomers*: (a) D-isomers , (b) L-isomers
2. *Geometrical isomers*: (a) cis-isomers, (b) trans-isomers

1. Optical isomers

These compounds differ only in their ability to rotate the plane of polarised light.

Dextrorotatory or (+) – *isomer*: Isomers which rotates the plane of polarised light to the right (clockwise direction).

Laevorotatory or (–) – *isomer*: Isomer which rotates the plane of polarised light to the left (anticlockwise direction).

Enantiomorphs: (Also called as optical antipodes or enantiomers) may be defined as optical isomers in which the atom or group about an asymmetric centre are arranged in such a manner that the two molecules differ only as does the right hand from the left.

- Enantiomers are stable, isolable compounds that differ from one another in three dimensional spatial arrangements.
- Enantiomers cannot be inter converted under ordinary conditions.
- Enantiomers rotate the plane of polarised light in equal amounts but in opposite directions.
- They are non-super imposable mirror images.
- Since there is no difference in physical properties between enantiomorphs, their difference in biologic activity must be due to their spatial arrangement or stereo chemistry.
- D and L denotes absolute configuration.
- d and *l* denotes rotation.

An oversimplified explanation of optical isomers can be stated as:

1. Atoms or groups surrounding asymmetric atom are given priorities according to atomic number (Highest atomic number is given highest priority).
2. Molecule is rotated in such a way that group with lowest priority is away from the viewer.
3. 'R' denotes clockwise rotation and
   'S' denotes counter clockwise rotation

e.g.

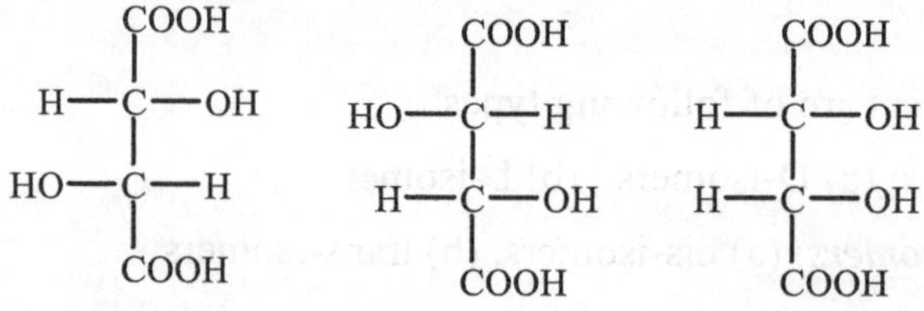

(+) (R, R) Tartaric acid **(–) (S, S) Tartaric acid** **Meso Tartaric acid**

Natural Compounds showing optical Isomerism

1. ***Sugars*:**

- Sugars are crystalline solids soluble in water, have a sweet taste and causes reduction of fehling's solution and other compounds (reducing agents) and give no colour with iodine solution.
- Sugar (sucrose) most widely occurring disaccharide in nature is manufactured from sugarcane and sugar beets.
- Soluble saccharides are used as nutritives, sweetening agents and vehicles for other medicines.
- They act as mild laxatives because of osmosis process.
- They are used in fermentation industries for manufacturing alcohol.
- If secondary alcohol group at the asymmetric carbon atom is to the right, it is called D-sugar (Dextro sugar) and if it is to the left position, it is called as L-sugar (Leavo sugar).

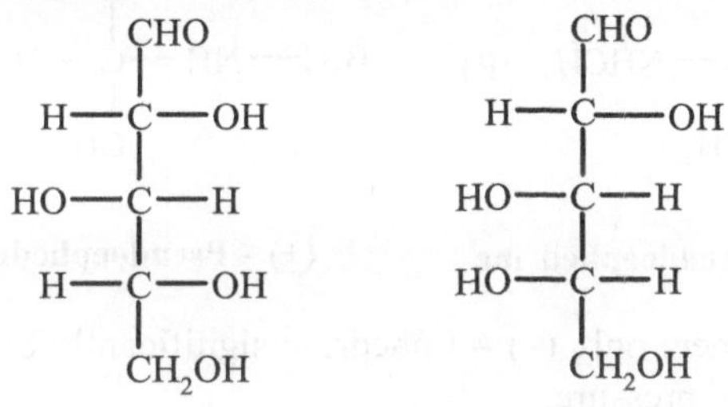

D-Arabinose **L-Arabinose**

2. ***Sympathomimetic agents*:**

- Epinephrine (Adrenaline) is isolated from adrenal (suprarenal) glands of certain mammals. It has two types of isomers as follows:

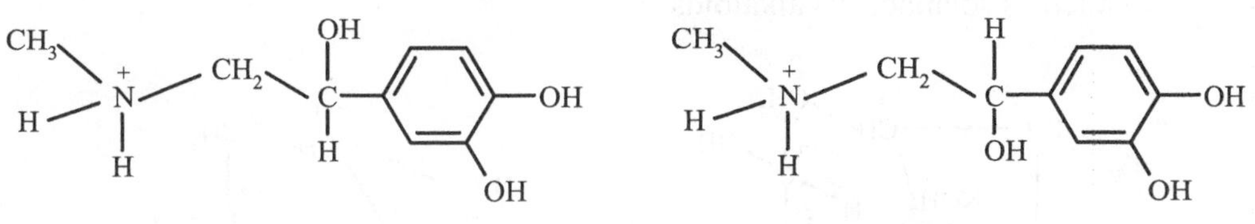

(+) – Epinephrine (Less active) **(–) – Epinephrine (More active)**

Ephedrine and Pseudoephedrine: Ephedrine obtained naturally from Ephedra species (*Ephedra gerardiana*). Pseudoephedrine is a diastereomer of Ephedrine.

Ephedrine structure has two asymmetric carbons having four optical isomers possible.

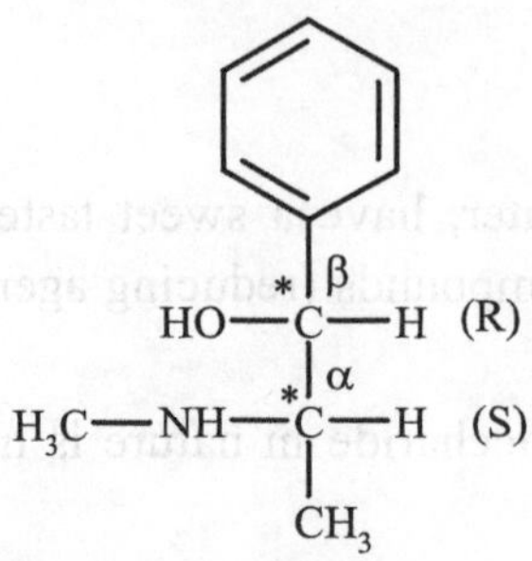

(–) – **Ephedrine**

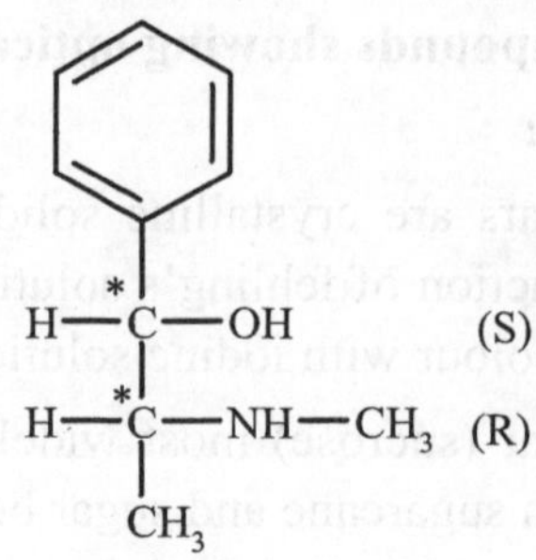

(+) – **Ephedrine**

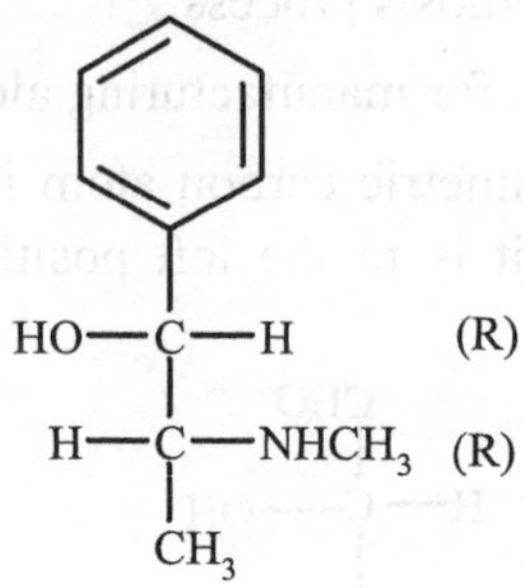

(–) – **Pseudoephedrine**

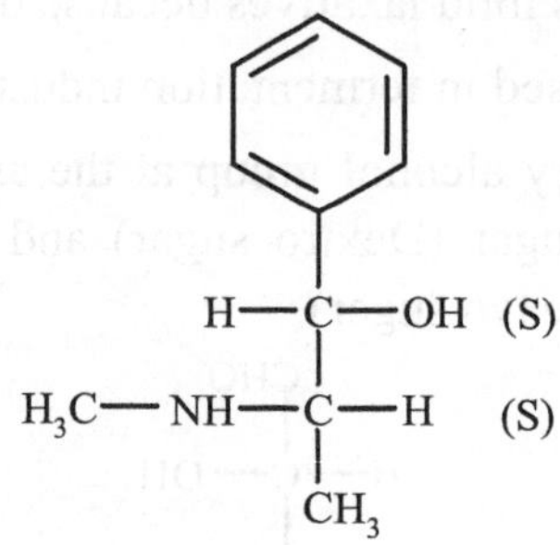

(+) – **Pseudoephedrine**

* In the above four isomers only (–) – Ephedrine significantly blocks β-adrenergic receptors thereby lowering blood pressure.

* For maximum activity of these molecules, β-center must be (R) and α-center must be (S) configuration.

3. Alkaloids

- Tropines, an alkaloid obtained from "*Atropa belladonna*" (Solanaceae); also called as solanaceous alkaloids.

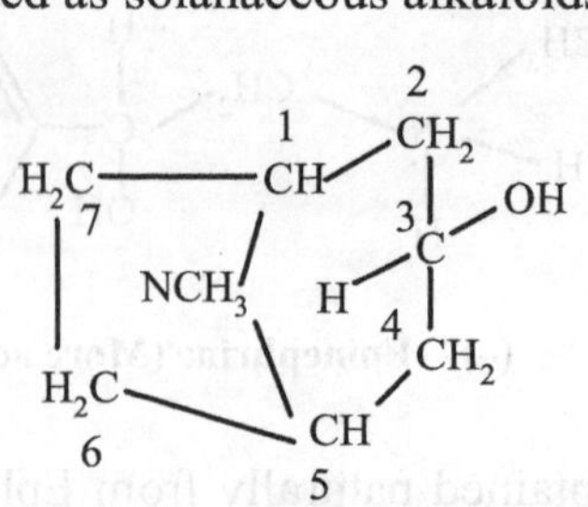

(a)

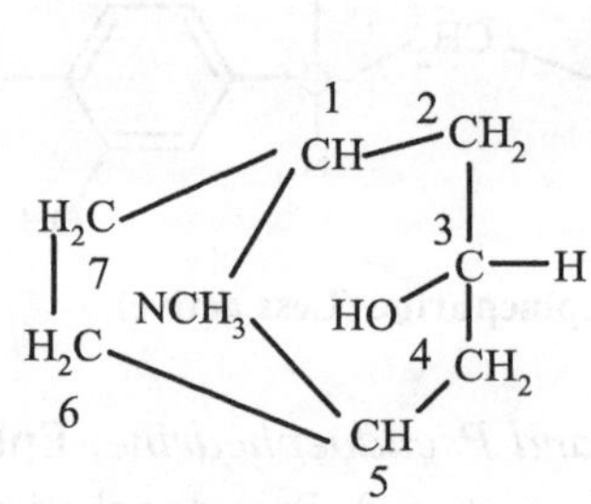

(b)

These are the two isomers or epimers of tropine – namely called as tropin and ψ-tropine (Pseudotropine). One epimer have the hydrogen atom on c-3 position on the same side of nitrogen bridge and the other has this hydrogen atom on the opposite side.

- ψ-tropine is the syn-compound (i.e., nitrogen bridge and hydroxyl groups are in cis-position) whereas
- Tropine is an anti-compound (i.e., nitrogen bridge and hydroxyl groups are in trans-position).

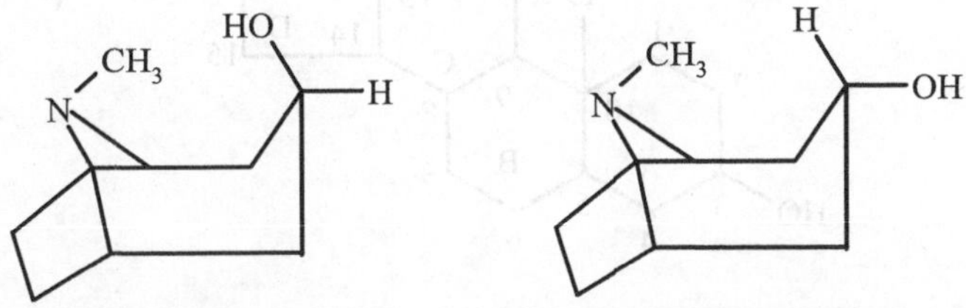

ψ- Tropine **Tropine**

- Tubocurarine, obtained from genes strychnos and found in extracts from "*Chondodendron tomentosum*".

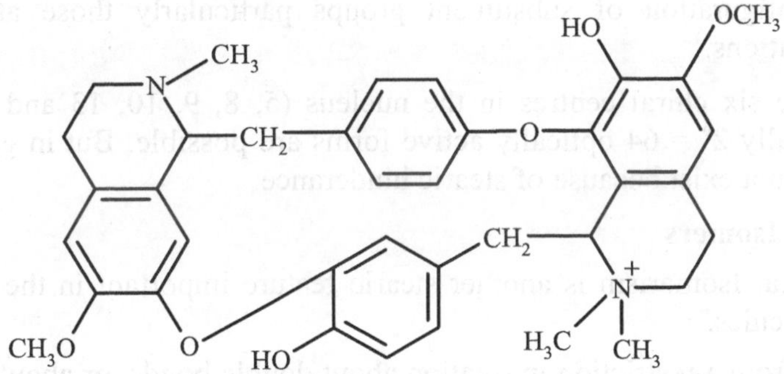

Tubocurarine chloride

- Tubocurarine chloride is used intravenously to produce skeletal muscle relaxation during surgical procedures.
- (+) – Tubocurarine, block the stimulating (nicotinic) action of acetyl choline on skeletal muscles and exerts little effect on autonomic ganglia.
- Methylation of free phenolic hydroxyl groups of (+) – tubocurarine increases the activity, whereas ethylation or butylation leads to less active or inactive derivatives.

4. *Steroids*

A fully saturated sterol contains 8 dissimilar chiral centres in the nucleus at carbon positions – 3, 5, 8, 9, 10, 13, 14, and 17. Hence there are ($2^8 = 256$) optical isomers possible of sterol.

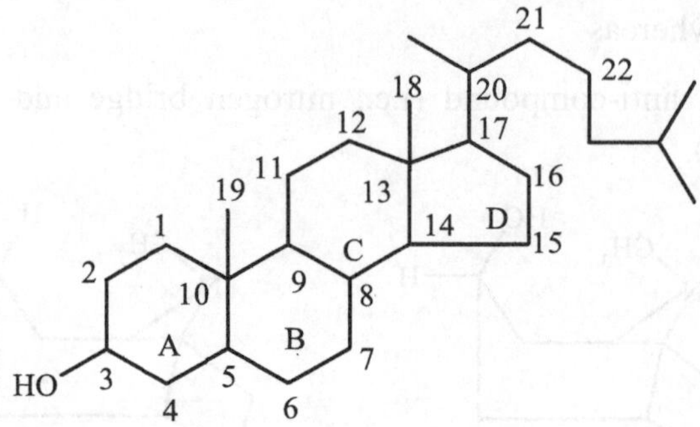

Sterol (Cyclopentenoperhydro phenanthrene Nucleus)

Stereoisomerism of steroids is classified into two types:

(i) The way in which the rings are fused together.

(ii) Configuration of substituent groups particularly those at c-3 and c-17 positions.

There are six chiral centres in the nucleus (5, 8, 9, 10, 13 and 14). Therefore, theoretically $2^6 = 64$ optically active forms are possible. But in general, many of these cannot exist because of stearic hinderance.

2. Geometrical Isomers

- Geometrical Isomerism is another stearic feature important in the action of many drug molecules.
- It results from a restriction in rotation about double bonds, or about single bonds in cyclic compounds.
- The term geometrical isomerism (or cis-trans isomerism) indicates a type of diastereoismers that occurs as a result of restricted rotation around a bond, as in olefinic compounds.
- The term 'cis' is used when identified groups are on the same side of the plane of the molecule and 'trans' is used when the groups are on the opposite sides of the plane of the molecule.
- Geometric isomerism does not necessarily impart optical isomerism to the compound.
- If the structure is asymmetric (or dysymmetric), however geometric isomers may exhibits optical activity.

- The trans isomers are more stable than the corresponding cis-isomers. This is because, in the cis-isomer, bulky groups are on the same side of the double bond. The stearic repulsion of groups makes the cis-isomer less stable than trans-isomer in which the bulky groups are far apart (as they are on the opposite sides of double bond).
- Geometrical Isomerism is possible only when each double bonded carbon atom is attached to two different atoms or groups.

Natural Compounds showing Geometrical Isomerism

Terpenoids

- Citral a colourless liquid (volatile oil) obtained naturally from "Lemon grass oil". Citral exhibits geometrical isomerism about the double bonded carbons carrying CH_3 and CHO groups. The cis-isomer is known as citral-a and trans-isomer is called as citral-b.

  Citral obtained from lemon grass oil contains = citral-a (90%) + citral-b (10%)

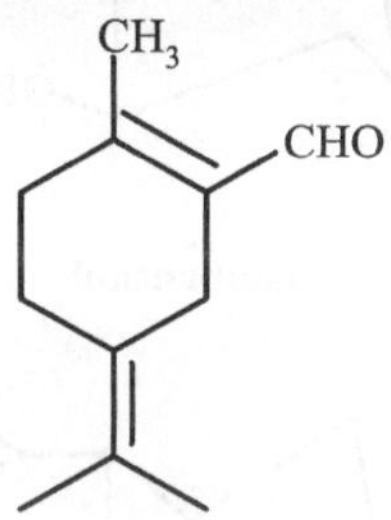

Citral-a (cis-isomer)
(Geraniol)

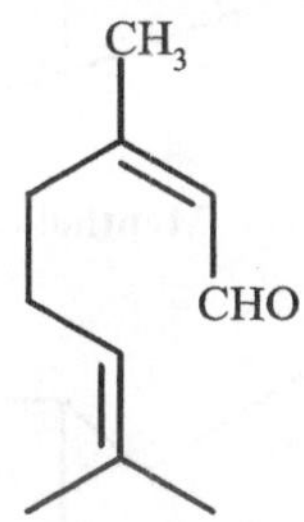

Citral-b (trans-isomer)
(Nerol)

- Geraniol, an acyclic terpene alcohol occurs in oils of rose, palm rosa, geranium, citronella, lemon grass and lavender.
- Geraniol exhibits geometrical isomerism and it is the cis-form.

  The trans-isomer is Nerol obtained from neroli oil.

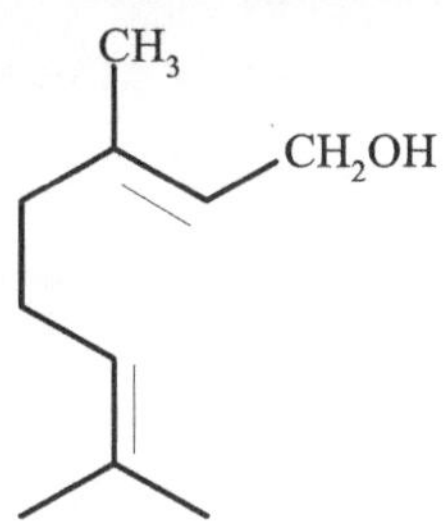

(Cis-form)

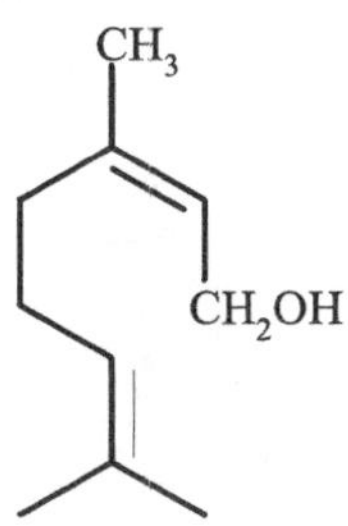

(Trans-form)

- Menthol, obtained naturally from plants of menta specias (*Mentha piperita*). It is a monocyclic monoterpene secondary alcohol having following structure:

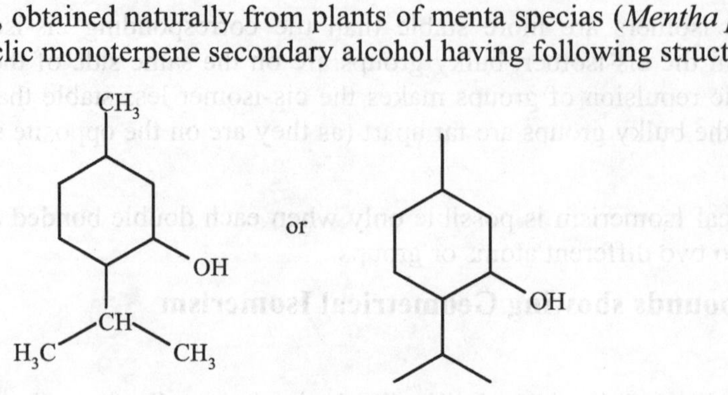

(±) Menthol, ↔ optically active compound

The chair conformations suggested for menthol isomers are:

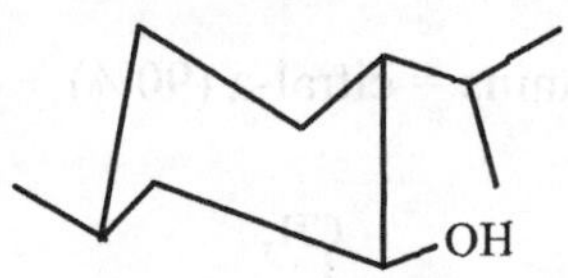

Menthol

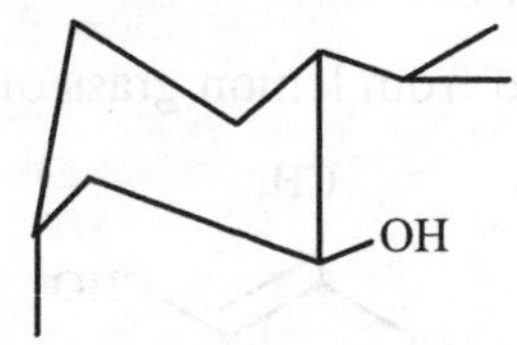

Isomenthol

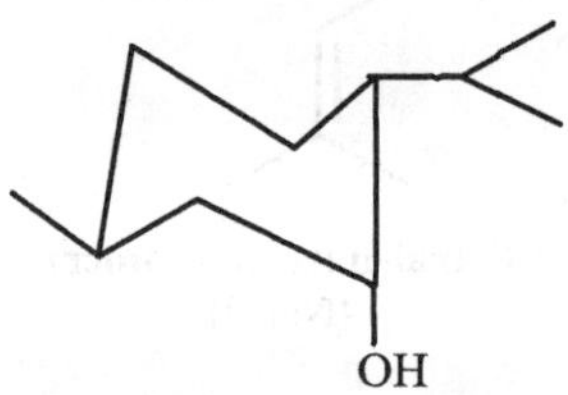

Neomenthol

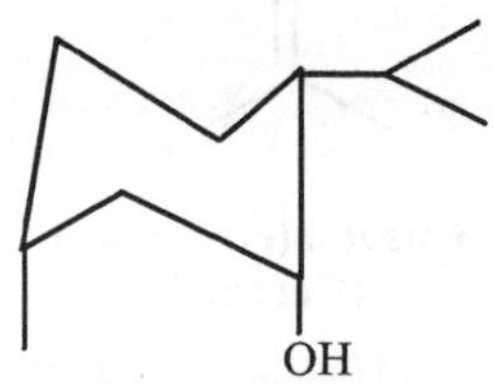

Neo-isomenthol

CHAPTER 11

PRODUCTION AND ANALYSIS OF VARIOUS PHYTOCONSTITUENTS

11.1 Introduction

Industrial production of a drug goes through a number of procedures before coming to the consumer market. Besides the routine methods of isolation, extraction, production and development of the product, new procedures are employed which are more compliable and has made in understanding the chemical complexity of tissues and their biogenetic behaviour.

Various steps involved in the industrial production are as follows:

(i) Selection or collection of desired herbs or parts.

(ii) Isolation of genuine raw material from the bulk.

(iii) Extraction of the desired active constituents from the raw material by employing various procedures.

(iv) Recent advancement in the field of industrial production of active constituents are "Tissue culture" and "Biogenetic pathways".

(v) Incorporation of desired active constituents into desired dosage form and large scale manufacturing or production.

(vi) Quality control of prepared dosage form and its analysis to ensure that it meets all required parameters.

(vii) Packaging and storage of the product.

(viii) Delivery to the consumer market.

11.2 General Methods of Isolation and Extraction employed in Industries

The choice of extraction procedure depends on the nature of the plant material and components to be isolated. Dried leaves materials are usually powdered before extraction, whereas fresh plants / leaves can be homogenized/macerated with alcohol.

Various methods for isolation and extraction are:

1. *Successive solvent' Extraction*: Various processes include–Infusion, Decoction, Maceration, Percolation, Digestion.
2. *Chromatographic Techniques*: This include techniques such as HPLC, TLC, GLC, partition chromatography, Electro-chromatography, capillary column chromatography, counter current chromatography.
3. Fractional Liberation
4. Fractional crystallization
5. Distillation
   (a) Fractional Distillation
   (b) Steam Distillation
6. Supercritical Fluid Extraction
7. Sublimation

11.2.1 Artemisine

Synonyms	:	Annual wormwood, sweet worm wood, sweet Annie, Quinghaosu.
Source	:	Isolated from leafs and other above ground parts of "*Artemisia annua*".
Family	:	Compositae/Asteraceae
Geo-Source	:	Grown as a weed in China, Eastern Asia, India, North America and Europe.

Extraction and Isolation

1. *Artemisia annua* is found predominantly in the temperate regions in the 0-50 cm precipitation zone, with southward extension towards the tropics.
2. Artemisinin is present in the leaves and flowering tops of the plant.
3. Yield of artemisinin in China ranges from 0.01 to 0.5% w/w, depending on the local climatic conditions as well as, season of harvesting.
4. The content of artemisinin is increased by 30% by applying growth regulator such as chlormequat before harvesting.

5. *In vitro production*: Artemisia annua is grown and propagated by micro cutting in a hormone-free medium from which artemisinin is isolated. Thus, Artemisinin produced by shoot cultures occur only in trace levels.
6. For research purposes, lyophilization is the most suitable method for drying the plant before extraction, since the moisture content of samples is easily controlled.
7. Artemisinin is extracted from air dried plants using ethyl ether, petroleum ether, and even gasoline as a solvent. Petroleum ether (30-60 ^{O}C) is the most satisfactory of various non-protic solvents, although extraction with lexane for several days at room temperature was also effective.

Chemical Structures: Following are the main active constituents of Artenisia annua:

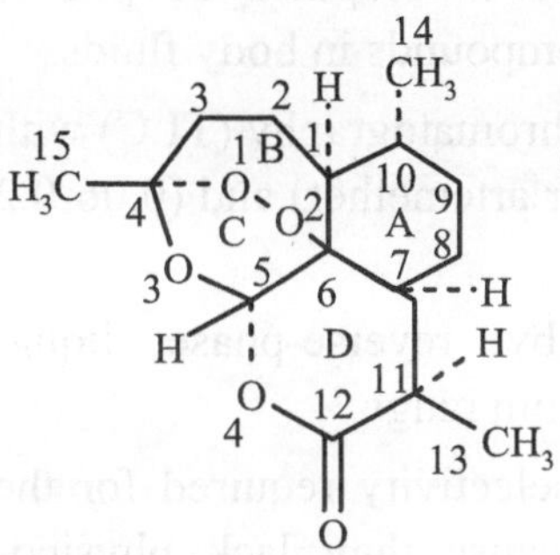

Artemisinin

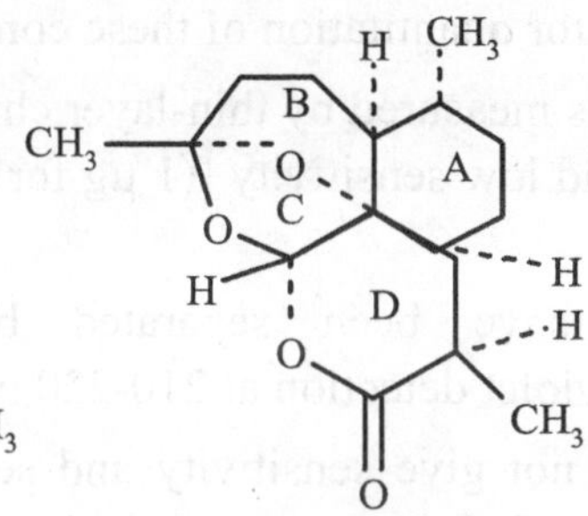

Deoxyartemisinin

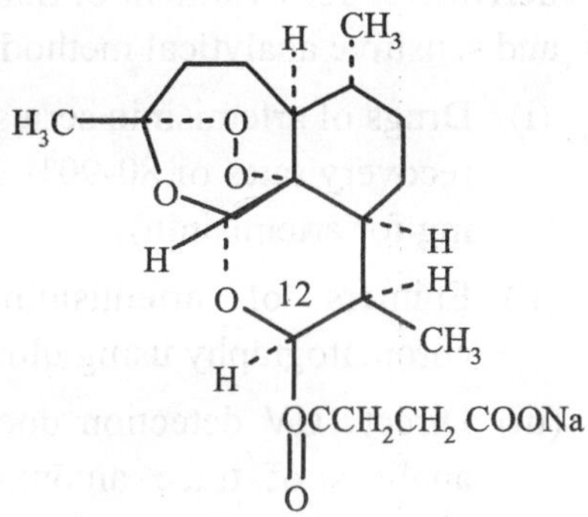

Sodium artesunate

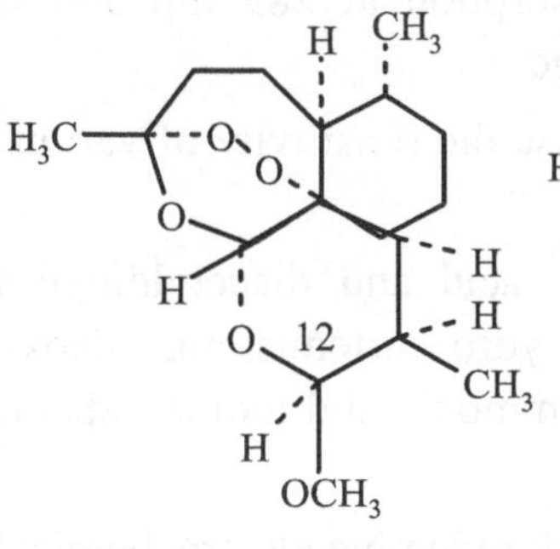

Artemether

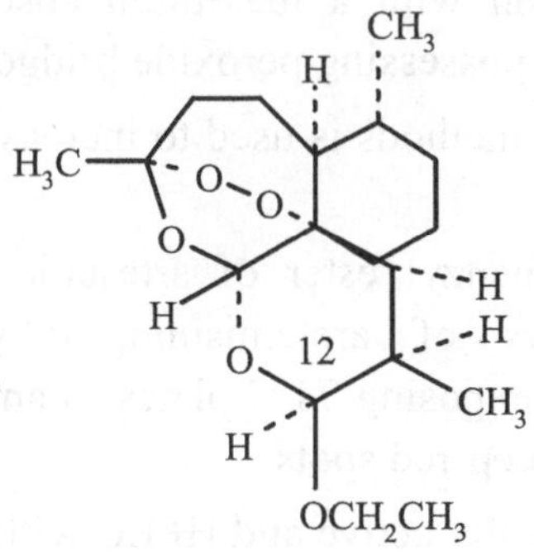

Arteether

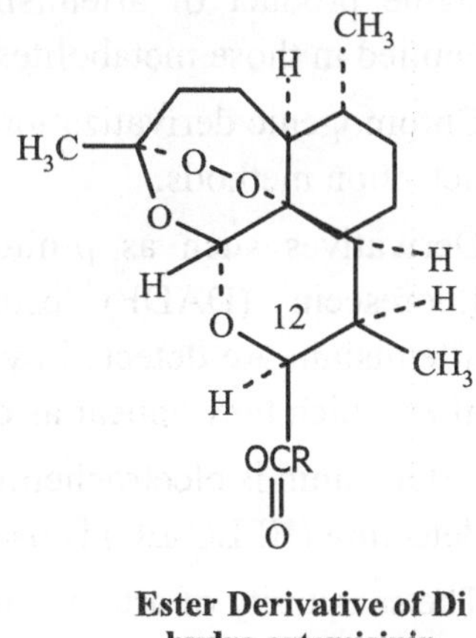

Ester Derivative of Di hydro artemisinin

Estimation and Analysis of Artemisinin

1. *Screening Methods used*

(i) Preliminary and double blind trials, have shown that injections or oral use of artemisinin or similar compounds rapidly and effectively cure people with malaria.

(ii) A human trial study showed that artemisinin reduced mortality due to malaria by 50% compared with treatment with a standard quinoline anti-malarial drug.

(iii) Test tube studies suggest that artemisinin can kill other parasites and bacteria possibly supporting the traditional notion of using it for parasite infections of the gastrointestinal tract.

2. The successful development of an optimum regimen of either artemisinin or one of its derivatives for treatment of malaria infections depends on the development of specific and sensitive analytical methods for quantitation of these compounds in body fluids.

(i) Drugs of artemisinin series is measured by thin-layer chromatography (TLC) with recovery rates of 80-90% and low sensitivity [(1 μg for artemether) and (0.06-0.2 mg for artemisinin)]

(ii) Epimers of artemisinin have been separated by reverse-phase liquid chromatography using ultraviolet detection at 210-220 nm range.

(iii) Direct UV detection does not give sensitivity and selectivity required for the analysis of trace amounts of these compounds because they lack physico-chemical properties.

(iv) The chromatographic column when treated with alkalis, used for detection of a stable product of artemisinin with a maximum absorption at 289 nm and is applied in those metabolites possessing peroxide bridge.

(v) Chromogenic derivatization methods is used to increase the sensitivity of various detection methods.

(vi) Derivatives such as p-nitobenzyl ester of artesunic acid and diacetyldihydro fluorescein (DADF) esters of aretemisinin, dihydro artemisinin, deoxy artemisinin are detected by exposing TLC plates to ammonia and iodine vapour, after which they appear as deep-red spots.

(vii) Artemisinin is electrochemically active and HPLC with reductive electrochemical detection (HPLC-EC) is used to measure artemisinin contents of plant extracts.

(viii) The sensitivity of artemisinin by:

1. Pulse Polarography Method – 0.6 μg/ml
2. Radio immune assay method – 2.3 ng/ml

Uses

(i) Artemisinin, its methyl ether derivative artemether and a hemisuccinyl derivative artensunate is used in clinical trials under the auspices of Ministry of Public Health of Peoples's Republic of China.

(ii) Endoperoxide bridge is essential for its anti-malarial activity. The compound is activated by intra-parasitic haeme to irreversibly decompose, generating free radicals that alkylate and oxidises proteins and lipids.

Note

- The promising antimalarial compound artemisinin has very low yield 0.01-0.18% and remains expensive and is hardly available on a global scale. Therefore, many research groups have directed their investigations towards the enhancement of artemisinin production in Artemisia annua cell cultures or whole plant in order to over produce artemisinin or one of its precursors.
- Chinese scientists have shown artemisinin (Quinghaosu) a novel antimalarial compound with the structure of a sesquiterpene lactone ring with an internal peroxide linkage.

11.2.2 Atropine

Biological source : Obtained from the roots and leaves of "*Atropa belladonna*", Datura species and Hyoscyamus.

Family : Solanaceae

Extraction and Isolation

Method I

(i) The powdered leaves are extracted with 95% alcohol (ethanol), which is removed by distillation process.

(ii) The syrupy mass thus obtained is treated with 1% HCl to remove the resinous matter.

(iii) Acid solution is purified by using light petroleum ether and made alkaline with ammonia, and extracted with chloroform.

(iv) The chloroform layer is shaken with dilute acid and separated.

(v) The separated solution is made alkaline with ammonia and re-extracted with chloroform.

(vi) The chloroform is evaporated and neutralized with oxalic acid to obtain oxalates of atropine and hyoscyamine.

(vii) These are separated by fractional crystallization method from acetone and ether, in which hyoscyamine oxalate is more soluble.

Method II

(i) Atropine is extracted either from Belladonna roots or from the juice of Datura plant.

(ii) These plant parts are extracted firstly with 95% ethanol.

(iii) This extract is treated and heated with potassium carbonate solution where hyoscyamine racemises to atropine.

(iv) This atropine is then extracted with chloroform.

(v) Chloroform is recovered by evaporation and the residue is then extracted with dilute H_2SO_4 acid.

(vi) The solution is made alkaline with potassium carbonate, where atropine is precipitated out.

(vii) The precipitated atropine is extracted with ether and then purified by converting it into oxalates or sulfates.

Estimation and Analysis of Atropine

1. *USP Assay for Belladonna Leaf*:

   - It is adapted for quantitative estimation of total alkaloids.

     The alkaloids are extracted by ether and purified by re-extracting into 0.5N H_2SO_4 acid (as sulphates) and then into chloroform (as free bases).

   - After evaporating the $CHCl_3$ extract to dryness, the alkaloidal residue is taken up with a definite quantity of standardized H_2SO_4 acid solution in slight excess of the quantity of acid required to form sulphate salts with all the alkaloids present.

   - The quantity of unreacted acid is determined by titration with standardized alkali.

   - Then the quantity of alkaloids is calculated from the molar quantity of acid which has reacted with alkaloids to form the salts of atropine.

2. *Assay for Atropine Methonitrate*:

   - 0.5 gm of atropine methonitrate was weighed accurately and dissolved in 50 ml of acetic anhydride.

   - This solution was titrated with 0.1N $HClO_4$ solution.

   - The end point was determined potentiometrically.

   - Then performed a blank determination and make up necessary corrections.

   - Each ml of 0.1N $HClO_4$ acid is equivalent to 0.036640 gm of atropine methonitrate.

3. *Assay of Atropine Sulphate*:
   - 0.1 gm of atropine sulphate was weighed accurately and dissolved in 50 ml of glacial acetic acid solution.
   - Then the solution was titrated with 0.1N $HClO_4$ solution.
   - The end point was determined potentiometrically.
   - A blank determination was performed and made up necessary corrections.
   - Each ml of 0.1N $HClO_4$ solution is equivalent to 0.06770 gm of atropine sulphate.

11.2.3 Calcium Sennosides

Synonyms : Senna leaf, Senae folium, cassia senna.

Source : Dried leaflets and pods of '*Cassia angustifolia*" (Indian Senna) and "*Cassia acutifolia*" (Alexandrian Senna)

Family : Leguminosae

Indian Senna contains not less than 2.0% of anthracene derivatives calculated as calcium sennoside-B.

Other sources of senna are:

Cassia sieberiana, Cassia obovata, Cassia podocarpa, Cassia sofora, Cassia alata, Cassia fistula.

Extraction of Sennosides: The Sennosides are extracted commercially as their calcium salts (called as calcium sennosides) from the leaves and pods of Indian and Alexandrian senna.

The extraction procedure is as follows:

Powder Drug Material (200 gm)

↓

Extracted with Benzene (600 ml) for 2 hours on an electric shaker

↓

Filtered under vacuum

↓ Distilled off the solvent

Dried the Marc obtained at room temperature

↓

Extracted with 10% Methanol (600 ml) and shaked well for about 6-8 hours

↓ Filtered under vacuum

Re-extracted the Marc with 400 ml of 70% Methanol for 2 hours

↓ Filtered it

Methanolic extract was combined to the filtrate

↓

Concentrated the solution to 1/8th volume and acidified to pH 3.2 with HCl acid with stirring

↓ Set aside for 2 hours

Filtered under vacuum

↓

To the filtrate, added anhydrous $CaCl_2$ (2 gm) in 25 ml of denatured spirit with continuous stirring.

↓

Adjusted the pH of solution to 8.0 by Ammonia solution

↓ set aside for 2 hours

Filtered under vacuum

↓

Dried the precipitate over phosphorus penta-oxide (P_2O_5) in a desiccator

↓

Dried powdered extract obtained

Isolation of Sennosides

(i) By the use of solution of non-ionic surfactants and polyethylene glycol in 70% ethanol, sennosides and other anthracene derivatives can be extracted.

(ii) For the isolation of sennosides, the use of non-polar synthetic resins with porous structure has been also proposed.

(iii) In another method, senna leaf powder is macerated with citric acid in methanol, followed by extraction with methanol-toluene mixture and ammonia. The extract product thus obtained is subjected to treatment with calcium chloride so as to get calcium salts of sennosides A and B.

Estimation and Analysis

1. Chromatographic Profile

Drug Sample : Senna fructus (methanolic extract 20 ml)
Senna folicum (methanolic extract 20 ml)

Reference compound	:	T_1 sennoside A T_2 sennoside B
Solvent System	:	n-propanol–ethyl acetate – water – glacial acetic acid (40 : 40 : 29 : 1)
Detection	:	HNO_3 – Potassium hydroxide reagent = visible range HNO_3 – Potassium hydroxide reagent = 365 nm range Sodium metaperiodate reagent = UV-365 nm range

2. Assay (For quality)

- Sennosides are assayed by chemical analysis methods such as TLC-spectro photometric and spectrocolometric based on quantitative elution of sennosides from silica gel G plates after separation.
- The analysis by high pressure liquid chromatography is also devised.
- The Biological assay method is based on the number of wet faeces produced by groups of mice in 24 hours after oral administration of drug suspension.

3. USP Assay Method

As per USP NF-24-2000, method of assaying sennosides is given as under:

- *pH 7.0 phosphate buffer*: Dissolve 4.54 gm of monobasic potassium phosphate in water to make 500 ml of solution. Dissolve 4.73 gm of anhydrous dibasic sodium phosphate in water to make 500 ml of solution. Mix 38.9 ml of monobasic potassium phosphate + 61.1 ml of dibasic sodium phosphate solution. Adjust drop wise if necessary with dibasic sodium phosphate solution to pH of 7.0.
- *Borate solution*: Dissolve 75.8 gm of sodium borate in water, diluted with water to 2000 ml and mix.
- *Sodium dithionite solution*: Prepare solution of 1.5 gm sodium dithionite in 100 ml of water.
- *Standard Preparation (SP)*: Dissolve about 25 mg of USP sennosides RS (accurately weighed) in pH 7.0 phosphate buffer in a 25 ml volumetric flask with the aid of an ultrasonic bath, dilute with pH 7.0 phosphate buffer to volume and mix.
- *Assay preparation (A.P)*: Dissolve about 25 mg of sennosides (accurately weighed) pH 7.0 phosphate buffer in a 25 ml volumetric flask with the aid of an ultrasonic bath dilute with pH 7.0 phosphate buffer to volume and mix.
- *Procedure*:

  25 Pippette out 1 ml of SP and AP into separate 100 ml volumetric flask, dilute with borate solution to volume and mix.

(ii) Transfer 5.0 ml of each of resulting solutions into separate low acitinic glass (50 ml volumetric flask) and add 15 ml of borate solution and 15 ml of sodium dithionite solution to it.

(iii) Pass nitrogen through the solutions, seal the flasks with nitrogen filled balloons and heat in a water bath for 30 minutes.

(iv) Cool the flask for 15 minutes in a water bath thermostatically controlled at 20 °C temperature. Dilute the solutions with Borate solution to volume and mix.

(v) Determine without delay the fluorescence intensities of resulting solutions in a fluorometer at an excitation wavelength of 392 nm range and an emission wavelength of 505 nm range.

(vi) The time elapsed between the additions of sodium dithionite solution and measurement being the same for the two solutions.

(vii) Calculated the quantity in mg, of sennosides in senna by using formula

$$25\,C\left(\frac{I_v}{I_s}\right)$$

where, C = concentration in mg/ml of USP sennosides RS, corrected for loss on drying in standard preparation.

I_v and I_s = fluorescence values observed for the solutions from the assay preparation and standard preparation respectively.

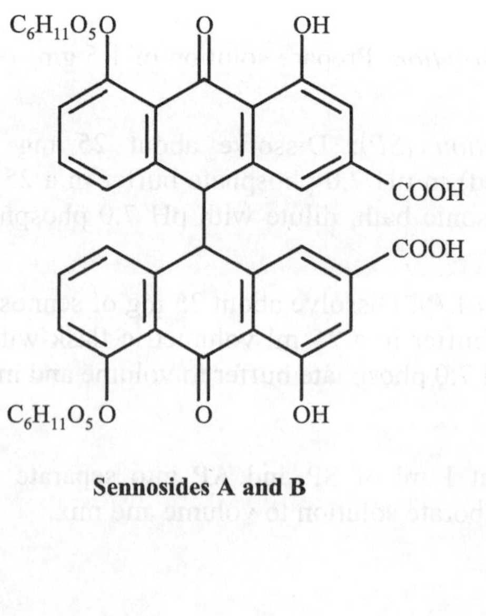

Sennosides A and B

11.2.4 Digoxin

Biological Source : Obtained from dried leaves of "*Digitalis Lanata*".

Family : Scrophulariaceae

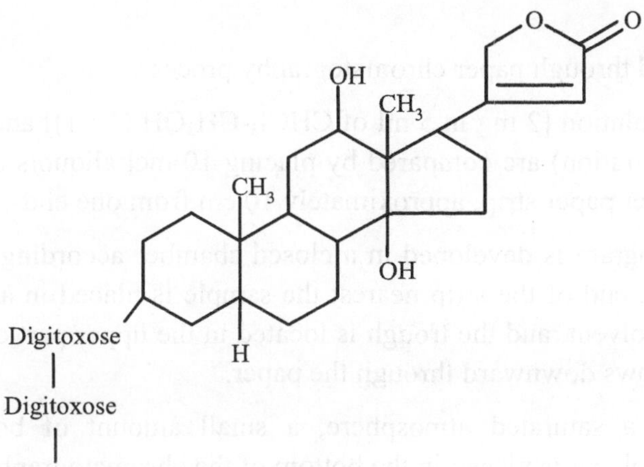

Digoxin

Extraction and Isolation: (by Stas-Otto Method)

Powdered drug of Digitalis lanata (10 gm)

↓

Extracted by continuous hot percolation with alcohol in soxhlate apparatus (During this process, enzyme glycosidase is deactivated)

↓

To the extract, lead acetate is added to precipitate tannins

↓

Filtered and passed H_2S gas to precipitate excess lead acetate as lead sulphide (PbS) or H_2SO_4 acid is passed to precipitate lead acetate as lead sulphate

↓

Filtrate is concentrated

↓

From crude glycoside fraction, the pure glycoside (digoxin) is obtained by fractional solubility, fractional crystallization and various chromatographic techniques.

Estimation and Analysis

1. A specific qualitative test for identification of digoxin utilizes a system composed of organic phase obtained by equilibrating 10 volumes of $CHCl_3$, 2 volumes of CH_3OH and 5 volumes of water.

Procedure

Digoxin is estimated through paper chromatography process.

(i) The sample solution [2 mg in 5 ml of $CHCl_3$-CH_3OH (1 : 1)] and standard solution (same concentration) are compared by placing 10 mcl aliquots of each as separate spots on a filter paper strip, approximately 10 cm from one end.

(ii) The chromatogram is developed in a closed chamber according to the descending technique i.e., end of the strip nearest the sample is placed in a trough containing equilibrated solvent, and the trough is located in the upper part of chamber, so that the solvent flows downward through the paper.

(iii) To maintain a saturated atmosphere, a small amount of both phases of the equilibrated solvent is placed in the bottom of the chromatographic chamber.

(iv) When the solvent reaches a point within 5 cm of the bottom edge of the strip, the chromatogram is allowed to remove and dried in the air.

(v) Location of glycosidic zones in both sample and standard is accomplished by spraying the strip with a 25% solution of trichloroacetic acid in methanol followed by heating at 100 °C temperature for 1 minute.

(vi) The presence of digoxin in the sample solution is established by the appearance of a greyish green spot, having R_f value same as in standard solution.

2. • Using Baljet picric acid reagent, digoxin is determined on paper chromatograms.
   • Using keller-killiani reagent (ferric chloride with sulfuric and glacial acetic acids), both digoxin and isodigoxin are determined.

3. *Standardization (For quality)*: TLC-densitometry is used as an alternative method to HPLC and GLC for the standardization of crude medicinal plant extracts of *Digitalis lanata*.

11.2.5 Digitoxin

Biological Source : obtained from dried leaves of "*Digitalis purpurea*"

Family : Scrophulariaceae

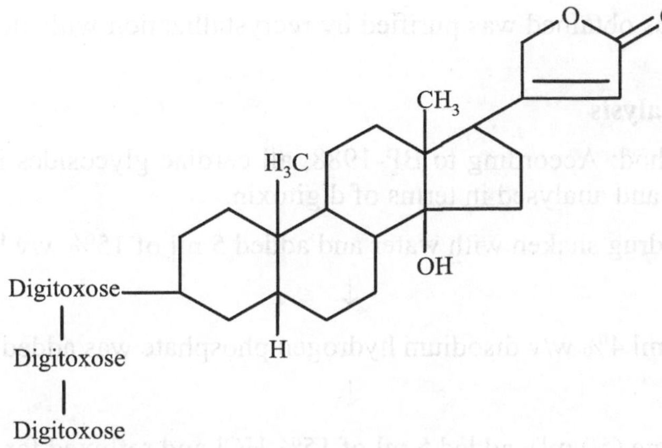

Digitoxin

Extraction and Isolation of Digitoxin

Powdered leaves of *Digitalis purpurea* are macerated with water at 45 °C temperature for 4-5 hours

↓

The leaves are again macerated with 20% methanol for 24 hours

↓

The aqueous and methanolic extract are mixed together

↓

The final extract was made alkaline with NaOH (for hydrolysis)

↓

Extracted with chloroform solution

↓

Evaporated $CHCl_3$ and extracted to dryness

↓

The residue obtained was chromatographed

↓

The column was packed with silica gel G and eluted by gradient technique initially with CCl_4, then with ethyl acetate and methanol

- CCl_4 fraction contains colouring pigments
- Ethyl acetate fraction contains flavones and anthraquinones.
- Methanol fraction contains digitoxin ($R_f = + 0.486$).

The digitoxin thus obtained was purified by recrystallization with alcohol and di-ethyl ether mixture (2:1).

Estimation and Analysis

1. *BP*-1988 method: According to BP-1988, all cardiac glycosides in digitalis leaves are estimated and analysed in terms of digitoxin.

Powdered drug shaken with water and added 5 ml of 15% w/v lead acetate

↓

To this 7.5 ml 4% w/v disodium hydrogen phosphate was added and filtered

↓

To the filtrate (50 ml), added 5 ml of 15% HCl and refluxed for 1 hour

↓

From aqueous (water) extract, drug was extracted with $CHCl_3$ (3 × 25 ml)

↓

Chloroform extract was dried over anhydrous sodium sulphate

↓

Evaporated to 40 ml and added 7 ml of 50% ethanol solution and 2 ml DNBA (3, 5 di-nitro benzoic acid) in 1 ml of 1M NaOH.

↓

Measured the absorbance at 540 nm range with reference blank reagent and calculated by comparing with digitoxin standard calibration curve.

2. *BP*-1990 *method*
   - Dissolved 40 mg powdered drug in ethanol to produce 50 ml solution.
   - Diluted 5 ml of solution to 100 ml with ethanol.
   - To 5 ml of above solution, added 3 ml alkaline trinitrophenol.
   - Allowed to stand for 30 minutes.
   - Measured the absorbance at 495 nm against reference blank reagent.
   - Calculated digitoxin content by measuring absorbance obtained from digitoxin RS.
3. *IP*-1996 *Method*
   - Weighed accurately about 40 mg of powdered drug and dissolved in ethanol and make up the volume to 100 ml.
   - To 5 ml of above solution, added 3 ml of alkaline picric acid solution.

- Allowed to stand for 30 minutes.
- Measured the absorbance against blank reagent at 495 nm.
- Calculated digitoxin content by repeating the procedure with digitoxin RS.

4. *USP*-1940 *method*:
   - *Reagents used*:
     (ii) Ethyl alcohol (95%)
     (ii) Sodium picrate reagent : 2 gm picric acid (containing about 10% moisture) is transferred into 100 ml volumetric flask with the aid of 50 ml C_2H_5OH. Then about 30 ml of water is added and mixture is shaken until all solid is dissolved. Then 5 ml of 10% NaOH solution is added and the solution is diluted to the mark with water. Thus, sample solution is prepared.

     Standard solution: USP reference standard digitoxin (dried for 1 hour at 105 °C), 0.2 mg/ml, in ethyl alcohol. The solution is stored in a refrigerator.

   Procedure:
   - A solution containing 0.2 mg of the sample per ml in ethyl alcohol is prepared from previously dried at 105 °C for 1 hour.
   - 3 ml of standard and sample solutions are transferred into separate 25 ml volumetric flasks and exactly 15 ml of sodium picrate reagent is added to each.
   - The mixture is diluted to the mark with ethyl alcohol.
   - A blank, containing only 15 ml of reagent diluted to 25 ml with ethyl alcohol is also prepared.
   - After 30 minutes from the addition of reagent to the sample, the absorbance of standard and sample are read out against blank reagent in a spectro photometer at 490 mμ range.

     Calculation:

$$\% \text{ purity of digitoxin} = \frac{[\text{A(sample)}]}{[\text{A(s tan dard)}]} \times 100$$

11.2.6 Diosgenin

Synonyms	:	Yam, Rheumatism root
Biological source	:	obtained from dried tubers of plants "*Dioscorea deltoidea*", "*Dioscorea composita*" and other species of Dioscorea
Family	:	Dioscoreaceae

Diosgenin occurs naturally in combined form as saponin glycoside and rarely in free state. It is present as rhamno-rhamno-glucoside called dioscin in tubers of commercial species of dioscorea.

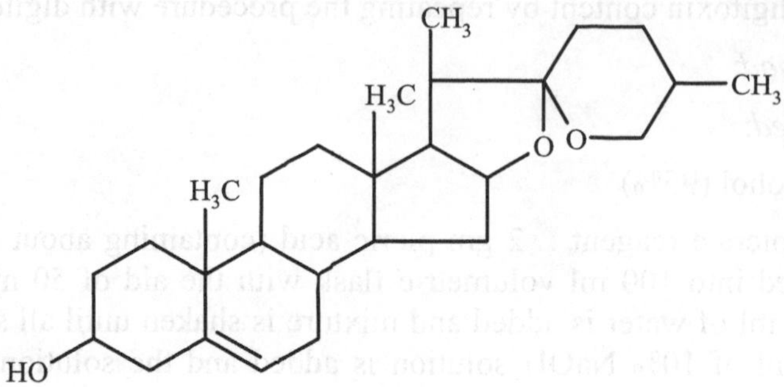

Diosgenin

Extraction and Isolation Method

Diosgenin can be extracted from fresh or dried tubers by three methods, namely:

(i) Alcoholic extraction of glycoside from the plant material, followed by acid hydrolysis.

(ii) Acid hydrolysis of total plant material, followed by extraction of liberated sapogenin with a hydrocarbon solvent.

(iii) Fermentation-cum-acid hydrolysis

Tubers dried in an oven at 80 °C or in the sun, and properly stored and handled under dry conditions do not lose diosgenin. Fresh tubers are used, if separated and processed soon after harvesting, as there is a rapid decrease in diosgenin content when the rotting proceeds. Dioscorea floriburda tubers are extremely susceptible to rotting.

***Method* I**

- 30 gm of plant material is hydrolyzed by autoclaving with about 200 ml of 2.5N H_2SO_4 for 1 hour, filter it, and washed with water.
- Then the solution was washed with 10% $NaHCO_3$ solution to remove acid.
- Dried the residue at 50 °C temperature overnight and extracted with 250 ml benzene for 6-8 hours.
- Benzene distilled off the residue.
- The residue so obtained is dissolved in chloroform and then concentrated and evaporated.
- The solution is re-crystallized with acetone.

***Method* II**

The powdered drug retain their pharmacological action after hydrolysis.

Powdered Drug refluxed with 2N HCl for 2 hours.

↓ Cool and filtered

Neutralized the residue by passing oil of ammonia

↓ Filtered

Dried the residue obtained on filter paper at 60 °C temperature for two hours

↓ React with HCl acid for hydrolysis, removed the sugar moiety and other impurities.

Extracted with petroleum ether in soxhlet apparatus

↓ (at 40-60 °C for 24 hours)

Reduced the volume and allowed to cool the residue

↓

Filtered the precipitate and recrystallized

After isolation, diosgenin is degraded to 16-dehydro pregnenolone acetate. This latter molecule is used as a precursor agent for synthesis of:

(i) Corticosteroids such as – Cortisone, hydrocortisone, prednisolone.

(ii) Pregnenes such as – progesterone, 17α-hydroxy progesterone

(iii) Androstanes such as – testosterone, methyl testosterone.

(iv) 19 – NOR steroids such as estrone.

These conversions are done with the help of microbial transformation reactions.

Another method for extraction is incubation-cum-acid hydrolysis method, which involves incubation of fresh plant material in water at 37 °C temperature for a period of a few hours to a few days before subjecting it to acid hydrolysis for obtaining diosgenin.

Estimation and Analysis

1. *By TLC method*:

The TLC profile is as given:

- Solvent system = $CHCl_3$: Ethanol (95 : 5)
  $CHCl_3$: Acetone (3 : 1)
  Ethyl Acetate
- Plates used = Silica gel plates
- Detecting agents = Antimony trichloride ($SbCl_3$)in chloroform

2. *By HPTLC method*:

   HPTLC profile is as follows:

   - Plates used = Silica gel G plates
   - Mobile phase = n-Hexane : Ethyl acetate (4 : 2)
   - Spraying reagent = 3 gm of $SbCl_3$ in 100 ml concentrated HCl acid
   - A green black colour is formed which is scanned by using densitometer.

11.2.7 Ephedrine

Biological source : Ephedrine is obtained in various species of Ephedra such as "*Ephedra gerardiana, Ephedra nebrodensis, Ephedra intermidia, Ephedra vulgaris, Ephedra sinica*

Family : Ephedraceae (Gnetaceae)

Ephedra contains not less than 1% of ephedrine as a total alkaloid.

Extraction and Isolation

Ephedrine is mainly extracted from more or less broken aerial stems which are woody and usually branched only at base.

- Drug in a powdered form containing alkaloidal salts is defatted with petroleum ether.
- The drug is moistened and rendered alkaline to free alkaloids as bases (with NH_3).
- The drug is extracted with aqueous alcohol solution or $CHCl_3$ (an organic solvent) in which alkaloidal salts are transferred.
- Now the alcoholic solution is evaporated to a thick syrup.
- After continuous extraction with organic solvent, aqueous phase is made alkaline with sodium carbonate.
- The basic aqueous solution is extracted and the alkaloid containing solution is dried, with sodium sulphate, filtered and evaporated to yield alkaloidal residue (ephedrine) with sodium sulphate, filtered and evaporated to yield alkaloidal residue (ephedrine).

Estimation and Analysis

1. *Ephedrine*: It is anhydrous and contains not more than one half volume of water of hydration. It contains not less than 98.5% and not more than 100.5% of ephedrine, calculated on anhydrous basis.

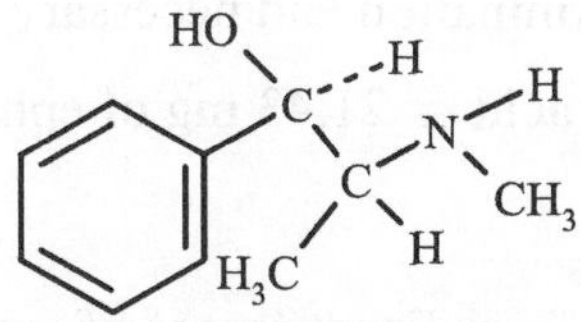

Ephedrine

Procedure: Weighed accurately about 100 mg and by burette added the exact volume of 0.1N H_2SO_4 acid determined in assay to neutralize it.

- Diluted with water in a volumetric flask to 25 ml.
- Mixed 2 ml of solution with 10 ml of alcohol and evaporated on a steam bath by passing current of air to dryness.
- Residue, thus obtained responds to identification test under Ephedrine sulphate.

Assay: Dissolved about 500 mg of ephedrine (accurately weighed) in 10 ml of neutralized alcohol and added 5 drops of Methyl Red TS and 40 ml of 0.1N HCl acid vs.

- Titrated the excess acid with 0.1 N NaOH vs and performed a blank determination.
- Each ml of 0.1N HCl acid ≅ 16.52 mg of Ephedrine.

2. *Ephedrine Sulphate*:

It is identified by:

a Infrared absorption

b A solution of ephedrine sulphate responds to test for sulphate.

Assay:

- Weighed accurately 300 mg of ephedrine sulphate and transfer it to a separator and dissolve it in about 10 ml water.
- Saturated the solution with NaCl (3 g) and added 5 ml of 1N NaOH and extracted with four 25 ml portions of $CHCl_3$.
- Wash combined chloroform extracts by shaking with 10 ml saturated solution of NaCl and filtered through chloroform saturated purified cotton into beaker.
- Extracted the washed solution with 10 ml of $CHCl_3$ and added to main chloroform extract.
- Added methylsed TS and titrated with 0.1N $HClO_4$ (Perchloric acid) in dioxane vs.

- Performed a blank determination and necessary corrections were made.
- Each ml of 0.1N $HClO_4$ acid ≅ 21.43 mg of ephedrine sulphate.

11.2.8 Ergometrine

Biological source : obtained from Ergot (ergot of rye), which is dried sclerotum of a fungus "*Claviceps purpurea*".

Family : Clavicipataceae/Hypocreaceae

It is also obtained from ovary of rye plant *Secale cereale* (Graminae)

There are three main groups of ergot alkaloids:

1. Ergometrine group : Ergometrine, Ergometrinine
2. Ergotamine group : Ergotamine, Ergotaminine, Ergosine, Ergosinine
3. Ergotoxine group : Ergocristine, Ergocristinine, Ergocryptine, Ergocryptinine, Ergocornine, Ergocorninine

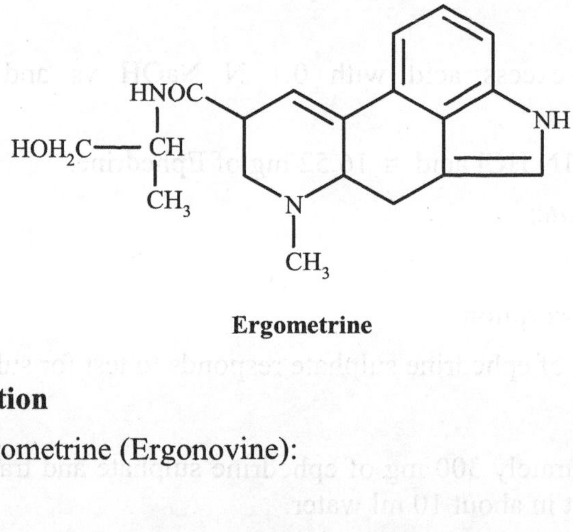

Ergometrine

Extraction and Isolation

1. Isolation of Ergometrine (Ergonovine):

***Method* I**

Powdered Ergot drug is defatted

↓

Extracted with hot dil. H_2SO_4 acid

↓

Acid extracted and treated with excess of Baryta ($BaSO_4$ solution))

↓

Excess Barium is removed by CO_2

↓ Filtered the solution

Filtrate | Marc (Residual matter)

Evaporation under reduced pressure

↓

Concentrated the above in vacuum

↓

Treated with alcohol (C_2H_5OH)

↓

Concentrated the ethanolic extract and made alkaline

↓

Extracted the above concentrate with $CHCl_3$

↓

Extracted $CHCl_3$ extract is extracted with dil. H_2SO_4

↓

The acidic solution is made alkaline with ammonia solution

↓

Saturated with sodium chloride and extracted with ether

↓

Solvent is removed leaving the alkaloidal residue from which ergometrine is crystallized from acetone.

***Method* II**

(i) Powdered Ergot drug is defatted by extraction with light petroleum and allowed to dry in air.

(ii) 15 gm of defatted powder is placed in 250 ml flask + 147 ml of reagent acetone + 3 ml of 10% ammonia solution, flask is stoppered and shaken on mechanical shaker for one hour.

(iii) Solution is filtered and 100 ml of filtrate is transferred to an evaporating dish.

(iv) Solution is evaporated and about 20 ml is transferred to a 125 ml separating funnel.

(v) 3 volumes of pure ether are added and solution is made acidic with 0.2 ml of 20% tartaric acid solution.

(vi) The acetone-ether solution is now extracted with four 10 ml portions of 1% tartaric acid solution, each portion being drawn off into a small round bottomed flask.

(vii) Traces of ether and acetone are removed at 40 °C temperature.

(viii) The solution is transferred to 50 ml volumetric flask.

(ix) Solution is made alkaline to a pH 8 with $NaHCO_3$ and volume made upto 50 ml with distilled water.

(x) Water insoluble Ergotoxine alkaloids are filtered off.

(xi) 45 ml filtrate is pipetted into separating funnel and shaken successively with two 50 ml portion of CCl_4 to remove traces of water insoluble alkaloids.

(xii) Discarded the CCl_4 extract and remove all traces of it from the aqueous fraction by evaporation at reduced pressure at 40 °C temperature.

(xiii) Transferred the aqueous solution to 125 ml separating funnel, saturated with NaCl, and shaken well with five successive portions of 50 ml ether.

(xiv) Combined ether extracts are evaporated to dryness under air current to get a residue of *ergometrine*.

2. *Isolation of Ergotamine*:

Powdered Ergot is defatted

↓

Thoroughly mixed with aluminium sulphate and water

↓

Continuous extraction with hot Benzene

↓ Removal of solvent

Residue obtained

↓

Stirred with several hours with a large volume of benzene made alkaline with ammonia gas

↓

Benzene extract is concentrated under reduced pressure, to about 1/50th of original volume

↓

Ergotamine crystallizes out

- A further quantity of ergotamine may also be crystallized from the mother liquor by treatment with petroleum ether
- The ergotamine crystals may be recrystallized from aqueous acetone

3. *Isolation of Ergotoxine Group*:

Powdered Ergot is extracted with ethanol and the solvent is then removed from the alcoholic extract

↓

Residue obtained is defatted by petroleum ether and then dissolved in ethyl acetate solution

↓

Extract obtained is shaken with 1-2% citric acid solution

↓

Sodium bromide is added to the acid solution to convert the alkaloidal salt to their hydro bromides which are then precipitated

↓

Made alkaline with dilute NaOH solution and extracted with ether

↓

Ether extract	Aqueous alkaline solution
↓	↓
Contains ergotinine and some traces of ergocristine	containing ergocryptine, ergocornine and some traces of ergocristine

↓

Neutralized and made slightly alkaline with Na_2CO_3 and extracted with ether

↓

Ether is removed by distillation

↓

Residue obtained is dissolved in 80% ethanol and a slight excess of phosphoric acid solution is added

↓ Stand for several days

Ergotoxin phosphate crystals precipitated out

↓

Separated and recrystallized from boiling 90% ethanol (50 ml for each gram of ergotoxine phosphate)

Estimation and Analysis

1. ***Method* – I:** Thin Layer Chromatography Method

   TLC profile is as follows:

   - *Drug sample*: *Secale Cornutum* (freshly prepared alkaloidal fraction)

     Secale Cornutum (stored alkaloid)
   - *Reference Compounds*:

     T_1 ergocristine T_2 ergotamine

     T_3 ergometrine T_4 ergometrine

     T_5 ergotamine T_6 ergocristin
   - *Solvent system*: Foluene : chloroform : ethanol (28.5 : 57 : 14.5)
   - *Detection*: UV = 254 nm (without any chemical treatment)

     Van urk reagent = visible range
   - *Evaluation*:

     Ergometrine $R_f = 0.05$

     Ergotamine $R_f = 0.25$

     Ergocristine $R_f = 0.45$
   - After treatment with Van urk reagent, the secale extract generates three blue zones of principal alkaloids (T_1-T_3) in the R_f range between 0.05-0.45.

2. ***Method* II:** Colorimetric Method

   - 4 ml ergot solution + 8 ml ergot reagent (0.125 gm p-dimethylamino benzaldehyde added to 0.1 ml of 5% solution of $FeCl_3$ + 65% v/v H_2SO_4 to make 100 ml) is mixed in a 25 ml volumetric flask.
   - Allowed to stand for 30 minutes, read the colour at 550 nm.
   - Prepared a standard curve using pure ergometrine.

3. ***Method* III:** Non-Aqueous Titrations (IP-1996 Method)

   - 0.15 gm of ergometrine maleate is dissolved in 40 ml of anhydrous glacial acetic acid.
   - 0.05M $HClO_4$ (perchloric acid) is used as a titrant and endpoint is determined potentiometrically.

4. ***Method* IV:** Colorimetric Method (USP-1995)

- Standard preparation : 40 μg/ml solution of USP ergometrine maleate RS in water
- Assay preparation : 40 μg/ml of sample in water
- Procedure : 5 ml of standard,assay, blank determination i.e., water and 10 ml paradimethylamino Benzaldehyde (PDAB). After 20 min take the absorbance at 555 nm against blank. Calculated quantity in mg by using formula

C(Au/As).

where, C = concentration in μg/ml of USP ergononine maleate Rs in standard preparation.

Au, As = absorbance of solution from assay and standard preparation respectively.

This method is generally *used* in obstetrics during child birth and also *used* to reduce incidence of postpartum haemorrhage (PPH).

5. ***Method* V:** Paper Chromatography Method

(i) This technique uses partition paper chromatography and the water soluble ergot alkaloids can be separated from water insoluble alkaloids.

(ii) *Solvent system used*: n-butanol : Acetic acid : water (4 : 1 : 5).

(iii) The water insoluble alkaloids passes down the paper (whatman paper no.1) with the solvent front and ergometrine (Rf = 0.59) and ergometrinine (Rf = 0.68) get separated on the paper.

(iv) After drying, examined under UV light when alkaloidal spot becomes visible.

11.2.9 Glycyrrhetinic Acid

Synonyms : Mulethi, liquorice root, glycyrrhizae radix

Biological source : Obtained from liquorice which consists of dried, peeled or unpeeled roots and stolon of "*Glycyrrhiza glabra*".

Family : Leguminosae

Liquorice should have a water soluble extractive not less than 20% w/w.

Extraction and Isolation

Liquorice root contains about 7% of glycyrrhizin (glycyrrhizic acid), a triterpenoid saponin, which is a potassium and calcium salts of glycyrrhizinic acid. On acid hydrolysis it yields glycyrrhetinic acid and mannuronic acid.

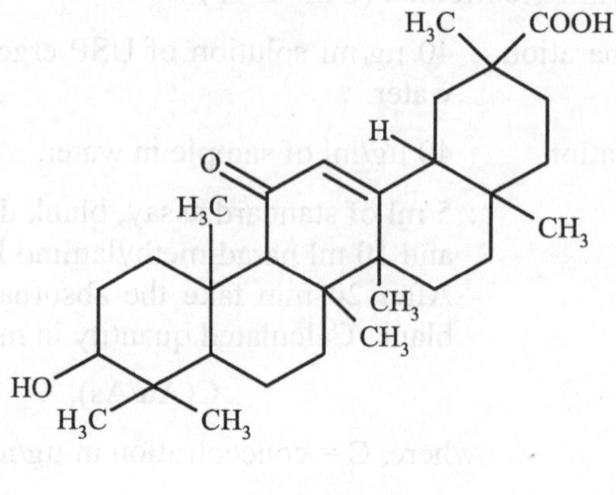

Glycyrrhetinic acid

1. ***Isolation of Glycyrrhetinic acid*:**

25 gm of powdered Liquorice root

↓

Adjust pH to 6.5-7.0 with dilute ammonia

↓

Centrifuged and evaporated to 75% of its volume under vacuum

↓

Supernatant liquid (Discarded)	Precipitated (crude Glycyrrhetinic acid)

↓

Suspended the solution in 25 ml of water

↓

Adjusted the pH to 4.0 with Na_2CO_3 solution

↓

Stirr continuously (2-3 hrs) and centrifuge.

↓

Suspended the residue in water

↓

Neutralize to pH = 6.0 with NH_3 solution

↓

Centrifuged and dried in an oven

↓

Calculated the percentage of glycyrrhetinic acid on the basis of air dried drugs

2. *Isolation and Extraction of Ammonium glycyrrhizinate*:

20 gm of powdered drug (Liquorice Root) + Acetone (50 ml) + dil. HNO_3 acid (2 ml)

↓ Mixed thoroughly in a flask

Flask was corked and macerated for about 2 hours

↓ Filtered

Filtrate | Marc + 20 ml acetone

Marc + 20 ml acetone ↓ Warmed on water bath and filtered → Filtrate

Filtrate + Filtrate (combined)

↓

Both filtrates concentrated under vacuum

↓

Dil. NH_3 solution is added to acetone extract (above filtrate) for precipitation of ammonium glycyrrhizinate

↓

Separated the precipitate by filtration and washed with 5 ml of acetone

↓

Product obtained was dried

↓

Yield of ammonium glycyrrhizinic acid (ammonium glycyrrhizinate) should be approx. 4.5% w/w.

3. ***Isolation of Glycyrrhizin***:

Glycyrrhizin is isolated by two methods:

(i) Acid Precipitation Method

(ii) Alcohol precipitation Method

(i) *Acid Precipitation Method*

Principle: Glycyrrhizin gets precipitated from aqueous solution on addition of conc. H_2SO_4 or conc. HCl at pH = 2.8. The Glycyrrhizin gets extracted by:

- Using root powder
- Using concentrate aqueous extract

Using Root Powder:

Powdered root 100 gm + boiling water 100 ml

↓ Moistened and wet the powder

Further added 200 ml hot water

↓ Shaken well and allowed to stand for 20 min

Supernatant liquid was decanted off and remaining solution was filtered

↓

Filtrate + super natant liquid + conc. H_2SO_4 acid (for adjustment of pH to 2.8)

↓

Glycyrrhizin precipitated (as brown mass)

↓

Mass collected on filter paper

↓

Washed with ice cold water to free it from acid

↓

Residue collected in a tared china dish

↓

Heated for water evaporation

↓

Calculated the percentage yield of Glycyrrhizin obtained

Using conc. aqueous extract:

Preparation of conc. Aqueous extract: → To a weighed quantity of roots, aqueous solvent in the ratio of 1: 5 is added and subjected to reflux. The extract obtained was concentrated to about 30% volume of original volume.

20 gm of conc. aqueous extract + 60 ml boiling water

↓ Shaken well to dissolve the conc. extract

Clear solution obtained

↓

To this, added H_2SO_4 acid drop wise to get pH = 2.8

↓

At this pH, glycyrrhizin gets precipitated

(ii) *Alcohol Precipitation Method*:

Principle: Glycyrrhizin is soluble in alcohol and practically insoluble in ether. The insolubility in other organic solvents was used to remove the interfering groups. Thus, alcoholic layer which contained glycyrrhizin was extracted successively with various solvents of increasing polarity. The alcoholic layer on concentration yields Glycyrrhizin. (Menthanol and Ethanol were used for isolation).

Estimation and Analysis of Liquorice Extract (Glycyrrhetinic acid/Glycyrrhizin):

I. *High Performance Thin Layer Chromatographic (HPTLC) Method*:

The HPTLC profile is as follows:

1. Instrumentation : A HPTLC system equipped with sample applicator device, TLC plate, development chamber, TLC plate scanner with software.
2. Drug sample : Liquorice (ethanolic extract 20 ml)
3. Reference compound : Glycyrrhizin, Glycyrrhetinic acid
4. HPTLC plate : Silica gel G-F_{254} (0.2 mm)
5. Mobile phase : Toluene : Ethyl Acetate : Glacial Acetic acid (12.5 : 7.5 : 0.5)
6. Wavelength : 254 nm
7. Visualization of spots : Anisaldehyde-Sulphuric acid
8. Standard Preparation : 5 gm of glycyrrhizin + 20 ml 0.5M H_2SO_4

↓ Reflux and cool

Extracted with $CHCl_3$ (2 × 10 ml)

↓ Evaporated the extract

Residue dissolved in chloroform : Methanol (1 : 1)

9. Sample Preparation : Powdered Drug (1 gm) + $CHCl_3$ (20 ml)

↓ Shaken for 15 minutes

Filtered and discarded the filtrate

↓

Reflux the marc for 1 hour with 30 ml of 0.5M H_2SO_4 and cool

↓

Shake the unfiltered mixture with $CHCl_3$ (2 × 20ml) and concentrated the combined extract

↓

Dissolved the residue in 1 ml of $CHCl_3$: CH_3OH (1 : 1)

II. *Thin Layer Chromatography (TLC) Method*:

The TLC profile is as given under:

1. Test Solution : Powdered Drug (1 gm) + $CHCl_3$ (20 ml)

↓ Shaken for 15 min

Filtered and discarded the filtrate

↓

Reflux the marc for 1 hour with 30 ml of 0.5M H_2SO_4 and cooled.

↓

Shake the unfiltered mixture with $CHCl_3$ (2 × 20 ml) and concentrated the combined extract

↓

Dissolved the residue in 1 ml of $CHCl_3$: CH_3OH (1 : 1)

2. Reference solution : 5 gm of Glycyrrhizin/Glycyrrhetin + 20 ml 0.5M H_2SO_4

↓ Reflux and cool

Extracted with $CHCl_3$ (2 × 10 ml)

↓ Evaporated and extract

Residue dissolved in $CHCl_3$: CH_3OH (1 : 1) mixture

3. Drug Sample : Liquorice (ethanolic/alcoholic extract 20 ml)
4. Reference compound : Glycyrrhetinic acid
5. Solvent system : Ethyl Acetate : Ethanol : water : Ammonia (65 : 25 : 9 : 1)
6. Procedure : Applied 5 ml each of test solution and reference solution in two different tracks on a precoated silica gel-G F_{254} plate (5 × 15 cm) of uniform thickness (0.2 mm). Developed the plate in solvent system to a distance of 12 cm.
7. Scanning : Scanned densitometrically at 254 nm both reference and test solution and recorded finger print profiles.
8. Visualization of spots
   - Under UV = 254 nm
   - Spray plate with Anisaldehyde-sulfuric acid reagent and heat at 110 °C temperature for 5-10 minutes.
9. Evaluation :
   - Under UV = 254 nm light (before spraying):
     Two spots (0.41, 0.45 = R_f value) exhibiting/quenching are visible in sample solution track. One of which (R_f = *0.41*) corresponds to glycyrrhetinic acid of reference track.
   - In Day light (After spraying):
     Glycyrrhetinic acid is visible as a dark violet spot in both reference and test solution tracks.
     Other spots visible in test solution includes : *two dark yellow spots* (R_f = 0.45, 0.49), two violet spots (R_f = 0.27, 0.70) and a *dark blue spot* running along with solvent front.

III. ***Assay Method*:**

Quantitative determination of Glycyrrhetinic acid in liquorice roots and extracts are assayed by TLC-Densitometry method.

1. TLC Plates : Kiesel gel 60 HF_{254}
2. Solvent system : n-butanol : acetic acid : distilled water (7 : 1 : 2)
3. Colour Reagent : 1% cerric surgatoin + 10% H_2SO_4 (105 °C temperature for 15 min)
4. Standard Preparation : Prepared a solution of known concentration (Range 0.5-2.0 µg/ml) of glycyrrhetinic acid in 50% ethanol.

5. Sample preparation :
   - Reflux for 1 hour, powdered root (1 gm) with 50% ethanol (50 ml) on a boiling water bath, cooled and filtered and then reflux (for 1 hr) the marc further with 50% ethanol (50 ml).
   - Evaporated the combined extract at 50 °C temperature and dissolved the residue in 50% ethanol solution (10 ml).
6. Procedure :
   - Apply 10 ml each of standard preparation and of sample preparation on TLC plate.
   - Developed plate on solvent system to a distance of 13-14 cm.
   - Scanned the plate in densitometer and integrated area of plates, corresponding to glycyrrhetinic acid.
   - Calculated the percentage yield of the above accordingly.

11.2.10 Morphine

Biological Source : It is present in the latex or milky exudates obtained by vertical incision of unripe capsules of "*Papaver somniferum*".

Family : Papaveraceae

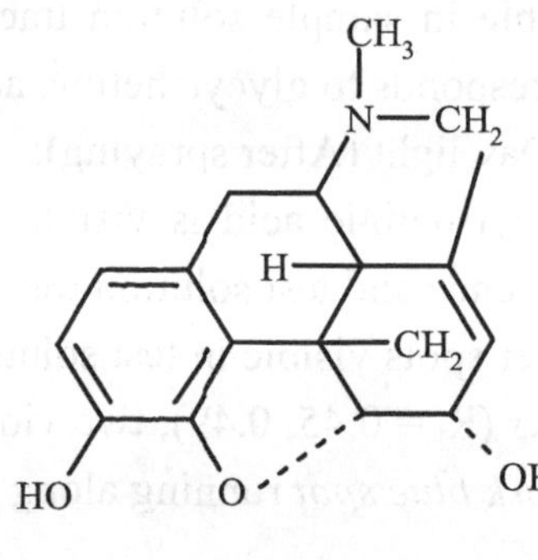

Morphine

Extraction and Isolation

Opium is obtained from milky exudates of incised unripe seeds and capsules of poppy plant. The milky juice is dried in the air which gets converted to a brownish gummy mass. It is further dried and is powdered to make official powdered opium containing well over a score of alkaloids. Alkaloids constitute only 25% by weight of opium.

The latex contains alkaloids, derived from amino acids such as phenyl alanine and tyrosine chemically placed under benzylisoquinoline and phenanthrene types.

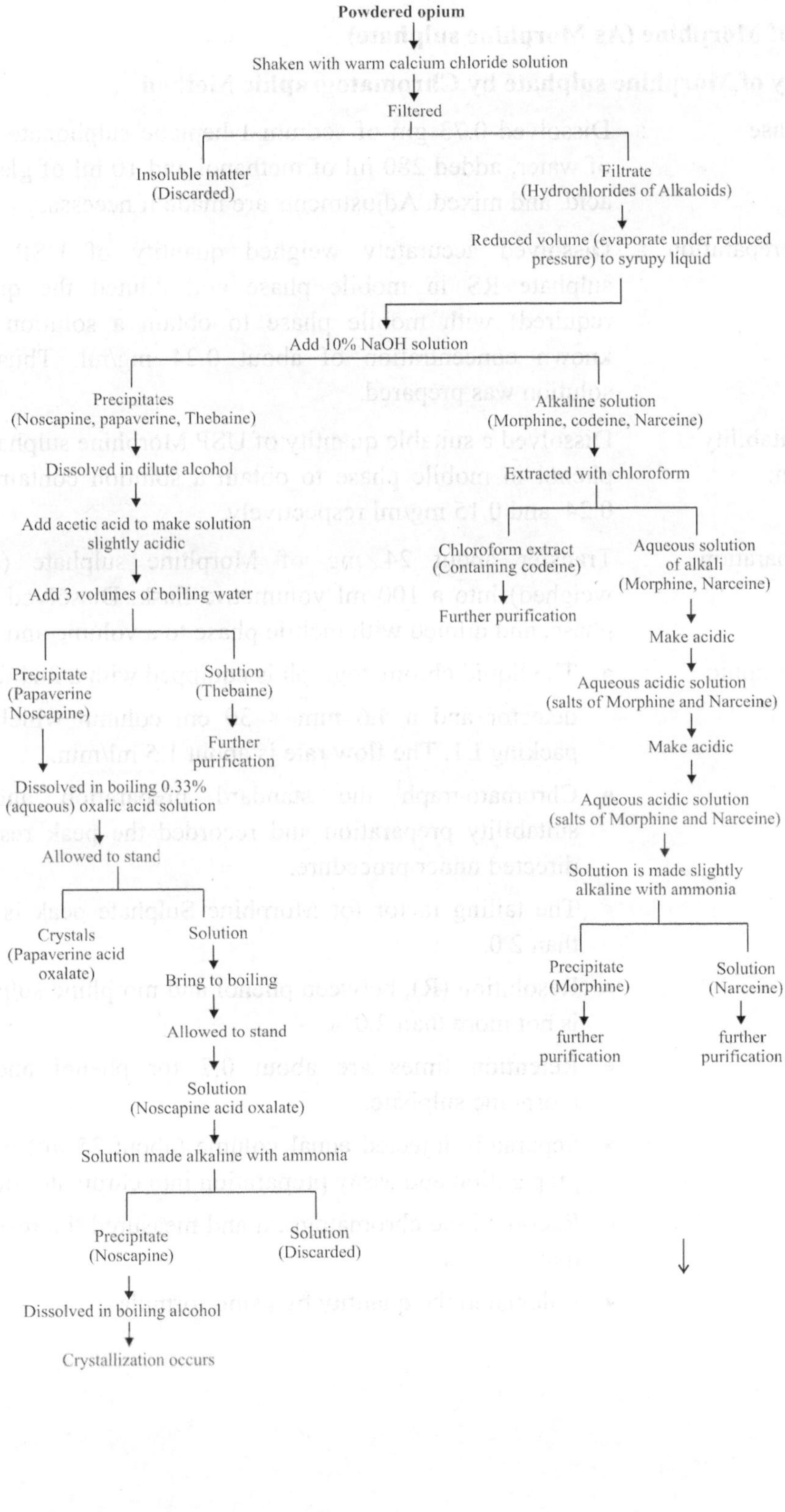
Powdered opium
Shaken with warm calcium chloride solution
Filtered
Insoluble matter (Discarded)
Filtrate (Hydrochlorides of Alkaloids)
Reduced volume (evaporate under reduced pressure) to syrupy liquid
Add 10% NaOH solution
Precipitates (Noscapine, papaverine, Thebaine)
Alkaline solution (Morphine, codeine, Narceine)
Dissolved in dilute alcohol
Add acetic acid to make solution slightly acidic
Add 3 volumes of boiling water
Precipitate (Papaverine Noscapine)
Solution (Thebaine)
Further purification
Dissolved in boiling 0.33% (aqueous) oxalic acid solution
Allowed to stand
Crystals (Papaverine acid oxalate)
Solution
Bring to boiling
Allowed to stand
Solution (Noscapine acid oxalate)
Solution made alkaline with ammonia
Precipitate (Noscapine)
Solution (Discarded)
Dissolved in boiling alcohol
Crystallization occurs
Extracted with chloroform
Chloroform extract (Containing codeine)
Further purification
Aqueous solution of alkali (Morphine, Narceine)
Make acidic
Aqueous acidic solution (salts of Morphine and Narceine)
Make acidic
Aqueous acidic solution (salts of Morphine and Narceine)
Solution is made slightly alkaline with ammonia
Precipitate (Morphine)
Solution (Narceine)
further purification
further purification

Analysis of Morphine (As Morphine sulphate)

USP Assay of Morphine sulphate by Chromatographic Method

Mobile phase : Dissolved 0.73 gm of sodium-1-heptane sulphonate in 720 ml of water, added 280 ml of methanol and 10 ml of glacial acetic acid, and mixed. Adjustments are made if necessary.

Standard preparation : Dissolved accurately weighed quantity of USP Morphine sulphate RS in mobile phase and diluted the quantity (if required) with mobile phase to obtain a solution having a known concentration of about 0.24 mg/ml. Thus, a fresh solution was prepared.

System suitability preparation: Dissolved a suitable quantity of USP Morphine sulphate and phenol in mobile phase to obtain a solution containing about 0.24 and 0.15 mg/ml respectively.

Assay preparation : Transfer about 24 mg of Morphine sulphate (accurately weighed) into a 100 ml volumetric flask. Dissolved in mobile phase, and diluted with mobile phase to a volume and mixed.

Chromatographic system :

- The liquid chromatograph is equipped with a 284 nm detector and a 4.6 mm × 30 cm column which contains packing L1. The flow rate is about 1.5 ml/min.
- Chromatograph the standard preparation and system suitability preparation and recorded the peak responses as directed under procedure.
- The tailing factor for Morphine Sulphate peak is not more than 2.0.
- Resolution (R), between phenol and morphine sulphate peak is not more than 2.0%.
- Retention times are about 0.7 for phenol and 1.0 for morphine sulphate.

Procedure :

- Separately injected equal volume (about 25 ml) of standard preparation and assay preparation into chromatograph.
- Recorded the chromatogram and measured the responses for major peaks.
- Calculated the quantity by using formula

$$100\,C\left(\frac{ru}{rs}\right)$$

where, C = concentration in mg/ml of anhydrous morphine sulphate in standard preparation as determined from conc. of USP morphine sulphate.

ru/rs = are peak responses obtained from assay preparation and standard preparation respectively.

11.2.11 Podophyllotoxin

Biological source : Obtained from dried rhizomes and roots of "*Podophyllum hexandrum royle*" or "*Podophyllum emodi*".

Family : Berberidiaceae/Podophyllaceae

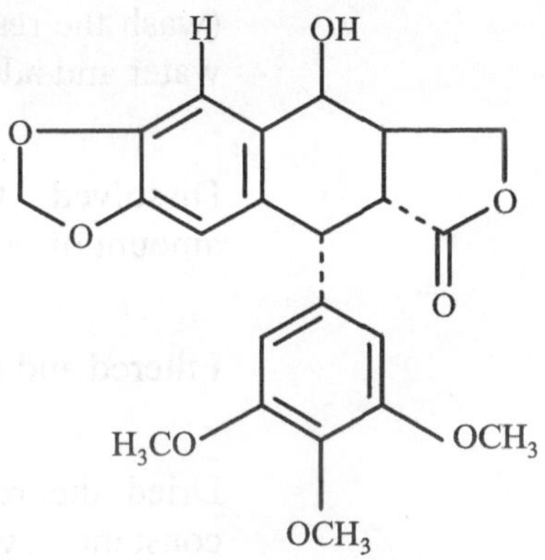

Podophyllotoxin

Extraction and Isolation

Podophyllum consists of dried roots and rhizomes of *Podophyllum peltatum emodii.* It yields not less than 5% of podophyllum resin (podophyllotoxin). Soxhlation method is used for its extraction.

100 gm of powdered drug

↓ Alcohol (90%) in soxhlate apparatus (4 hours)

Remove alcohol by distillation

↓

Evaporated the extract to syrupy consistency

↓

Poured it into a mixture of 200 ml of water + 2 ml of HCl with continuous stirring

↓ Cooled below 5 °C temperature.

Allowed the mixture to stand for 2 hours below 5 °C temperature

↓

Filtered under vacuum

↓

Filtrate (Discarded) | Residue

Residue

(wash the residue with 50 ml of acidified water and added below 5 °C temperature)

↓

Dissolved the residue in sufficient amount of hot alcohol (90%)

↓

Filtered and evaporated the alcohol

↓

Dried the residue (Resinous matter) to constant weight at about 80°C temperature

Specification of Indian Podophyllum Resin

Add 400 mg to 3 ml of 60% alcohol and the add 0.5M of 1N KOH solution and shake well the mixture gently and then allowed to stand for 2 weeks. It doesn't gelatinize.

Estimation and Analysis

***Method* I Thin Layer chromatography Method**

Test solution : Powdered drug (1 gm) + Methanol (50 ml)

↓ Reflux for ½ an hour

Evaporated the filtrate to dryness

↓

Dissolved residue in methanol (5 ml)

Reference solution	:	Dissolved podophyllotoxin (1 mg) in methanol (2 ml)
Solvent system:		Toluene : Ethyl acetate (5 : 7)
Procedure	:	Apply test and reference solution (5 ml each) in two different tracks on a precoated silica gel G plate (5 × 15 cm) of uniform thickness (0.2 mm). Develop the plate in a solvent system at a distance of 10 cm.
Scanning	:	Scanned densitometrically at 280 nm for both reference and test solution tracks and recorded finger print profiles. Compared the profile of test solution with that given (spray with sulphuric acid reagent heated at 120 °C for 10 min)
Evaluation	:	*In day light.* A spot (R_f = 0.39, violet coloured) corresponds to podophyllotoxin is visible in both reference and test solution tracks. A dark brown spot remains at application site.

Method II (*Used for Absence of Peltatins*)

Test solution	:	Heated the powdered drug (1 gm) under reflux for 10 min with methanol (10 ml). Filtered and evaporated the filtrate up to 3 ml.
Solvent System	:	Chloroform : Methanol (90:10) – upto 6 cm and then, Toluene : acetone (65:35) – up to 15 cm distance
Procedure	:	Apply 20-30 ml of test solution on a precoated silica gel G_O plate of uniform thickness and run plate in a solvent system.
Visualization	:	Spray the plate with fast blue salt reagent.
Evaluation	:	• Red brown tailing zones due to presence of tannins (R_f value up to 0.6 or above) • Absence of Red brown zones (due to absence of peltatins) • If α and β peltatins are present (*podophyllum peltatum*) red brown zones at R_f = 0.65 and R_f = 0.80 will be visible.

Method – III HPLC determination of Podophyllotoxin

Column	:	Cis-symmetry 4.6 × 150 mm of 5μ
Mobile phase	:	Methanol : water (62 : 38)
Flow rate	:	1.0 ml/min
Detection	:	UV at 280 nm

Standard preparation : Prepared a solution of known concentration of podophyllotoxin in methanol so as to lie it within linearity range (20 µg-2 µg)

Sample preparation :
- Reflux for 1 hour, the powdered sample (2 gm) with methanol (50 ml) cooled and filtered
- Reflux for 1 hour, the marc further with methanol (50 ml)
- Combined the filterate obtained from two cycles of refluxes and evaporated to dryness under vacuum
- Dissolved the residue in methanol (20 ml) and make up volume up to 50 ml with same solvent

Procedure : Inject known volume (5.0 ml) of each of standard and sample preparation to HPLC on triplicate and recorded the peak areas corrresponding to podophyllotoxin.

Calculated its yield in percentage in the sample.

11.2.12 *Quinine*

Biological Source : It is a quinoline alkaloid present in bark of "*Cinchona officinalis, Cinchona succirubra, Cinchona ledgeriana, cinchona calisaya*".

Family : Rubiaceae

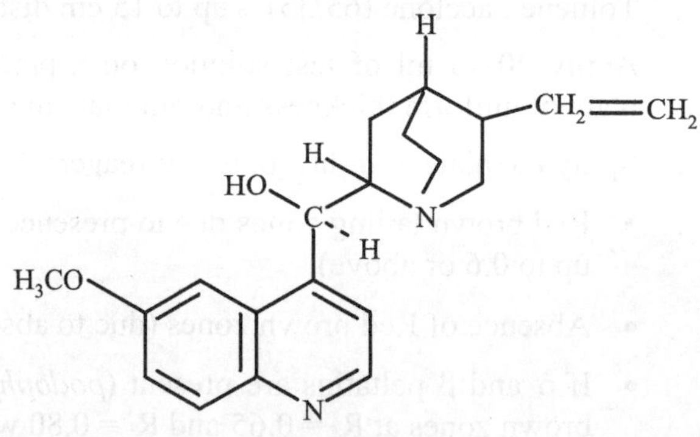

Quinine

Extraction and Isolation of total Cinchona alkaloids:

Dried powdered bark (15-20 gm)

↓

Mixed well with $Ca(OH)_2$ (30% of its weight)

↓

5% NaOH solution to make paste

↓

Allowed to stand for few hours

↓

Extraction with Benzene (Soxhlate continuous extraction process)

↓

Shake the above extract with three successive portion of 5% H_2SO_4 acid

↓

Aqueous acidic extract basified with ammonia solution (pH = 8.5)

↓

Shaken well with chloroform solution

↓

Chloroform extract obtained

↓

Distilled and transferred to a tared beaker

↓

Residue dried at 100 °C temperature to a constant weight (contains quinine, quinidine, and Cinchonine Cinchonidine)

Isolation of Individual Alkaloids

Aqueous acid extract obtained from previous process of extraction of total alkaloids.

Aqueous acid extract

↓

Adjusted to pH = 6.5 with dil. NaOH

↓

Cool and stand

↓

Crystals of neutral quinine sulphate

↓

(i) Repeated re-crystallization from hot water to free the quinine salt from cinchonine and cinchonidine

(ii) Removed the colouring matter by activated charcoal

↓

Mother Liquors (Quinidine, cinchonine, cinchonidine)

↓

Made slightly alkaline with ammonia

- Liquid (Discarded)
- Precipitate

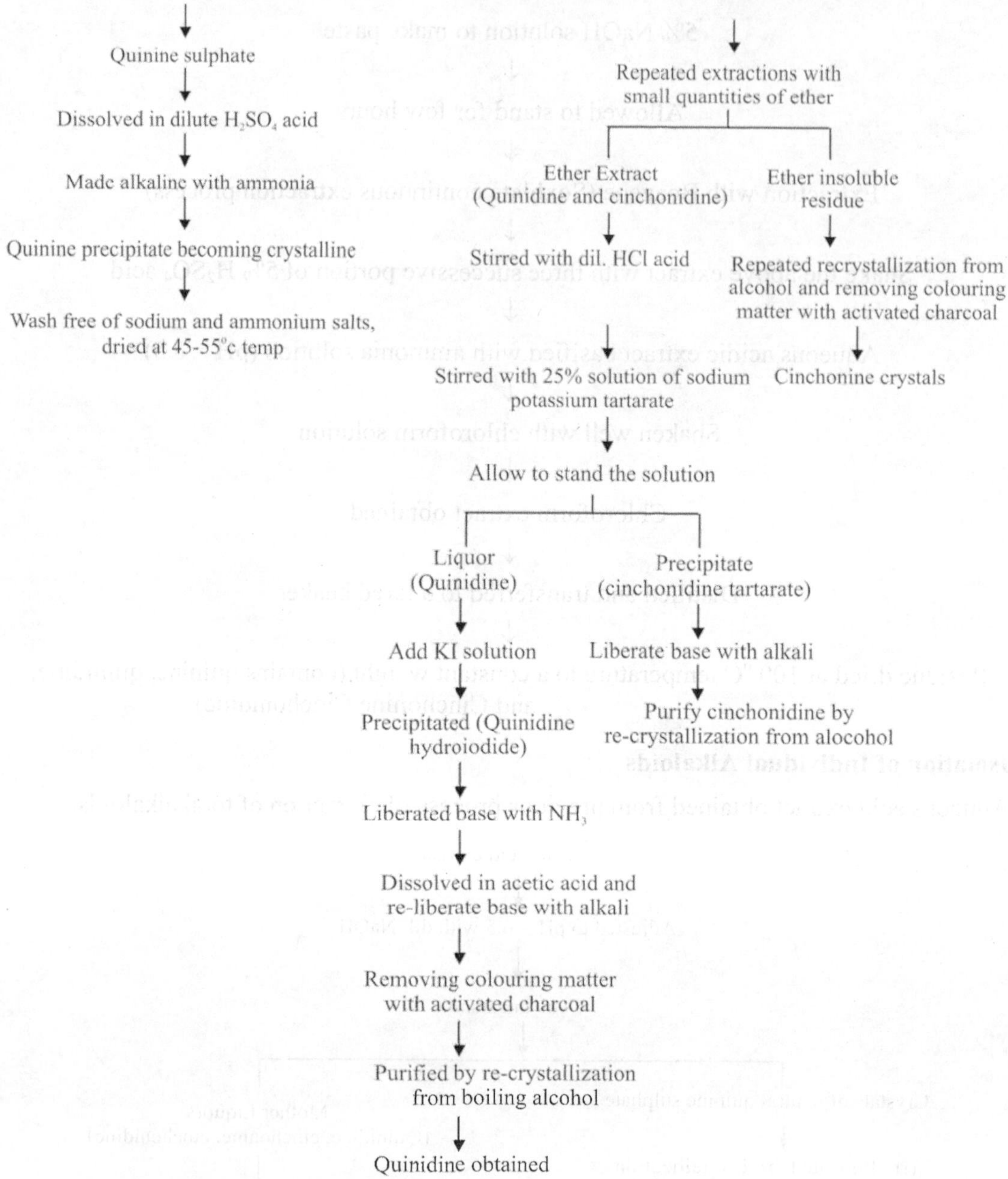

Estimation and Analysis

1. ***By Non-aqueous Titration Method*:**
   - Weighed accurately about 0.2 gm of quinidine sulphate/quinine sulphate and dissolved it in mixture of $CHCl_3$ (50 ml) and acetic anhydride (20 ml).

- Equivalence point is determined by potentiometrically by using 0.1M HCl acid.
- Plot the graph of potential v/s volume of titrant consumed.
- Each ml of 0.1M perchloric acid ≅ 0.02490 gm of quinidine/quinine.

2. ***By Fluorimetry Method*:**
   - Stock the solution of quinidine sulphate prepared by dissolving 10 mg in 1000 ml of 0.1N H_2SO_4 in a volumetric flask.
   - Prepared a serial dilution using 0.1N H_2SO_4 solution.
   - Measured the fluorescence and plotted a graph of fluorescence intensity v/s concentration of quinidine sulphate.
   - Quinidine shows maximum intensity 250 nm.

3. ***TLC Method*:**

Drug sample	:	*Cinchona calisaya* and *cinchona succirubra* (20 ml)
Reference compound	:	*TC cinchona alkaloidal mixture contains*: T_1 = Quinine (violet-brown) T_2 = Cinchonidine (violet-grey) T_3 = Quinidine (weak red-violet) T_4 = Cinchonine (prominent brown red zone)
Solvent system	:	$CHCl_3$: Diethylamine (90 : 10)
Detection	:	• 10% ethanolic H_2SO_4 = UV 365 nm 10% H_2SO_4 followed by Iodoplatinate reagent
Evaluation	:	• Treated with Iodoplatinate reagent and this results in eight mostly red-violet zones in the R_f range of 0.05-0.65 (visible). • The violet brown zones of quinine is followed by grey-violet zone of cinchonidine, weak red violet zone of quinidine and the most prominent brown red zone of cinchonine.

11.2.13 Taxol

Biological source	:	Taxol, a naturally occurring diterepenoid, initially called as paclitaxel, was isolated from the barks of genus taxus called as "*Taxus brevifolia, Taxus cuspidata*", "*Taxus Canadensis*". Taxus genus is also called as 'Yews"
Family	:	Taxaceae

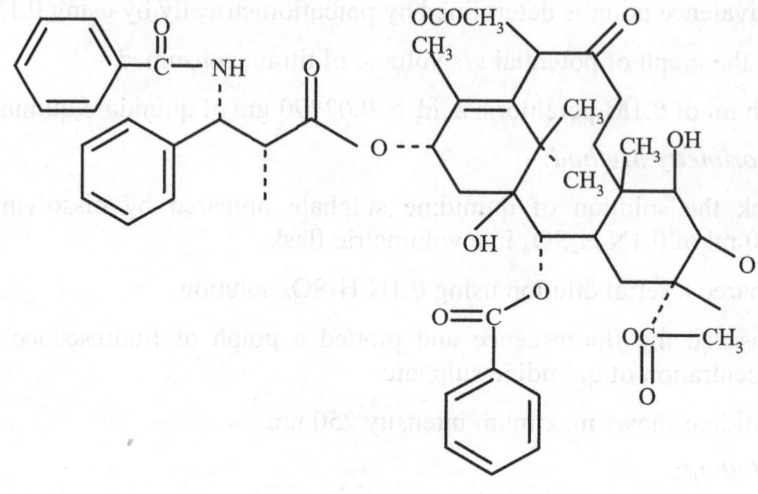

Taxol (Paclitaxel)

Immobilized Cell system for Taxol Production

1. *Callus culture method*: It is an induction method for cultured yew plant cells. Callus culture is started from needles and young stems. The agar culture media used for production is *Gamborg's* B-5 medium.
2. Perfusion culture method: Because, a considerable amount of paclitaxel is released into suspension culture medium, hence a perfusion culture is performed in a 300 ml *Erlenmeyer Flask* with a mesh net separator.
3. *Continuous Production System*:
   - For better productivity, a high dilution rate of the medium is very important.
   - For economical production at high dilution rates, medium must be reused after removing taxanes.

Continuous Production system

↓

Production Sub-system	Separation sub-system
↓	↓
Using yew cell immobilized particles	Taxane removal using extraction/absorption method

- The medium is recycled between the two systems with the addition of small amount of fresh medium into production side.

- This process is now being scaled up for the mass production of paclitaxel (Taxol)

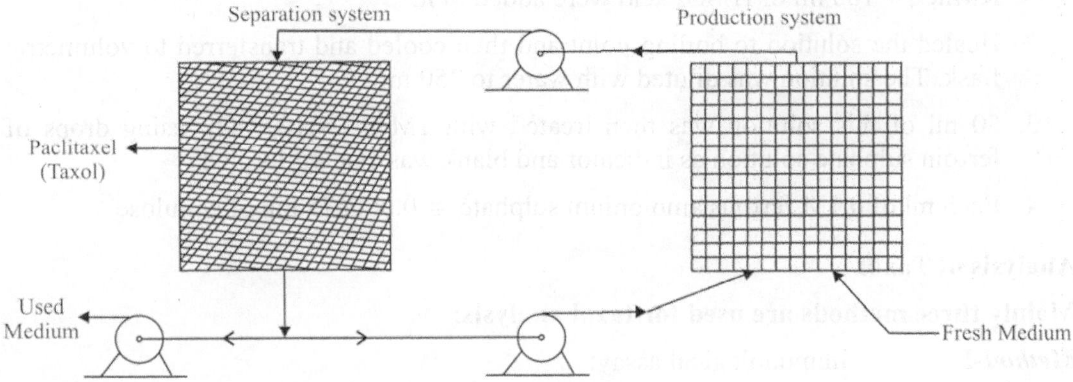

A Continuous Production System

Isolation of Taxol

1. *From Taxus brevifolia*:
   - Air dried plant (100 gm) is extracted with methanol for 16 hours.
   - Filter it and the filtrate is dried at 40 °C.
   - The residue obtained is extracted with methanol for 16 hours.
   - Filtered it, and evaporated to dryness.
   - The residue is extracted with CH_2Cl_2 and water, filtered and centrifuged.
   - Combined the CH_2Cl_2 layer and evaporated to dryness under vacuum.
   - The residue obtained is treated with methanol and CH_2Cl_2 (1 : 1) ratio, filtered and evaporated.
   - The residue thus formed is TAXOL.
2. *From Taxus Cuspidata*:
   - Twigs and stems are extracted with n-Hexane for 12 hours, then filtered and discarded the filtrate.
   - Residue is extracted with CH_2Cl_2 : CH_3OH (1 : 1) for 12 hours.
   - Extract is evaporated and residue is extracted with CH_2Cl_2 and CH_3OH.
   - Filtered the solution and residue is taken for chromatography.
   - Preparative TLC is performed by using silica gel and solvent system used is CH_2Cl_2 : CH_3OH (95 : 5).
   - R_f of Taxol = 0.37.

Estimation of Taxol

1. Take 0.125 gm of drug in 250 ml conical flask + 25 ml water + 50 ml of 0.83M $KMnO_4$ + 100 ml of H_2SO_4 acid were added in it.
2. Heated the solution to boiling point and then cooled and transferred to volumetric flask. The solution was diluted with water to 250 ml.
3. 50 ml of this solution was then treated with 1M $Fe(NH_4)_2$ SO_4, using drops of ferroin sulphate solution as indicator and blank was also performed.
4. Each ml of 0.1M ferrous ammonium sulphate ≅ 0.000675 gm of cellulose.

Analysis of Taxol

Mainly three methods are used for taxol analysis:

***Method*-I** : Immunological assay:

- Basic aim is to develop Immuno-affinity columns to apply in the extraction of various types of samples which contain taxanes.
- Polyclonol antibodies against taxanes are isolated from animals and immobilized on an appropriate support.
- Samples with low taxane content could be easily extracted and subsequently analysed by HPLC diode assay using methods already developed.
- HPLC analysis can be simplified and prove more informative since numerous contaminants would already be discarded during immuno-assay.

***Method*-II** : Liquid chromatography – Mass spectrometer: (LC/MS)

- Traditional structure analysis protocols involves scale up, extraction and fractionation.
- Individual fraction spectroscopic analysis is performed more rapidly with LC/MS instrument.

***Method*-III** : High performance liquid chromatography-mass spectrometry: (HPLC-MS):

In this method Taxol concentration is determined by comparison with an authentic standard.

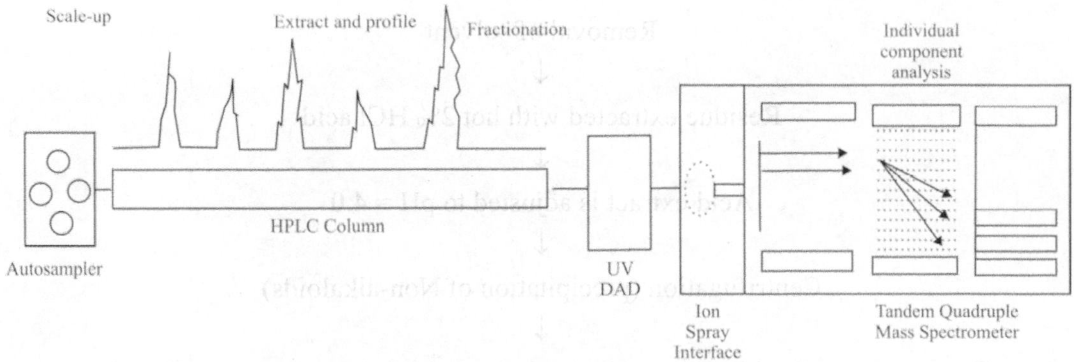

HPLC-MS

11.2.14 Vincristine

Biological source : Obtained from dried whole plant of "*Catharanthus roseus*". Also known as vinca rosea

Family : Apocynaceae

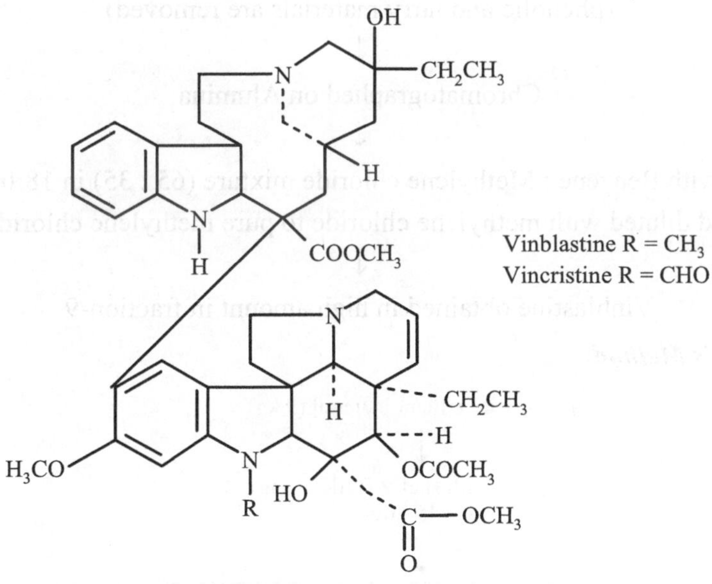

Extraction and Isolation

1. *Isolation of Vinblastine (Beer's Method)*:

Leaves (Dried) + Hot mixture of $C_2H_5OH : H_2O : CH_3COOH$ (9 : 1 : 1)

↓ Extraction process

Removal of solvent

↓

Residue extracted with hot 2% HCl acid

↓

Acid extract is adjusted to pH = 4.0

↓

Centrifugation (precipitation of Non-alkaloids)

↓

To supernatant liquid, aqueous acid solution is added to adjust the pH to 7.0

↓

Extracted the above with benzene and evaporated

↓

Dried residue obtained (containing vinblastine and other alkaloids)

↓

Residue washed with dilute alkali
(phenolic and tarry materials are removed)

↓

Chromatographed on Alumina

↓

Eluted with Benzene : Methylene chloride mixture (65 : 35) in 18 fractions
and diluted with methylene chloride to pure methylene chloride.

↓

Vinblastine obtained in high amount in fraction-9

4. ***Svoboda's Method***:

Ground whole Plant material (9 kg)

↓

Extracted with skelly-B (defatting)
(2 × 45 litres)

↓

Skelly extract	Defatted Plant Material
↓	↓

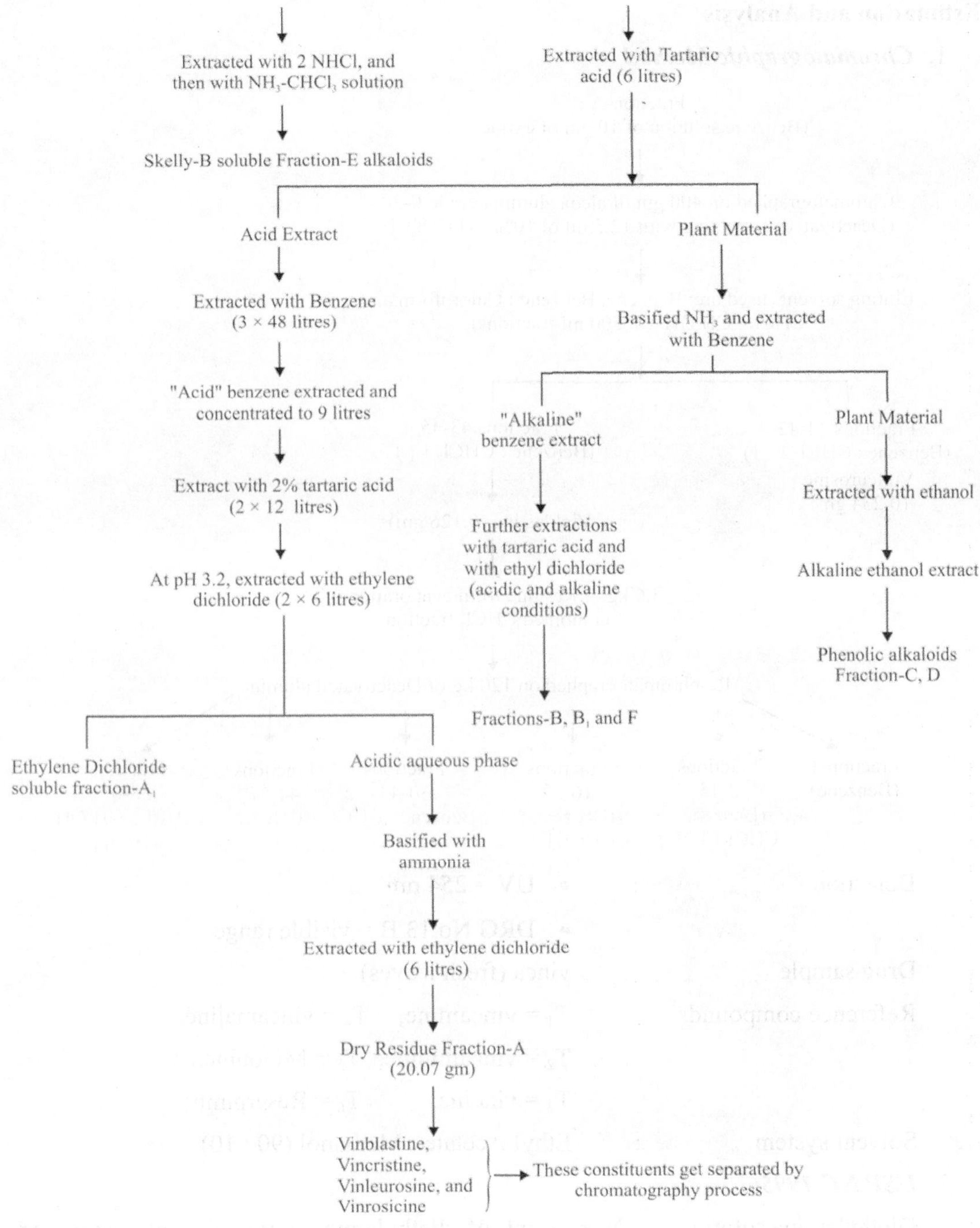
Extracted with 2 NHCl, and then with NH_3-$CHCl_3$ solution
Skelly-B soluble Fraction-E alkaloids
Extracted with Tartaric acid (6 litres)
Acid Extract
Plant Material
Extracted with Benzene (3 × 48 litres)
Basified NH_3 and extracted with Benzene
"Acid" benzene extracted and concentrated to 9 litres
"Alkaline" benzene extract
Plant Material
Extract with 2% tartaric acid (2 × 12 litres)
Extracted with ethanol
Further extractions with tartaric acid and with ethyl dichloride (acidic and alkaline conditions)
At pH 3.2, extracted with ethylene dichloride (2 × 6 litres)
Alkaline ethanol extract
Phenolic alkaloids Fraction-C, D
Fractions-B, B_1 and F
Ethylene Dichloride soluble fraction-A_1
Acidic aqueous phase
Basified with ammonia
Extracted with ethylene dichloride (6 litres)
Dry Residue Fraction-A (20.07 gm)
Vinblastine, Vincristine, Vinleurosine, and Vinrosicine
These constituents get separated by chromatography process

Estimation and Analysis

1. ***Chromatographic Method***

Fraction-A
(Benzene solution of 10 gm of extract)

↓

Chromatographed on 400 gm of alcoa alumina grade F-20
(Deactivated by treating with 12.5 ml of 10% CH_3COOH)

↓

Eluting solvents used are: Benzene, Benzene : Chloroform and
$CHCl_3$: CH_3OH (in 500 ml fractions)

↓

Fractions 34-42 (Benzene : $CHCl_3$ 1 : 1) Vinleurosine (0.234 gm)

Fractions 43-45 (Benzene : $CHCl_3$ 1 : 1)

↓

Vinblastine (0.126 gm)

↓

3.6 kg of Residue from evaporation of combined $CHCl_3$ fractions

↓

Re-chromatographed on 120 kg of Deactivated alumina

Fraction-1	Fractions 2-15	Fractions 16-29	Fractions 30-43	Fractions 44-57	Fractions 58-67
(Benzene)	(Benzene : $CHCl_3$ (3 : 1))	(Benzene : $CHCl_3$ 1:1)	(Benzene : $CHCl_3$ 1 : 3)	($CHCl_3$)	($CHCl_3$: CH_3OH) (19 : 1)

Detection : • UV = 254 nm
• DRG No.13 B = visible range

Drug sample : vinca (fresh leaves)

Reference compounds : T_1 = vincamine, T_4 = vincamajine
T_2 = vincaminine, T_5 = Minouincine
T_3 = vincine, T_6 = Reserpinine

Solvent system : Ethyl Acetate : Methanol (90 : 10)

2. ***USP NF-1995:***

Diethylamine solution : Mix 5 ml of diethylamine with 295 ml water and adjusted pH with phosphoric acid to 7.5.

Mobile phase	:	Prepared a filtered and degassed mixture of methanol and diethyamine solution (70 : 30)
Standard preparation	:	Dissolve accurately weighed quantity of USP vincristine sulphate Rs in water to obtain a concentration of 1 mg/ml.
Assay preparation	:	• Equilibrate a portion of vincristine sulphate for 30 min with an ambient humidity. • Transferred about 10 mg (accurately weighed) to 10 ml volumetric flask • Dissolved in water to volume make up and mix
System suitability Preparation	:	• Transferred 5 mg of USP vincristine sulphate and 5 mg of vinblastine sulphate Rs (each accurately weighed), into a 5 ml volumetric flask. • Dissolved in water, diluted with water to volume and mix.
Chromatographic system		
Column	:	4.6 mm × 25 cm analytical column containing L7 packing. 2.5 cm guard column containing L1 packing
Flowrate	:	1.5 ml/min
Detector	:	297 nm
Procedure	:	• 10 ml of each of standard and assay preparation are injected into the chromatograph and the peak responses recorded. • Calculated the quantity in mg of vincristine sulphate by using formula 10 C (ru/rs) where, C = concentration (mg/ml) of USP vincristine sulphate RS in standard preparation ru, rs = peak responses obtained from assay and standard preparations respectively.

11.2.15 Papain

Biological source : A mixture of proteolytic enzymes derived from the latex of unripe fruit of "*Carica Papaya*".

Family : Cariaceae

Extraction and Isolation

Latex of fruits of papaya collected in aluminium trays

↓

To this, added potassium metabisulphite (5 g/kg of latex)

↓

Extraneous matter is cleared out by passing through sieves

↓

Latex dried in vacuum shelf drier (55-60 °C temperature)

↓

Dried latex is called Papain

- Papain is also processed by spray-drying method.
- One NF (National formulary) unit of papain represents the activity which releases equivalent of 1 μg of tyrosine from a standard casein substrate.

Analysis of Papain

TLC Determination method:

Plates used ⇒ Sephadex G-100

Solvent system ⇒ 0.02M Na_3PO_4 buffer solution containing 0.2M NaCl.

Reagents used ⇒ Naphthalene Black

CHAPTER 12

CHEMISTRY, BIOGENESIS AND PHARMACOLOGICAL ACTIVITY OF NATURAL PRODUCTS

12.1 Artemisine/Artimisinin

Biological Source : It is obtained from leafs and other aerial parts of "*Artemisia annua*".

Family : Asteraceae/Compositae

Quinghaosu, an antimalarial principle is available as parent compound artemisinine.

Chemistry

1. Artemisinine possess the structure of a sesquiterpene lactone ring with an internal peroxide linkage.
2. The structure of artemisinin is determined by using Infra Red spectroscopy (IR), Nuclear Magnetic Resonance (NMR) and X-ray diffraction.
3. The Infrared spectrum showed the presence of δ-lactone ring and a peroxide group.
4. The peroxide group presence is verified by quantitative reaction of artemisinin with triphenylphosphine while the lactone structure is confirmed by oxine formation.

5. H^1-NMR and C^{13}-NMR spectra indicates the presence of three methyl groups (one tertiary and two secondary), an acetal function and various aliphatic carbon atoms.

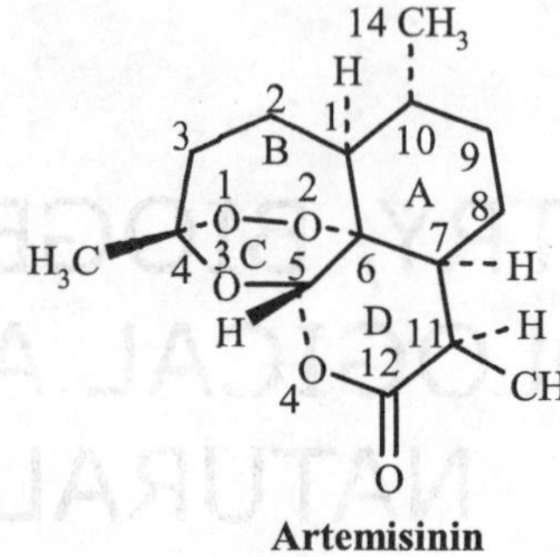

Artemisinin

6. X-ray diffraction analysis confirms the structure unambiguously, as well as its relative configuration, showing that 15 carbon and 5 oxygen atoms in the artemisinin molecule formed four correlating rings:
   - A ring is a chair-shaped cyclohexane ring.
   - B and C rings are both saturated oxyhetero cyclic rings.
   - D-ring is a δ-lactone ring that assumes dissorted chair shape.
7. Artemisinine contains all five oxygen atoms on the same side of the molecule.
8. C-O bonds are of alternating long and short lengths, thus giving molecule stability and accounting for its antimalarial action.

Biogenesis

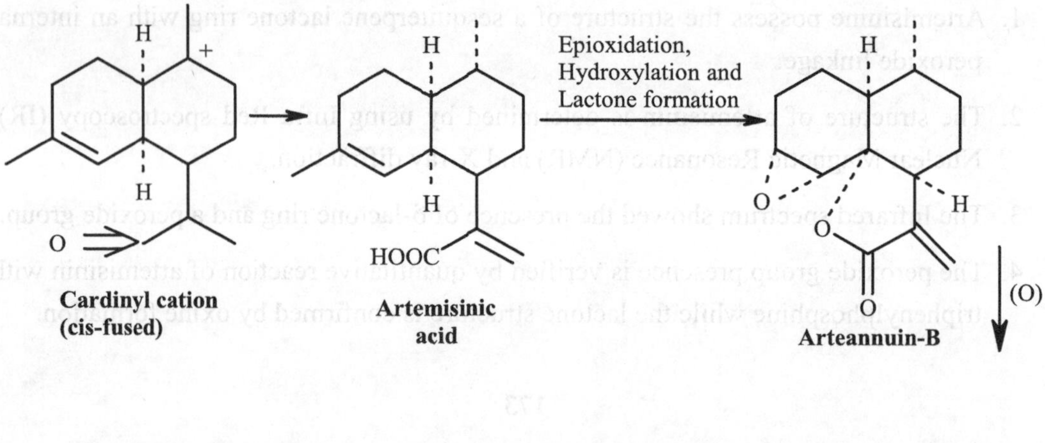

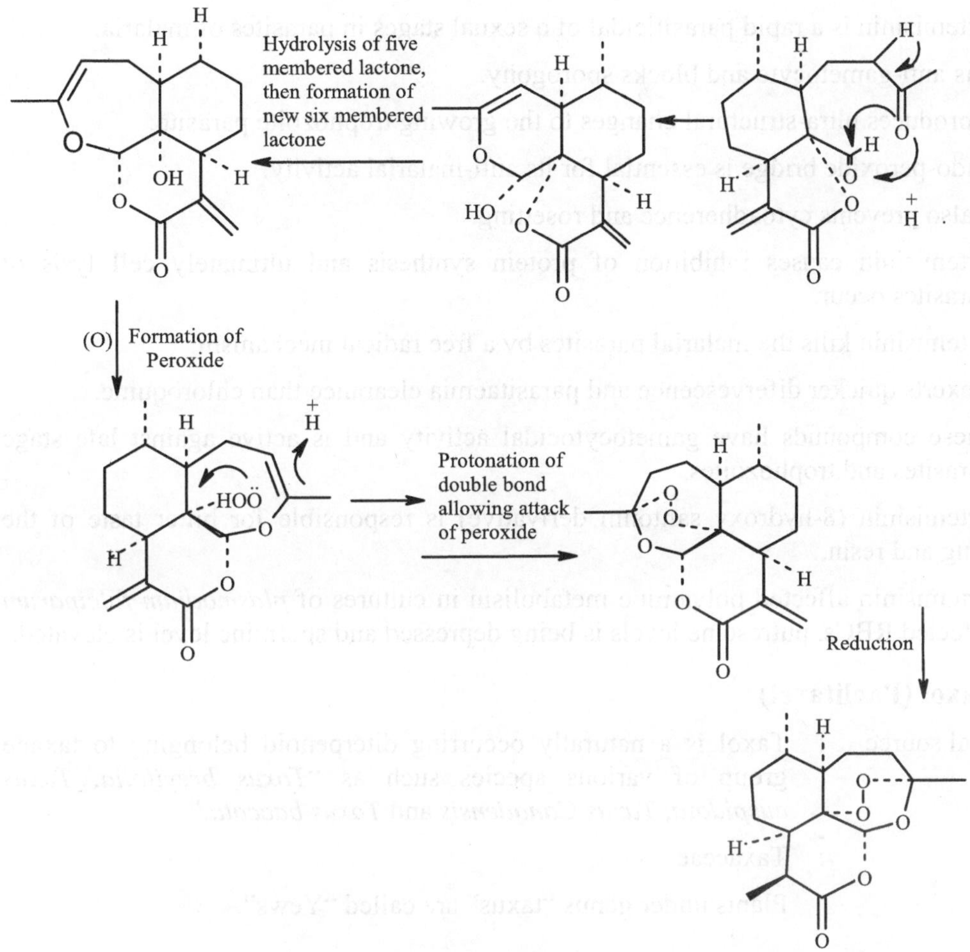

Artemisinin (Quinghaosu)

Biogenetic Pathway of Artemisinin

Pharmacological Activity

Artemisinin possess following pharmacological activities:

1. Artemisinine is a safe and effective alternative to quinine in the treatement of falciparum malaria.
2. Derivatives of artemisinine such as artesunate, artemether, artether etc., used to treat multi-drug resistant malaria.
3. Useful in cerebral malaria and act mainly as schizontocides.

4. Artemisinin is a rapid parasiticidal of a sexual stages in parasites of malaria.
5. It is anti-gametocyte and blocks sporogony.
6. It produces ultra-structural changes to the growing trophozoite parasite.
7. Endo-peroxide bridge is essential for its anti-malarial activity.
8. It also prevents cytoadherence and rosetting.
9. Artemisinin causes inhibition of protein synthesis and ultimately cell lysis of parasites occur.
10. Artemisinin kills the malarial parasites by a free radical mechanism.
11. It exerts quicker difervescence and parasitaemia clearance than chloroquine.
12. These compounds have gametocytocidal activity and is active against late stage parasites and trophozoites.
13. Artemisinin (8-hydroxy santonin derivative) is responsible for bitter taste of the drug and resin.
14. Artemisinin affected polyamine metabolism in cultures of *plasmodium falciparum* infected RBCs, putrescine levels is being depressed and spermine level is elevated.

12.2 Taxol (Paclitaxel)

Biological source : Taxol is a naturally occurring diterpenoid belonging to taxane group of various species such as "*Taxus brevifolia*, *Taxus cuspidata*, *Taxus Canadensis* and *Taxus baccata*."

Family : Taxaceae

Plants under genus "taxus" are called "Yews".

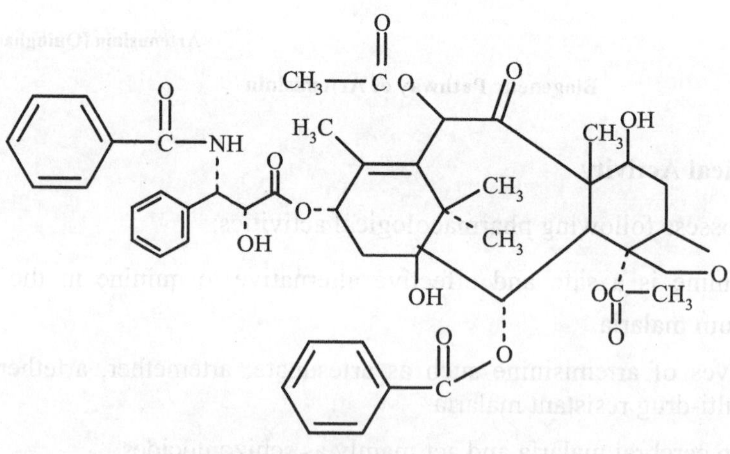

Paclitaxel (Taxol)

Chemistry

1. Taxol (Paclitaxel) is prepared as a non-aqueous solution in poly-oxymethylated cator oil and dehydrated alcohol.
2. Taxol is a novel diterpenoid (C_{20}) alkaloidal drug.
3. The nitrogen atom is not incorporated into diterpene skeleton.
4. The side-chains in taxol contain aromatic rings derived from shikimic acid via phenylalanine.
5. Taxol is a member of a small group of compounds possessing a four membered oxetane ring and a complex ester side-chain in their structures, both of which are essential for antitumour activity.

Biogenesis

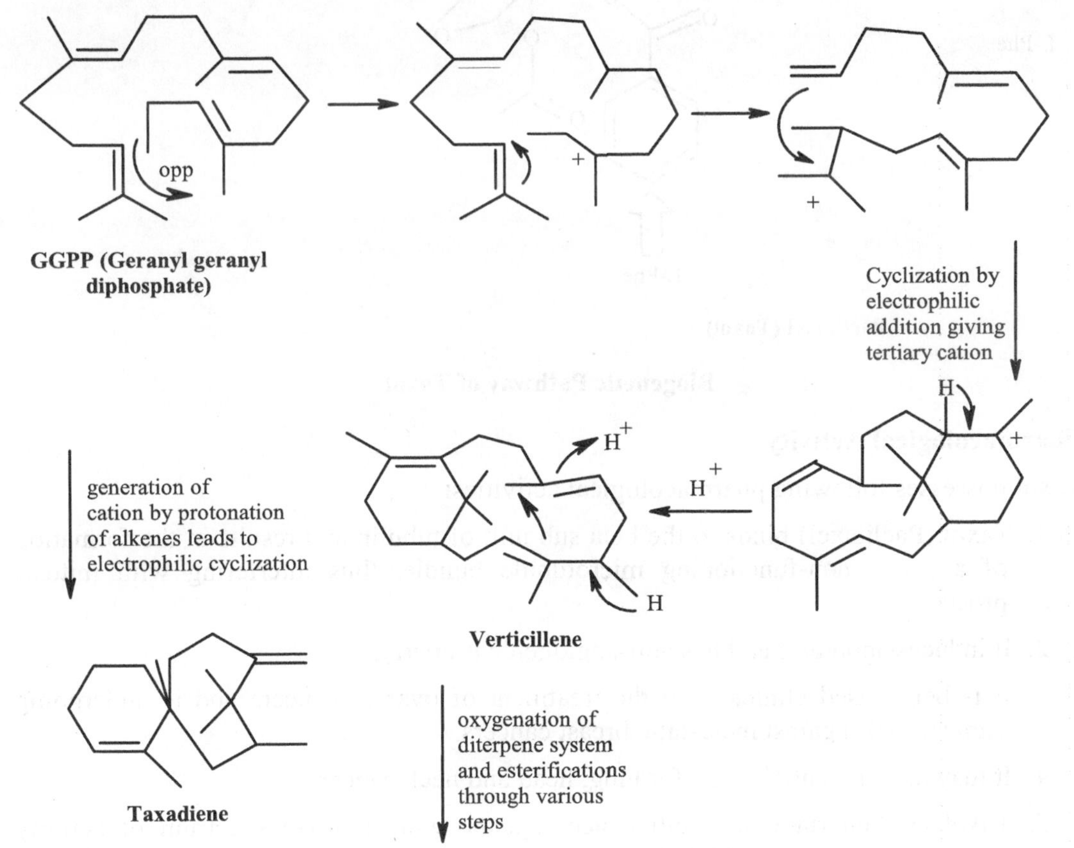

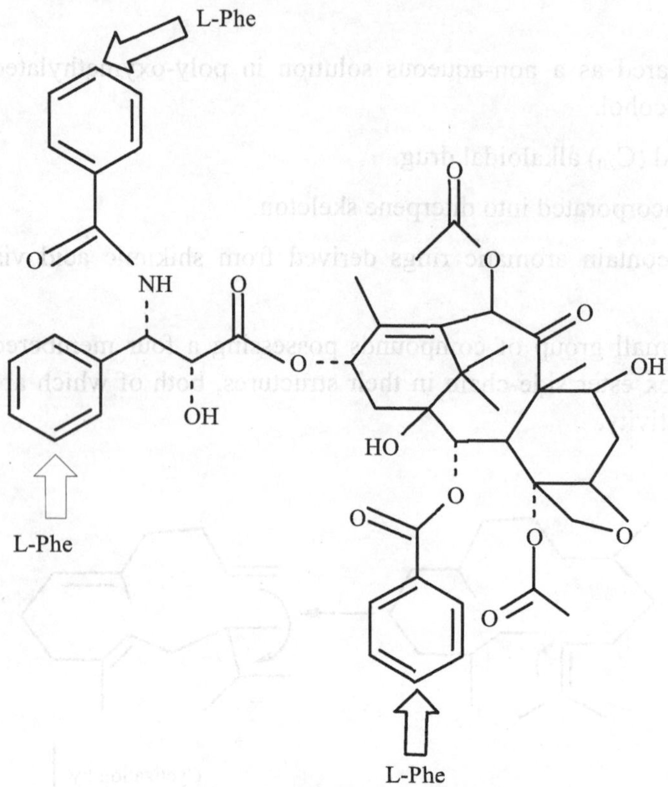

Paclitaxel (Taxol)

Biogenetic Pathway of Taxol

Pharmacological Activity

Taxol possesses following pharmacological activities:

1. Taxol (Paclitaxel) binds to the beta sub unit of tubulin and results in the formation of a stable non-functioning microtubule bundle, thus interfering with mitosis process.
2. It induces apoptosis and has anti-angiogenic property.
3. It is being used clinically in the treatment of ovarian cancers and is undergoing clinical trials against metastatic breast cancers.
4. It may have potential value for lung, head and neck cancers.
5. Taxol an important new anti cancer agents, with a broad spectrum of activity against some cancers which do not respond to other agents.

12.3 Atropine

Biological Source : It is obtained from dried leaves or leaves and other aerial parts of "*Atropa belladonna/Atropa acuminata*".

Family : Solanaceae

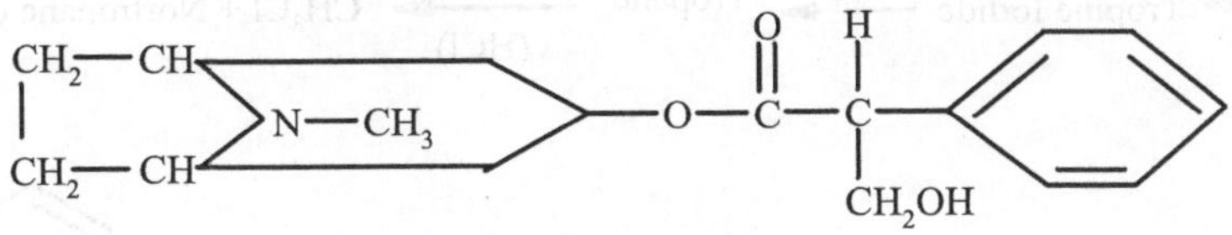

Atropine (Tropine (±) - Tropate)

Chemistry

1. Its molecular composition is $C_{17} H_{23} O_3 N$.
2. On hydrolysis, atropine gives an alcohol called as tropine ($C_8 H_{15} NO$) and (±) tropic acid ($C_9H_{10}O_3$) indicating that atropine is an ester i.e., tropine-tropate.

$$\underset{\text{(Atropine)}}{C_{17} H_{23} O_3N} + H_2O \rightarrow \underset{\text{(Tropine)}}{C_8H_{15}NO} + \underset{\text{(Tropic acid)}}{C_9H_{10}O_3}$$

Hence, the constitution of atropine is resolved into two parts:

1. Structure of Tropic acid
2. Structure of Tropine

1. *Constitution of Tropic acid*:
   - Tropic acid ($C_9 H_{10} O_3$) is found to possess one alcoholic and one carboxylic group by usual tests.
   - On strong heating, it looses a molecule of water to form atropic acid ($C_9H_8O_2$), which on oxidation yields benzoic acid.

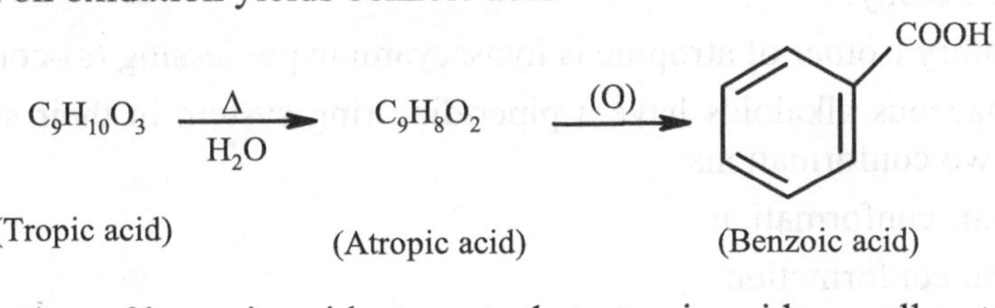

(Tropic acid) (Atropic acid) (Benzoic acid)

The formation of benzoic acid suggests that atropic acid as well as tropic acid, both contains a benzene ring with one side chain.

2. *Constitution of Tropine (Tropanol)*:

Tropine ($C_8 H_{15} NO$), is found to be a saturated secondary alcohol group having tertiary nitrogen in the form of N-CH_3 group.

Tropine on treatment with hydroiodic acid (HI) gives tropine iodide which on reduction with zinc and HCl, gives tropane hydrochloride which on distillation followed by zinc dust distillation yields 2-Ethyl pyridino through nor-tropane.

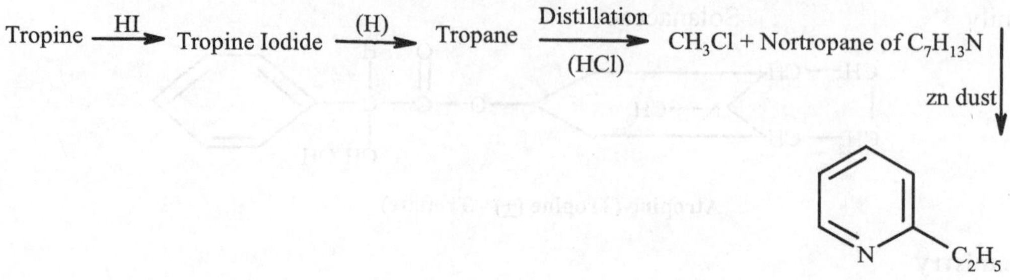

2-Ethyl pyridino

These reactions proposed that tropine is a reduced pyridine derivative.

3. The solanaceous alkaloids (atropine) are the esters of bicyclic amino alcohol-3-tropanol (tropine) with tropic acid.

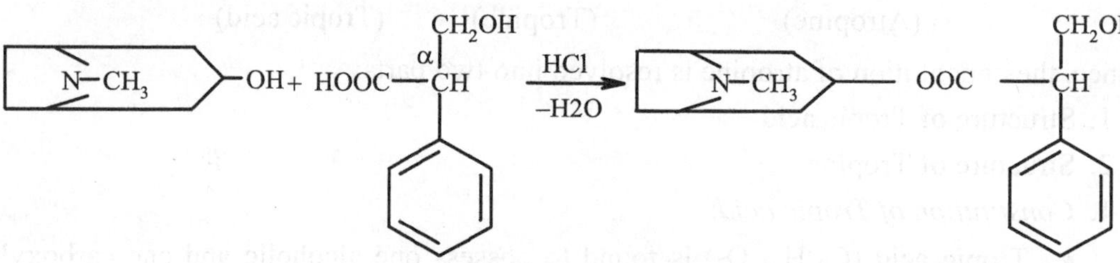

Tropine **Tropic acid** **Atropine**

4. The carbon-α to the carboxylic acid group of tropic acid is asymmetric and can be racemised easily.
5. Leavorotatory isomer of atropine is hyosscyamine possessing (s)-configuration.
6. The solanaceous alkaloids have a piperidine ring system in their structures which exists in two conformations:
   (a) Chair conformation
   (b) Boat conformation

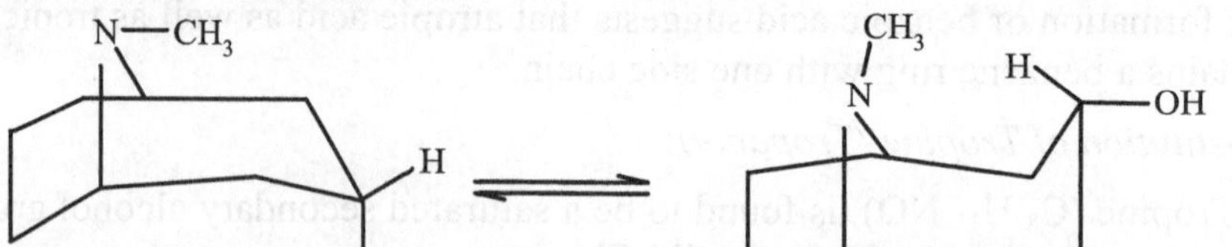

(Chair) **Tropine** **(Boat)**

Chair conformation is commonly accepted due to its lowest energy requirement

Biogenesis

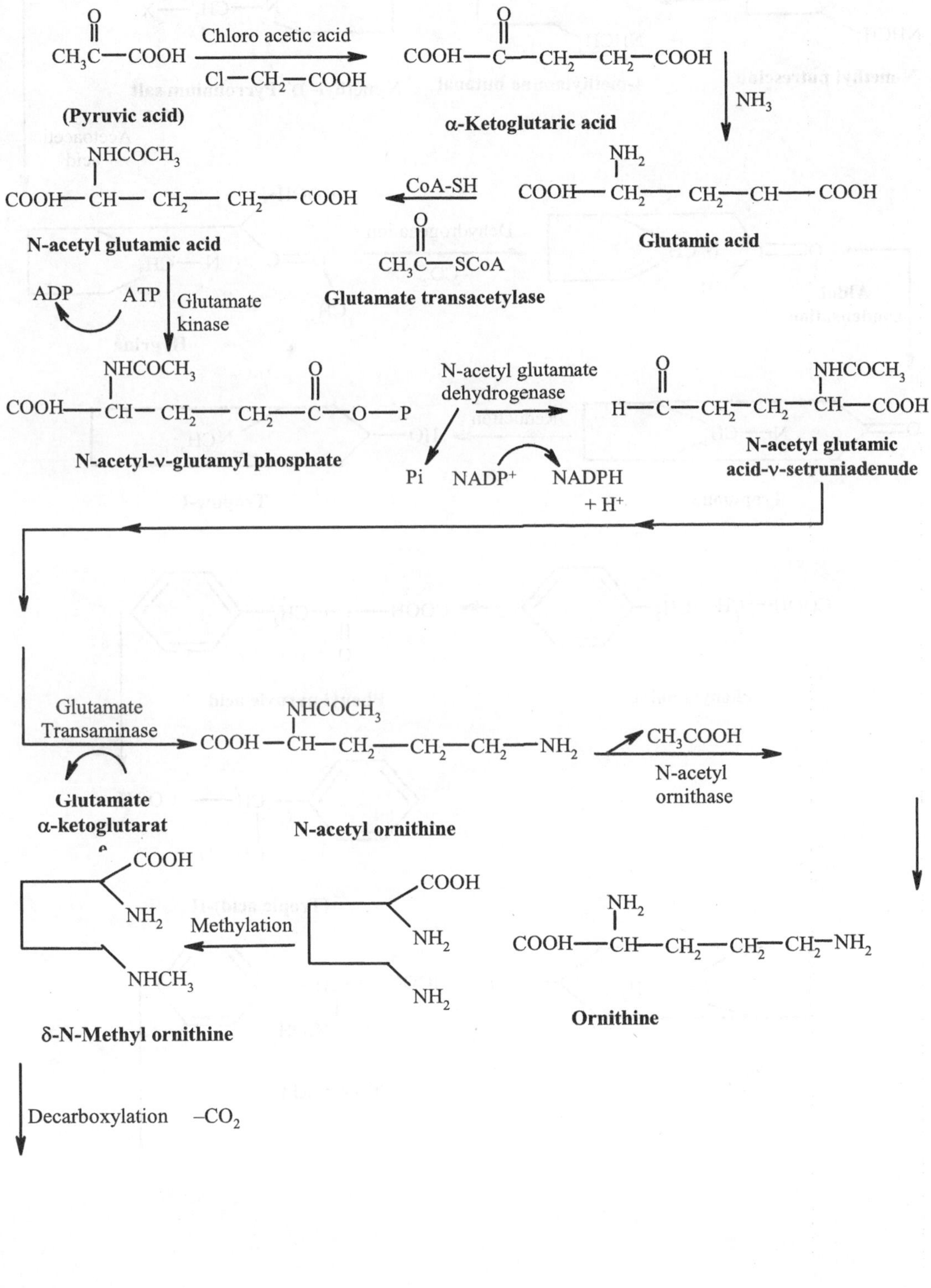
Chloro acetic acid
(Pyruvic acid)
α-Ketoglutaric acid
NH3
CoA-SH
Glutamic acid
N-acetyl glutamic acid
Glutamate transacetylase
ADP
ATP
Glutamate kinase
N-acetyl glutamate dehydrogenase
N-acetyl-ν-glutamyl phosphate
Pi
NADP+
NADPH + H+
N-acetyl glutamic acid-ν-setruniadenude
Glutamate Transaminase
Glutamate
α-ketoglutarate
N-acetyl ornithine
CH3COOH
N-acetyl ornithase
Methylation
Ornithine
δ-N-Methyl ornithine
Decarboxylation –CO2

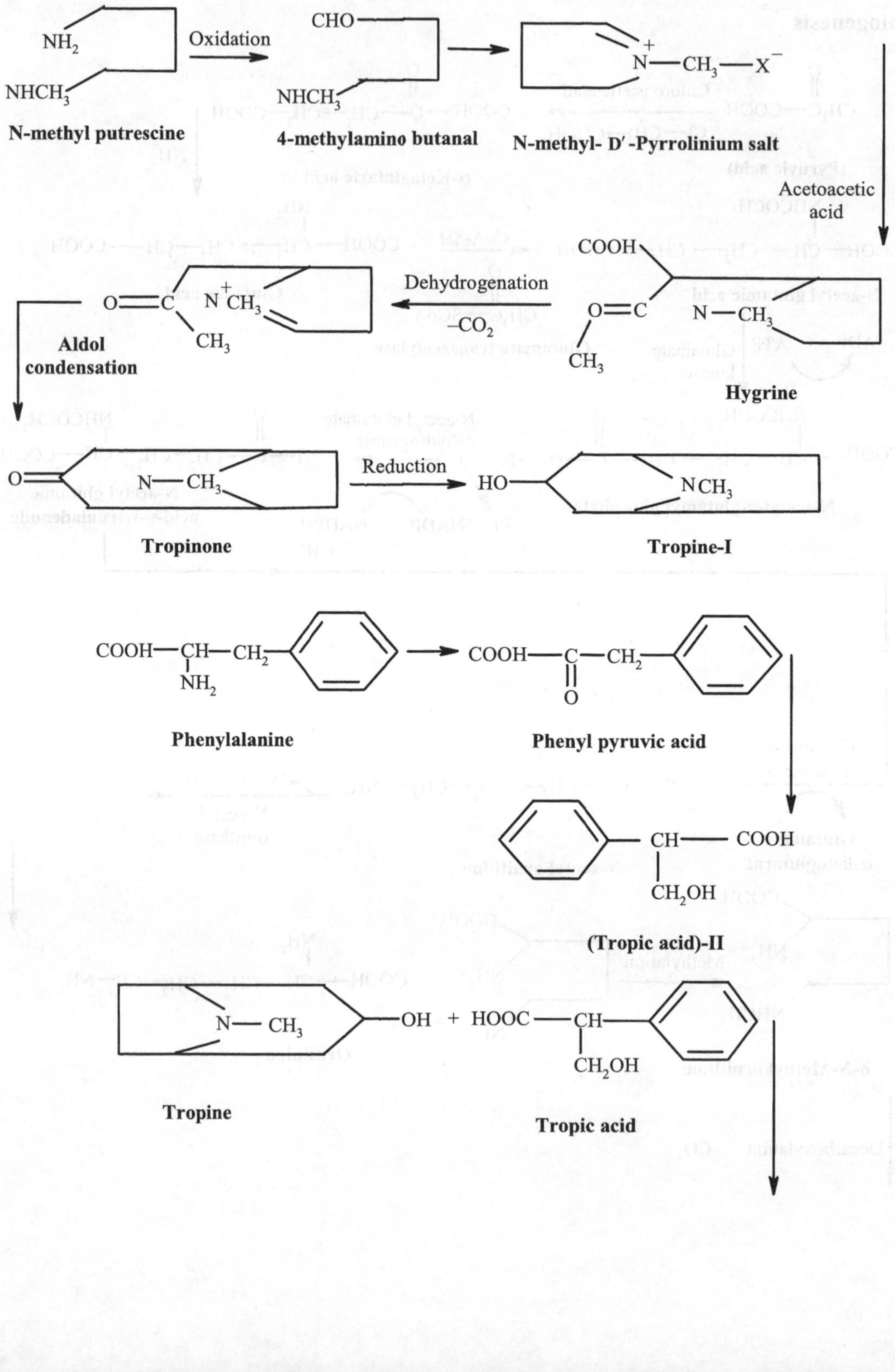

Oxidation
N-methyl putrescine
4-methylamino butanal
N-methyl- D′-Pyrrolinium salt
Acetoacetic acid
Hygrine
Dehydrogenation
$-CO_2$
Aldol condensation
Tropinone
Reduction
Tropine-I
Phenylalanine
Phenyl pyruvic acid
(Tropic acid)-II
Tropine
Tropic acid

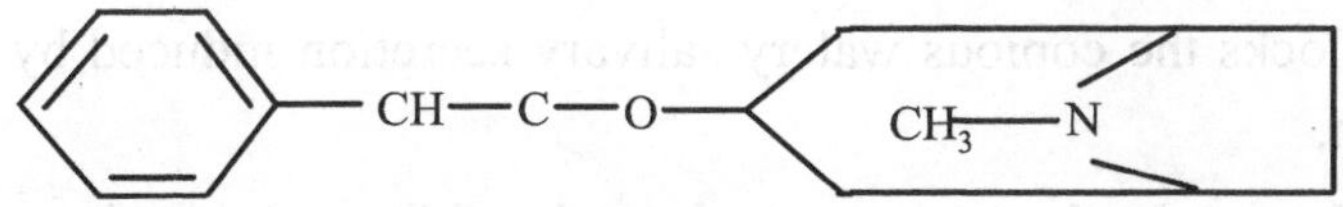

Atropine (Hyoscyamine)

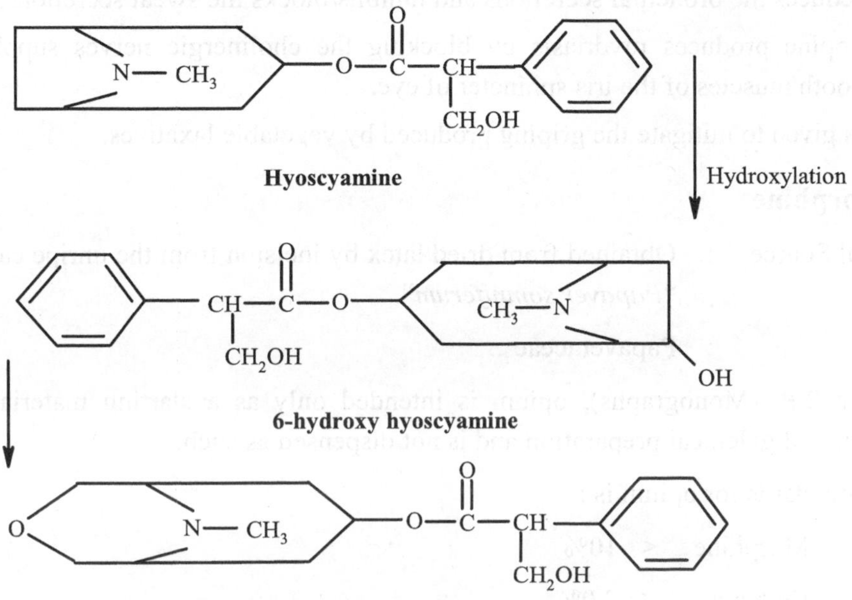

Biogenetic Pathways of Atropine

Pharmacological Activity

1. Atropine, an antimuscarinic alkaloid possesses both central and peripheral actions. It exerts firstly a stimulatory and then a depressant action on the CNS.
2. In diagnosis of heart diseases, atropine find its use to stop extra systoles and complete heart block.
3. It has depressant action on the nerve endings of CNS, especially on certain motor mechanism in symptomatic treatment of parkinsonism.
4. Highly effective in counteracting the muscarine symptoms and higher dose antagonizes the central effects.
5. It has antispasmodic action on smooth muscles. It reduces the tone of smooth muscles.

6. Atropine blocks the copious watery salivary secretion induced by parasympathetic stimulation.
7. Atropine decreases the volume and total acidity of gastric acid secretion by reducing the secretion of mucin and gastric enzymes.
8. It reduces the bronchial secretions and inhibits/blocks the sweat secretions.
9. Atropine produces mydriasis by blocking the cholinergic nerves supplying the smooth muscles of the iris sphincter of eye.
10. It is given to mitigate the griping produced by vegetable laxatives.

12.4 Morphine

Biological Source : Obtained from dried latex by incision from the unripe capsules of "*Papaver somniferum*".

Family : Papaveraceae

As per B.P. (Monographs), opium is intended only as a starting material for the manufacture of galenical preparation and is not dispensed as such.

B.P. standards for opium is :

Morphine	<	10%
Codeine	<	2.0%
Thebaine	=	3.0%

Chemistry

1. Its molecular formula is $C_{17}H_{19}NO_3$.
2. Morphine takes up one mole of methyl iodide to form quarternary ammonium salt showing that the nitrogen is present as tertiary one. The tertiary nature of nitrogen is conformed by Hofmann's degradation of codeine derivative which further indicates that nitrogen is in the ring.
3. It exhibits characteristics of phenol group (namely, coloration of morphine with $FeCl_3$ solution and solubility in an aqueous NaOH solution to form monosodium salt which is re-converted into morphine by passing CO_2 gas, hence one of the hydroxyl group must be phenolic one.

4. Morphine on acetylation or benzoylation gives diacetyl morphine (heroine, DAM) or dibenzoyl derivatives, which indicates the presence of two hydroxyl groups.
5. On treatment with halogen acids, morphine forms monohalogeno product indicating that an alcoholic hydroxyl group is present in morphine.
6. When morphine or its hydrochloride is heated at 140 °C temperature, under pressure (in a sealed tube) with HCl acid, apomorphine is formed.
7. Morphine is laevorotatory in nature. (i.e., (–)-Morphine).
8. The structure of morphine is composed of five fused rings and the molecule has five chiral centres with an absolute stereo chemistry 5(R), 6(S), 9(R) 13 (S) and 14 (R), and is monoacidic in nature.

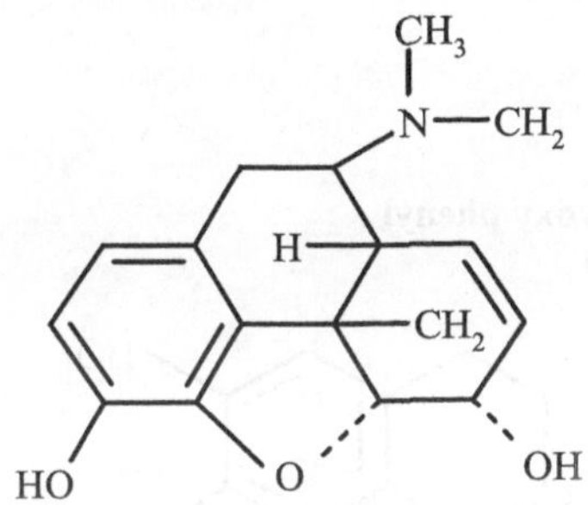

Morphine

9. Opium contains about 30 alkaloids which combines with meconic acid (a dibasic acid).

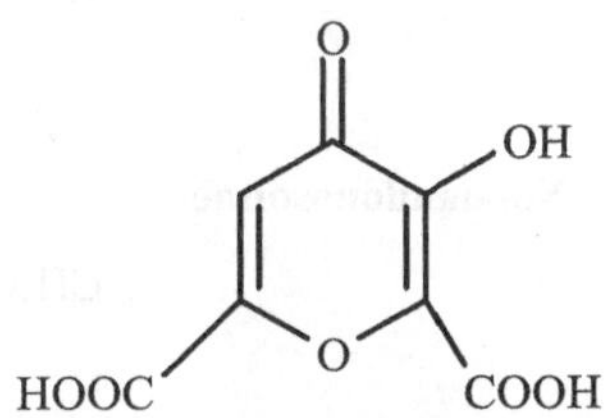

Meconic acid

10. The opium latex contains alkaloids derived from amino acids such as phenylalanine and Tyrosine.
11. Chemically alkaloids are placed under two categories:
    (a) Benzyl isoquinoline type (*e.g.* Narcotine (Noscapine), Narceine, Papaverine
    (b) Phenanthrene type (*e.g.* Morphine, codeine, Thebaine)
12. Due to the presence of phenolic hydroxyl group, morphine is soluble in alkali hydroxides except ammonium hydroxides.

Biogenesis

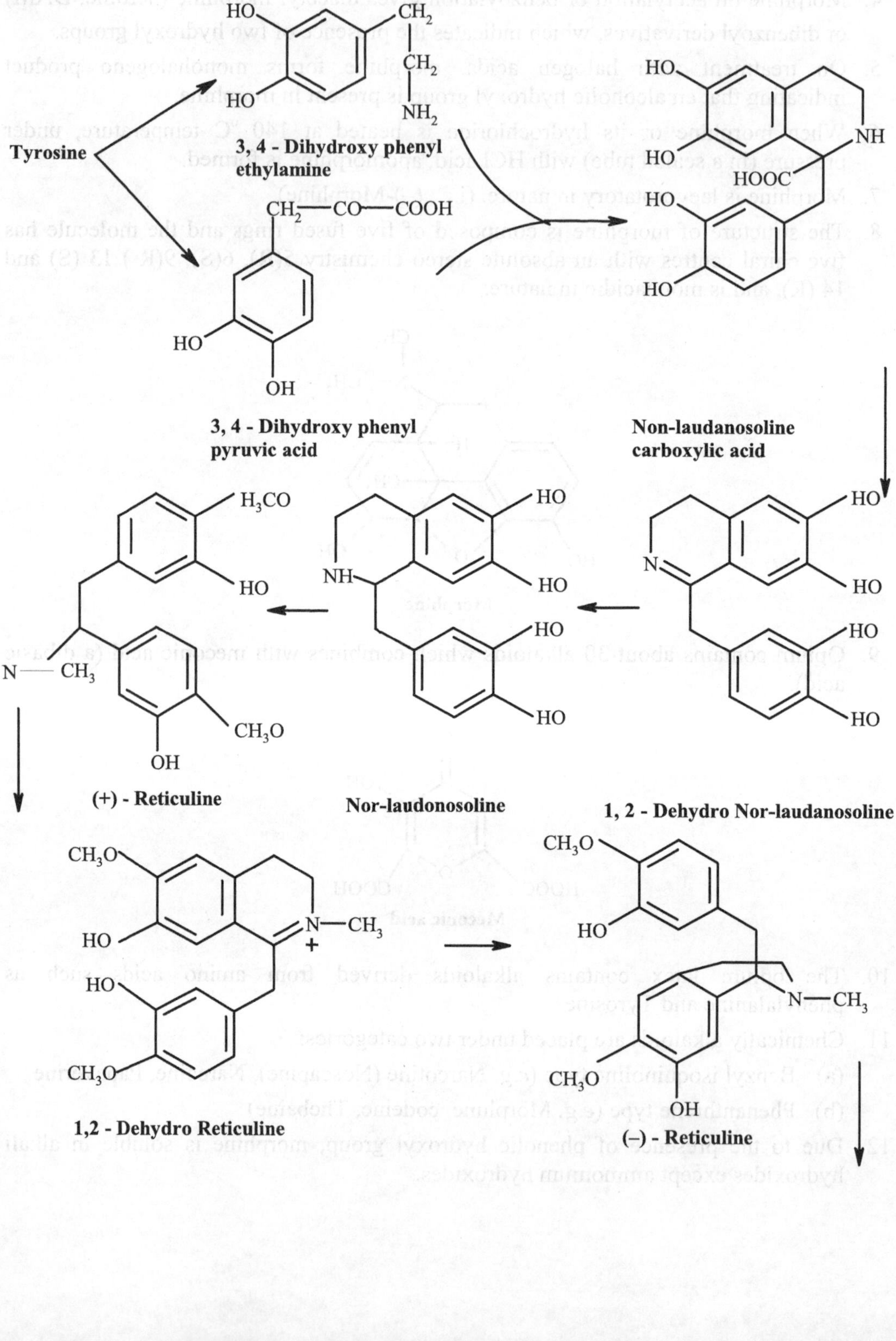
Tyrosine
3, 4 - Dihydroxy phenyl ethylamine
3, 4 - Dihydroxy phenyl pyruvic acid
Non-laudanosoline carboxylic acid
1, 2 - Dehydro Nor-laudanosoline
Nor-laudonosoline
(+) - Reticuline
1,2 - Dehydro Reticuline
(–) - Reticuline

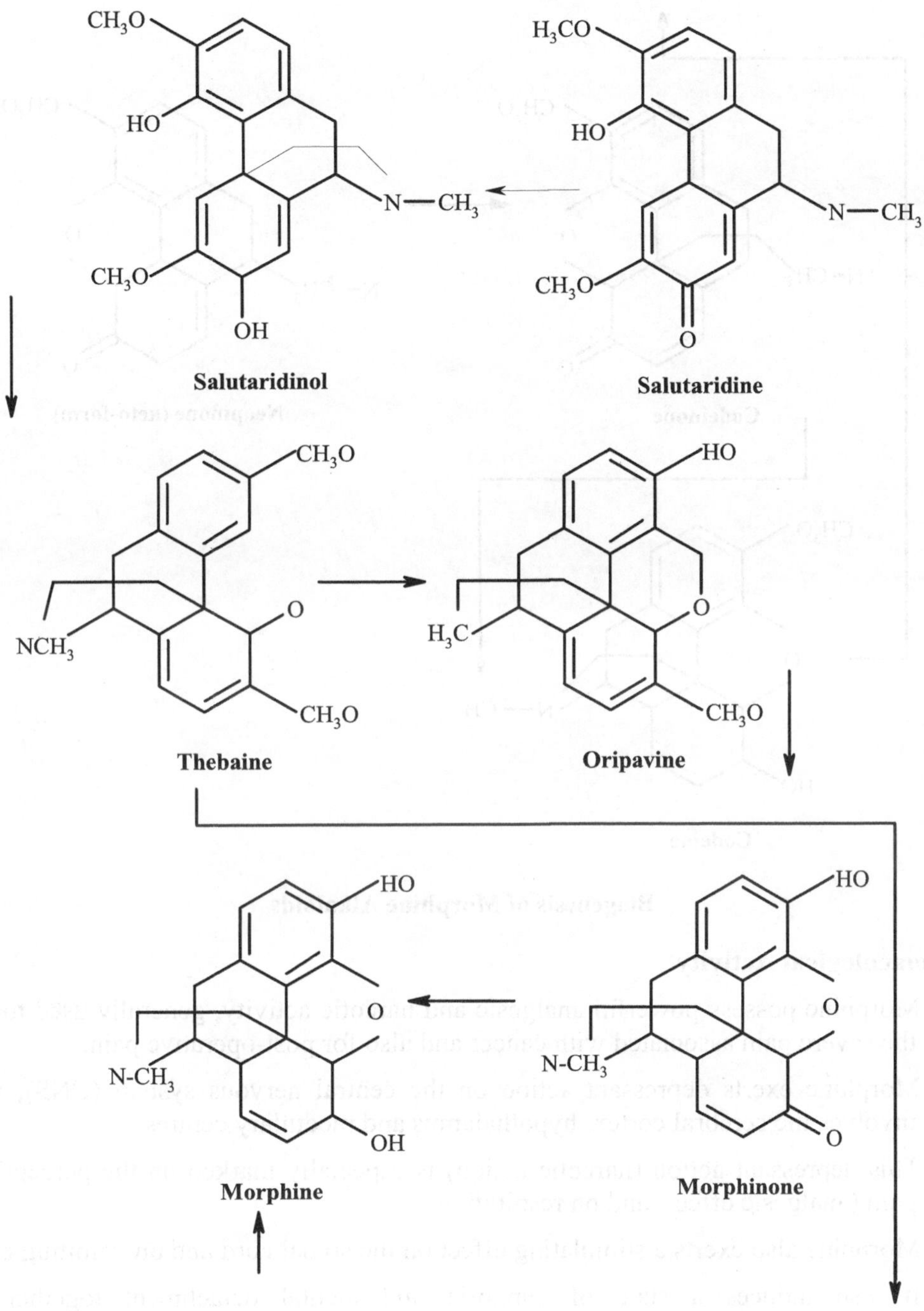

Salutaridinol, Salutaridine, Thebaine, Oripavine, Morphine, Morphinone

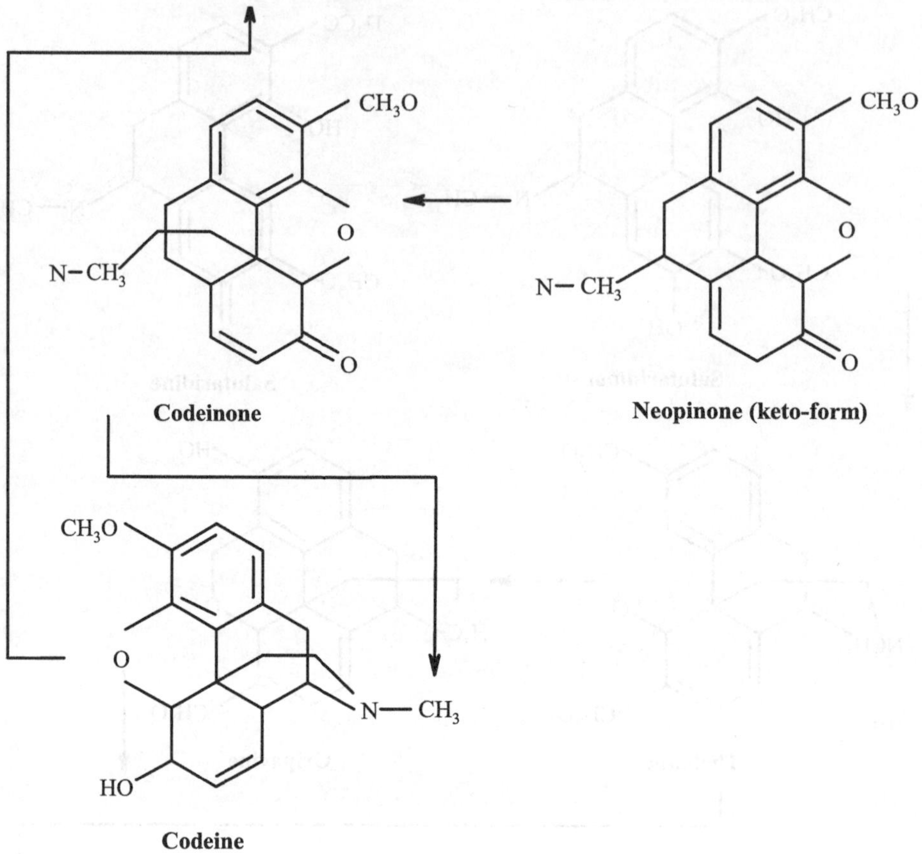

Biogenesis of Morphine Alkaloids

Pharmacological Activity

1. Morphine possess powerful analgesic and narcotic activity, generally used to relief the severe pain associated with cancer and also for post-operative pain.
2. Morphine exerts depressant action on the central nervous system (CNS), which involves the cerebral cortex, hypothalamus and medullary centres.
3. This depressant action (narcotic action) is especially marked on the perception of pain (analgesic effect) and on respiration.
4. Morphine also exerts a stimulating effect on the spinal cord and on vomiting centre.
5. It also induces a state of euphoria and mental detachment together with constipation, tolerance and addiction.

   Morphine reduces intestinal motility and is used in the treatment of diarrhoea.

6. Morphine produces a depression of respiration partly:
   - By direct depressant action on the brain stem respiratory centre and
   - By reducing the sensitivity of medullary respiratory centre to increased plasma CO_2 concentration.
7. Morphine depresses cough reflex, induces bradycardia and increases vigorous spasm of the smooth muscle of gut, ileocholic and anal sphincters.
8. Morphine in therapeutic doses produces an increase in intra biliary pressure by producing a spasm of sphincter of oddi.

12.5 Quinine

Biological source : Obtained from dried bark of stem or of the root of "*Cinchona succirubra*", *cinchona calisaya, cinchona ledgeriana* or *cinchona officinalis*.

Family : Rubiaceae

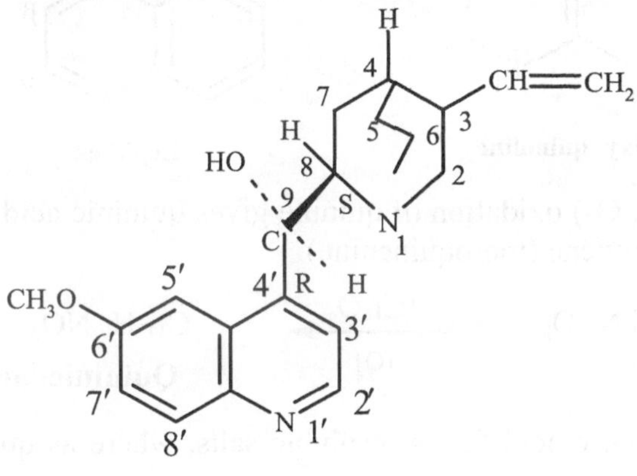

Quinine

Chemistry

1. Its molecular composition is $C_{20}H_{24}N_2O_2 . 3\ H_2O$.
2. Quinine has a methoxy group attached to the quinoline heterocyclic ring and a vinyl group attached to the quinuclidine ring. It has 4 chiral centres at C_3, C_4, C_8 and C_9 respectively.
3. Quinine shows specific optical rotation of 165° at 20°.
4. Quinine and cinchonidine has 8S, 9R configurations where as Qunidine and cinchonine possess 8R, 9S configurations.

5. It forms two series of quarternary salts by absorbing two moles of CH_3I, suggesting that it has two alike tertiary nitrogen atoms.
6. Quinine may be mono-acetylated, mono-benzylated and converted into mono-chloro derivative indicating the presence of hydroxyl group.

   Furthermore, quinine on oxidation gives a ketone (quininone), which suggests that hydroxyl group is secondary alcohol in nature.

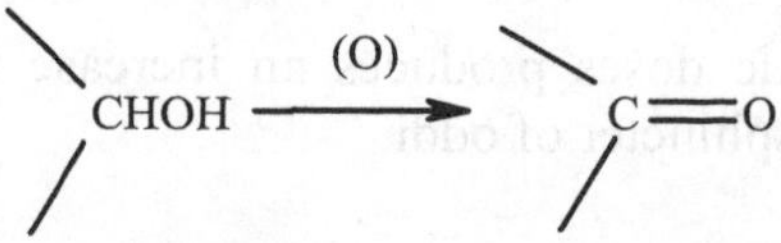

(alcohol) **(Ketone)**

7. On fusion with conc. KOH solution, quinine yields 6-methoxy quinoline and ν-methyl quinoline (Lepidine) along with other products.

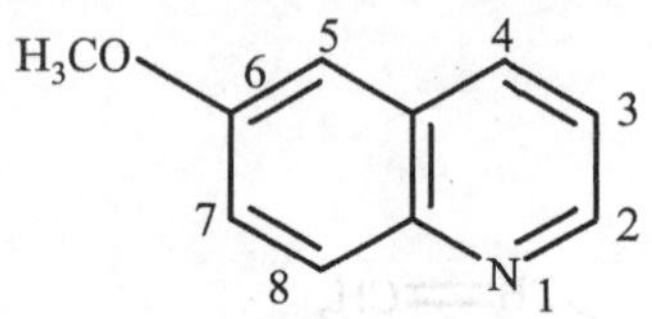

6-Methoxy quinoline

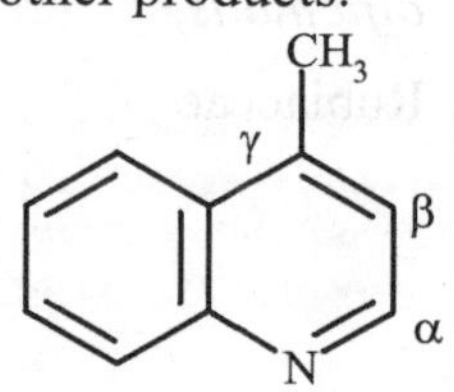

Lepidine

8. Chromic acid ($C_r O_3$) oxidation of quinine gives quininic acid and other component known as meroquinene (meroquinenine).

$$C_{20} H_{24} N_2 O_2 \xrightarrow[\text{[O]}]{[Cr\ O_3]} C_{11} H_9 NO_3 + C_9H_{15}NO_2$$

Quininic acid **Meroquinene**

9. Quinine with tartaric acid forms insoluble salts, where as quinidine forms soluble salts.

Biogenesis

The Quinine is biosynthesized in four steps:

Step – I: Formation of Tryptamine

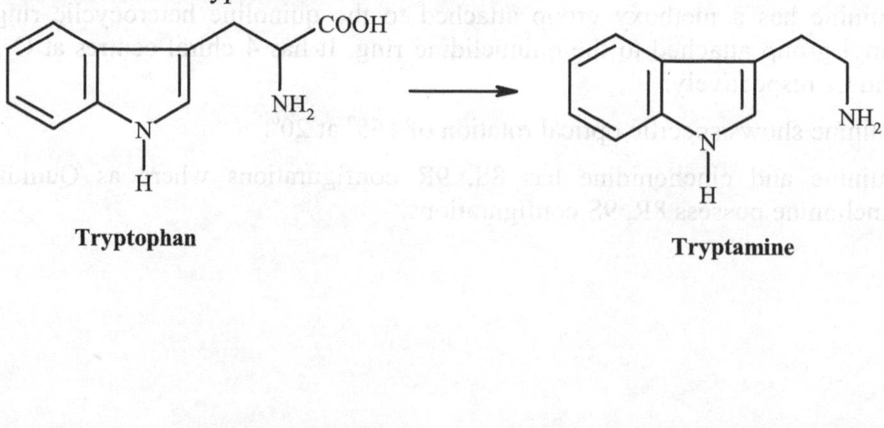

Tryptophan **Tryptamine**

Step-II: Formation of secologanin

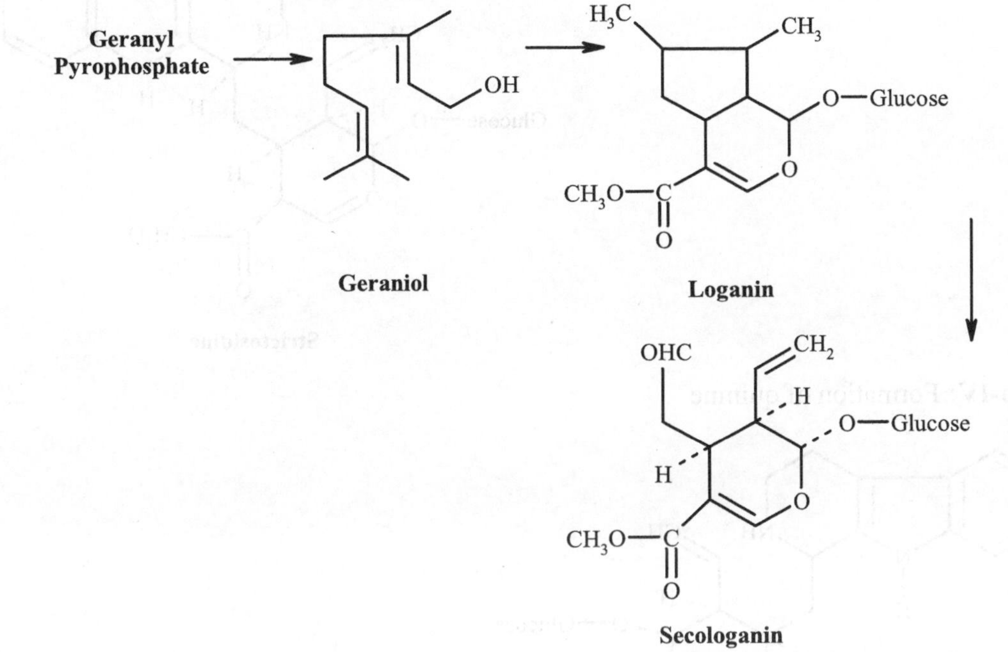

Step-III: Formation of Strictosidine

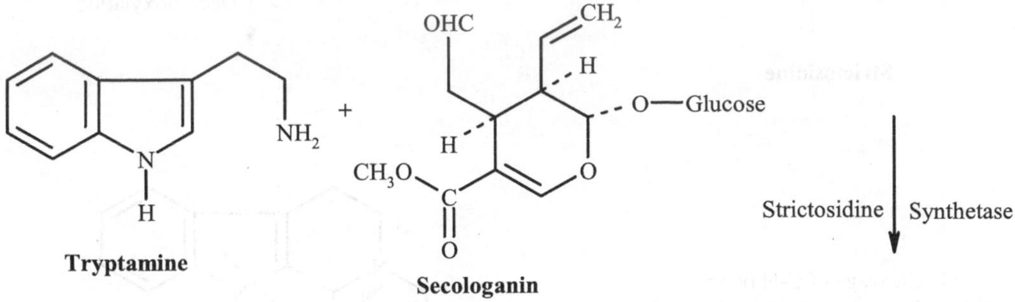

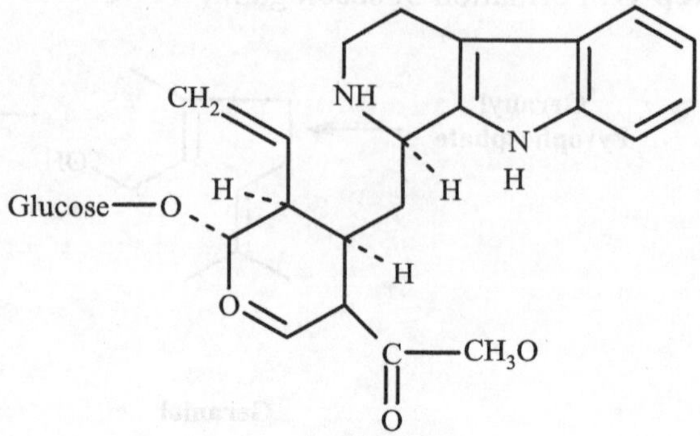

Strictosidine

Step-IV: Formation of quinine

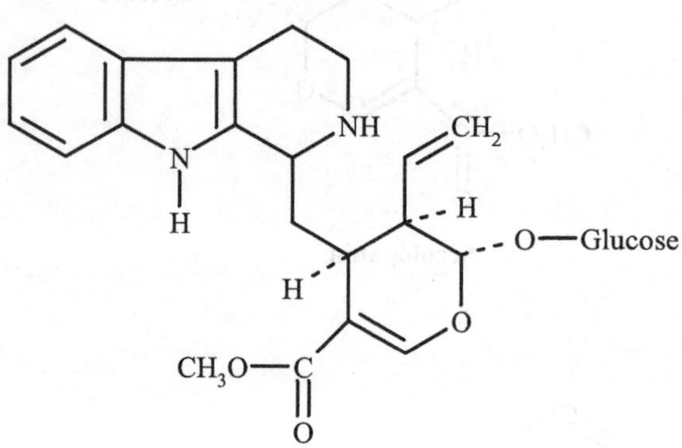

Strictosidine

Hydrolysis
and
Decarboxylation

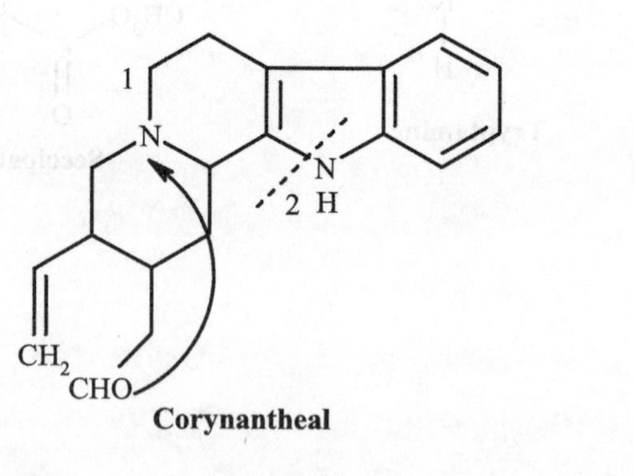

Corynantheal

(1) Cleavage of C-N bond
and then formation of new C-N bond

(2) Cleavage of Indole C-N bond

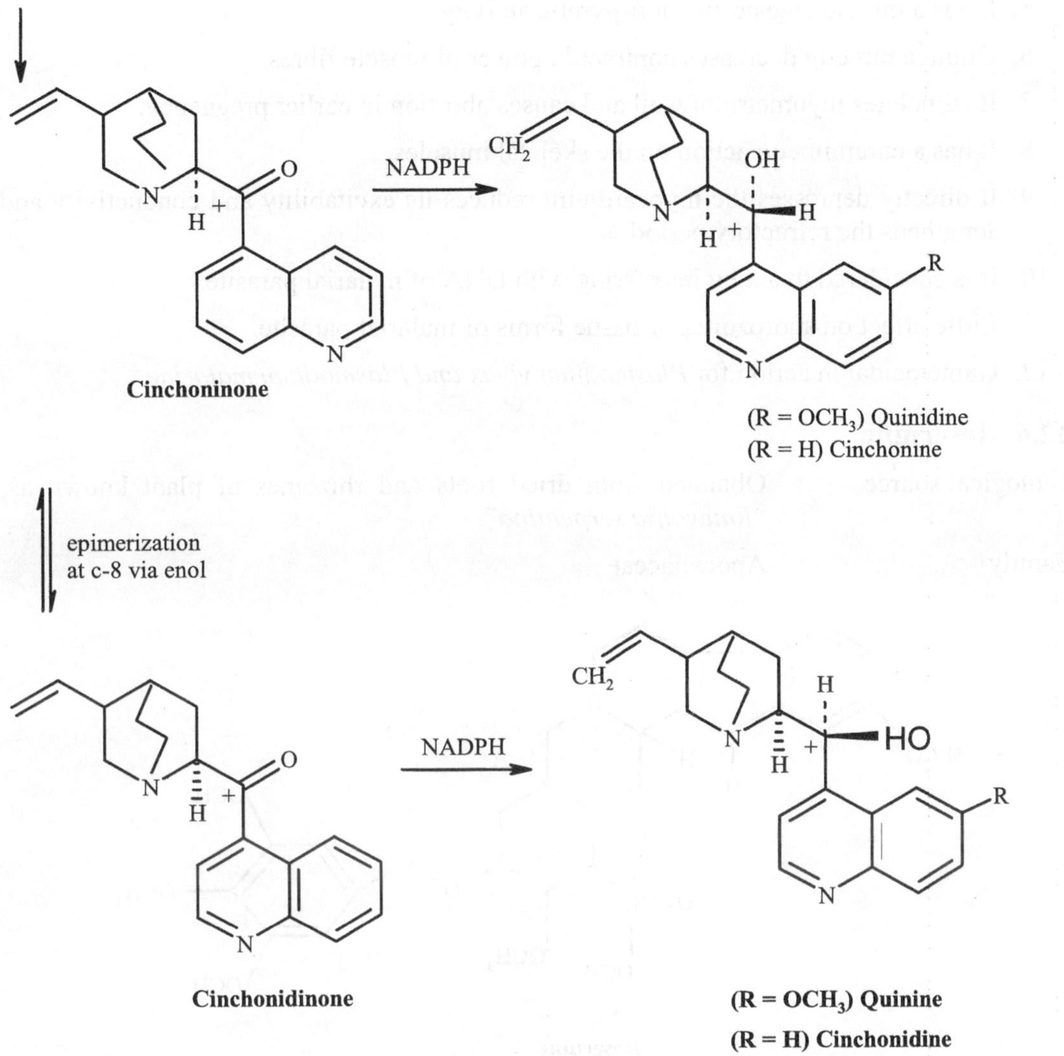

Biogenetic pathways of Quinine and its related alkaloids

Pharmacological Activity

1. Quinine and its salts are used in the treatment of malaria. Quinine is a protoplasmic poison especially for protozoa.
2. Quinine is schizontocidal in action and hence, is used as a suppressive agent.
3. Infusion of quinine eliminates the risk of sudden death.
4. It increases gastric secretion (due to its bitter taste).

5. It has a mild analgesic and anti-pyretic activity.
6. Quinine directly decreases contractile power of muscle fibres.
7. It stimulates myometrium wall and causes abortion in earlier pregnancy.
8. It has a curamimetic action on the skeletal muscles.
9. It directly depresses the myocardium, reduces its excitability and conductivity and lengthens the refractory period.
10. It is considered to act by interfering with DNA of malarial parasite.
11. Little effect on sporozoites or tissue forms of malarial parasite.
12. Gametocidal in action for *Plasmodium vivax and Plasmodium malariae.*

12.6 Reserpine

Biological source : Obtained from dried roots and rhizomes of plant known as, "*Rauwolfia serpentina*".

Family : Apocynaceae

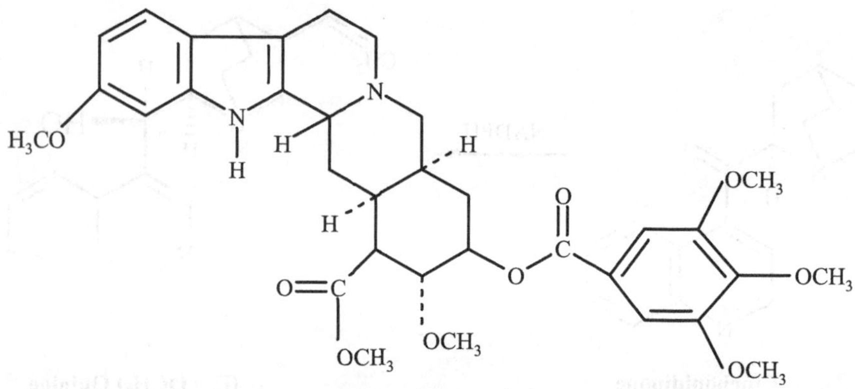

Reserpine

Chemistry

1. Reserpine is an indole alkaloid derivative.
2. It is an ester compound.
3. On controlled alkaline hydrolysis, reserpine yields reserpic acid.
4. Reserpine is metabolized by the liver and intestine to methyl reserpate and 3, 4, 5-trimethoxy benzoic acid.
5. Reserpine and other related alkaloids (rescinnamine, deserpidine and ajmalicine) are weak bases.

6. Reserpine forms a white or pale buff to slightly yellowish crystalline powder, practically insoluble in water and in solvent ether but freely soluble in chloroform.
7. Alkaloid reserpine is chemically named as methyl o-(3, 4, 5-trimethoxy benzoyl) reserpate, corresponding to the carboxylic acid named reserpic acid.

Biogenesis

The non-tryptophan portions of alkaloids mainly reserpine is derived from monoterpenoid precursor coryanthe type.

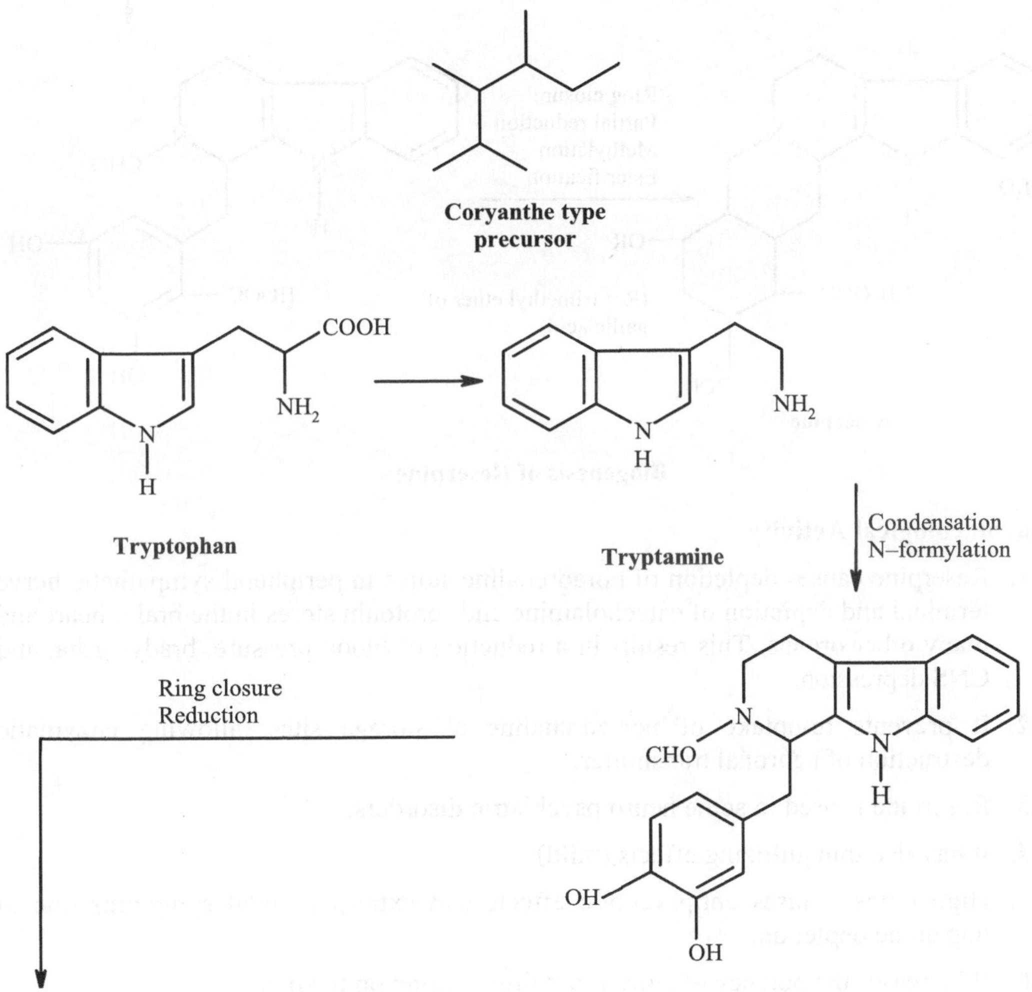

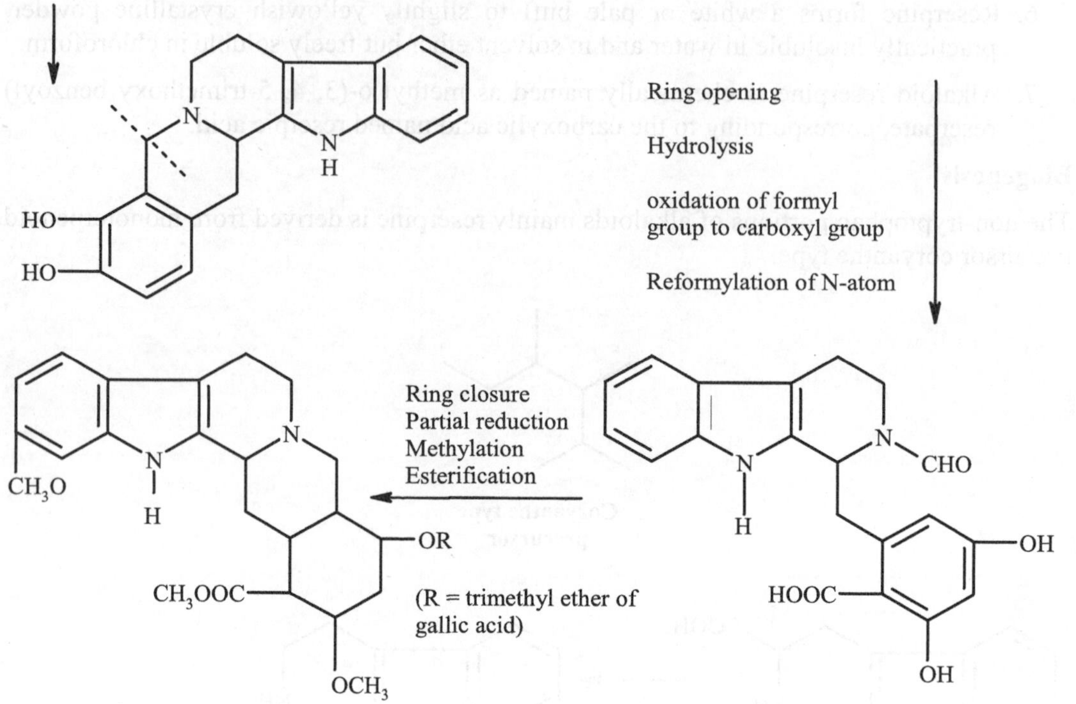

Biogenesis of Reserpine

Pharmacological Activity

1. Reserpine causes depletion of noradrenaline stores in peripheral sympathetic nerve terminal and depletion of catecholamine and serotonin stores in the brain, heart and many other organs. This results in a reduction of blood pressure, bradycardia, and CNS depression.
2. It prevents re-uptake of nor-adrenaline at storage sites, allowing enzymatic destruction of neuronal transmitter.
3. Reserpine is used in some neuro psychiatric disorders.
4. It has also tranquillizing effects (mild).
5. Higher dose causes antipsychotic effects and extra-pyramidal symptoms due to dopamine depletion.
6. It increases the potency of convulsant drugs acting on the brain.
7. It acts synergistically with other hypotensive agents such as diuretics.
8. Reserpine causes increased gastric acid secretion and augmentation of peristalsis.

9. The drug is also used to induce experimental peptic ulceration in animals.
10. Reserpine has also been suggested to play a role in the promotion of breast cancers.

12.7 Sennosides

Biological source : Obtained from dried leaflets of "*Cassia angustifolia*".

Family : Leguminosae

Senna leaves contains not less than 2% of anthracene derivatives calculated as calcium sennoside-B.

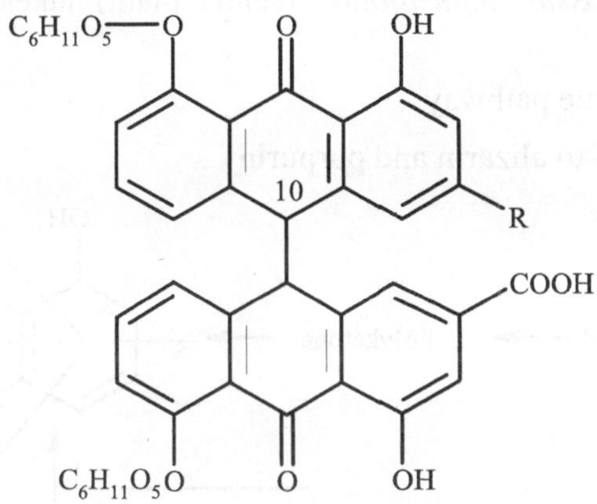

Sennosides

R	10 - 10′	Glycosidal content
COOH	trans	Sennoside-A
COOH	meso	Sennoside-B
CH_2OH	Trans	Sennoside-C
CH_2OH	meso	Sennoside-D

Chemistry

1. Sennoside is an anthracene derivatives having formula $C_{42}H_{33}O_{20}$.
2. The two main principles of senna namely: sennoside A and B differs principally in the manner of linkage of glucose to aglycone fraction.
3. Both sennoside-A and sennoside-B are phenolic glycosides of a stereoisomers of rhein dianthrone 10, 10′ – bis (9, 10-dihydro-1, 8-dihydroxy-9-oxoanthracene-3-carboxylic acid).

4. The aglycone of sennoside-A is dextro-rotatory while that of sennoside-B is meso-form.
5. The sugar moiety of glycoside acts as transporter of active aglycone, enabiling it to reach the large intestine.
6. The sugar moiety of glycoside also acts as a protector which prevents oxidation of aglycone to the relatively inactive anthraquinone in the mouth.
7. It is assumed that primary compounds are slowly changed into less active secondary glycoside which gave the same chemical assay.

Biogenesis

The biosynthesis in "*Cassia angustifolia*" (senna plant) takes through two different pathways.

1. Acetate polymalonate pathway
2. From shikimic acid to alizarin and purpurin

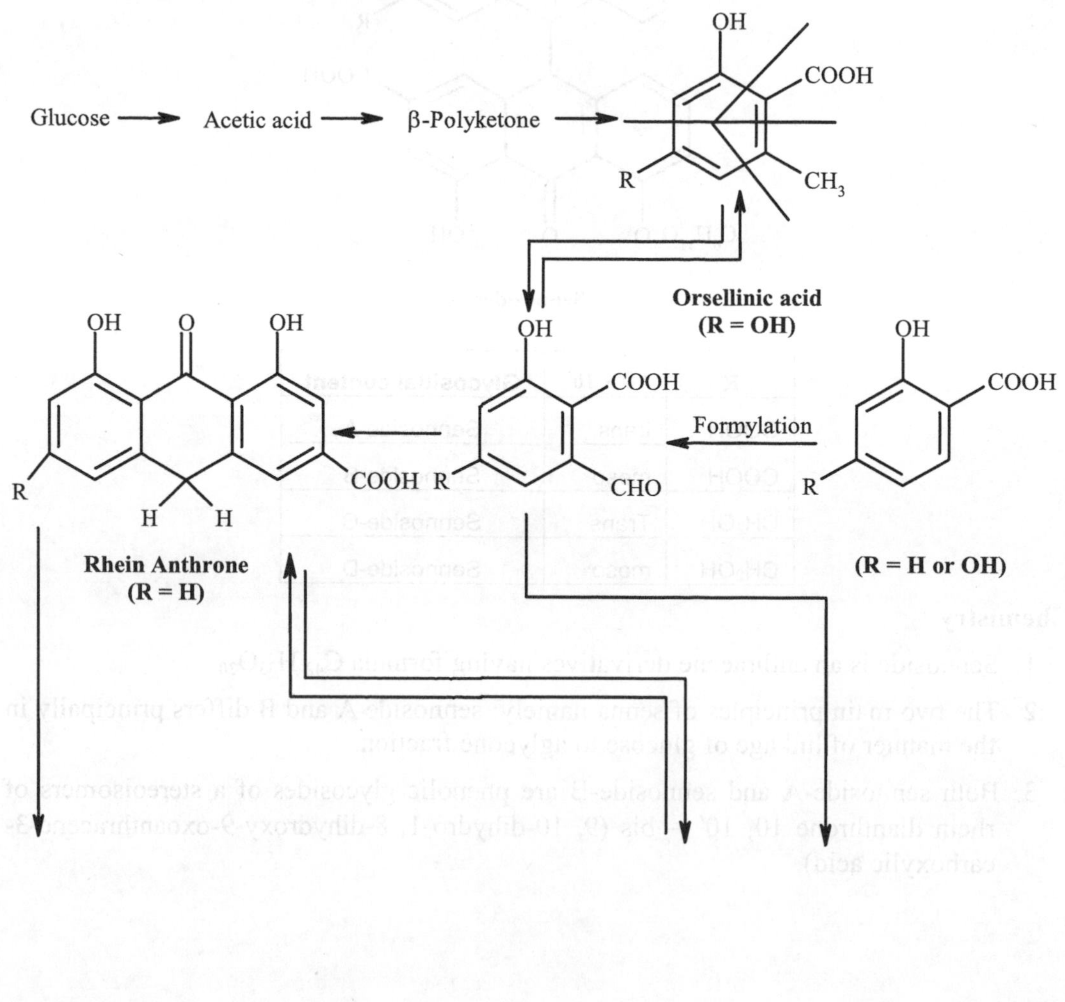

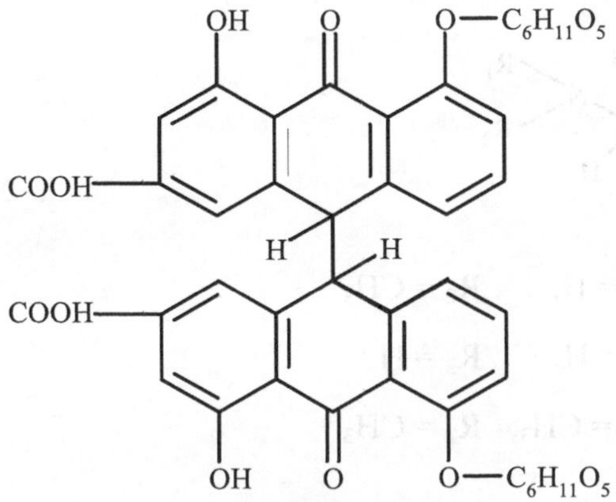

Sennosides A and B

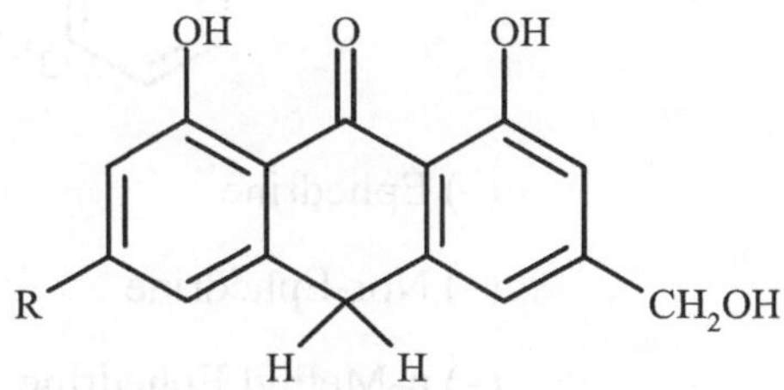

Aloe-emodinanthrone (R = H)

Biogenetic Pathways of Sennosides

Pharmacological activity

1. The action of sennosides is chiefly on the lower bowel and is suitable for habitual constipation.
2. The glycosides are absorbed from the intestinal tract and active anthraquinones are liberated in the course of their breakdown.
3. These drugs stimulate and increase peristaltic movements of colon by its local action upon the intestinal wall, which results in decreased absorption of water and thereby a bulkier and softer faecal mass.
4. They are excreted in milk during lactation which produces diarrhoea in breast-fed infants.
5. They do not produce any effect in stomach and small intestines.
6. Senna extract and sennoside-A have synergistic action and is used as a laxative.

12.8 Ephedrine

Biological source : It is obtained from dried aerial parts of "*Ephedra gerardiana*", "*Ephedra sinica*", "*Ephedra nebrodensis*" and other various species.

Family : Ephedraceae/Gnetaceae

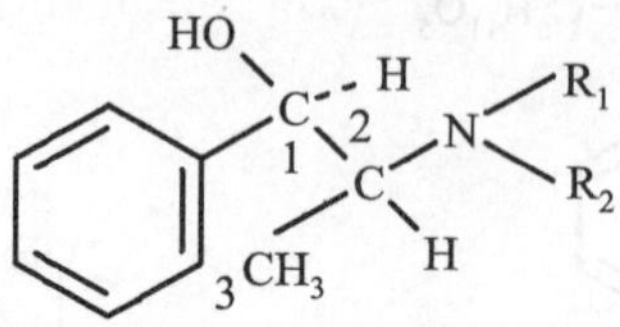

(–) Ephedrine	$R_1 = H$,	$R_2 = CH_3$
(–) Nor-Ephedrine	$R_1 = H$,	$R_2 = H$
(–) n-Methyl Ephedrine	$R_1 = CH_3$,	$R_2 = CH_3$

Chemistry

1. Structurally, Ephedrine ($C_{10}H_{15}NO$) is 1-phenyl-1-hydroxy-2-methyl amino propane.
2. Along with amino alkaloids, macrocyclic alkaloids called ephedradines are present in roots.
3. It decomposes when exposed to air.
4. Ephedrine is an amino alkaloid, as it is biosynthesized through phenyl alanine (an amino acid).
5. Ephedrine contains a hydroxyl group on β-carbon, which decreases their central stimulating action because of lower lipid solubility of such compounds.
6. The presence of a substituent on α-carbon (carbon next to the amino group) blocks the oxidative deamination of ephedrine.
7. Lacking hydrogen bonding phenolic substituents, ephedrine is less polar than the other compounds.
8. Ephedrine does not have any phenolic substituents on the phenyl ring and possess good oral activity because it is not a substrate for COMT.
9. Ephedrine structure has two asymmetric carbon atoms, hence there are four optical isomers possible namely:

   (–) – Ephedrine, (+) – Ephedrine,

   (–) – Pseudoephedrine, (+) – pseudo ephedrine
10. Naturally occurring ephedrine has IR, 2S configuration and has erythro form.

Biogenesis

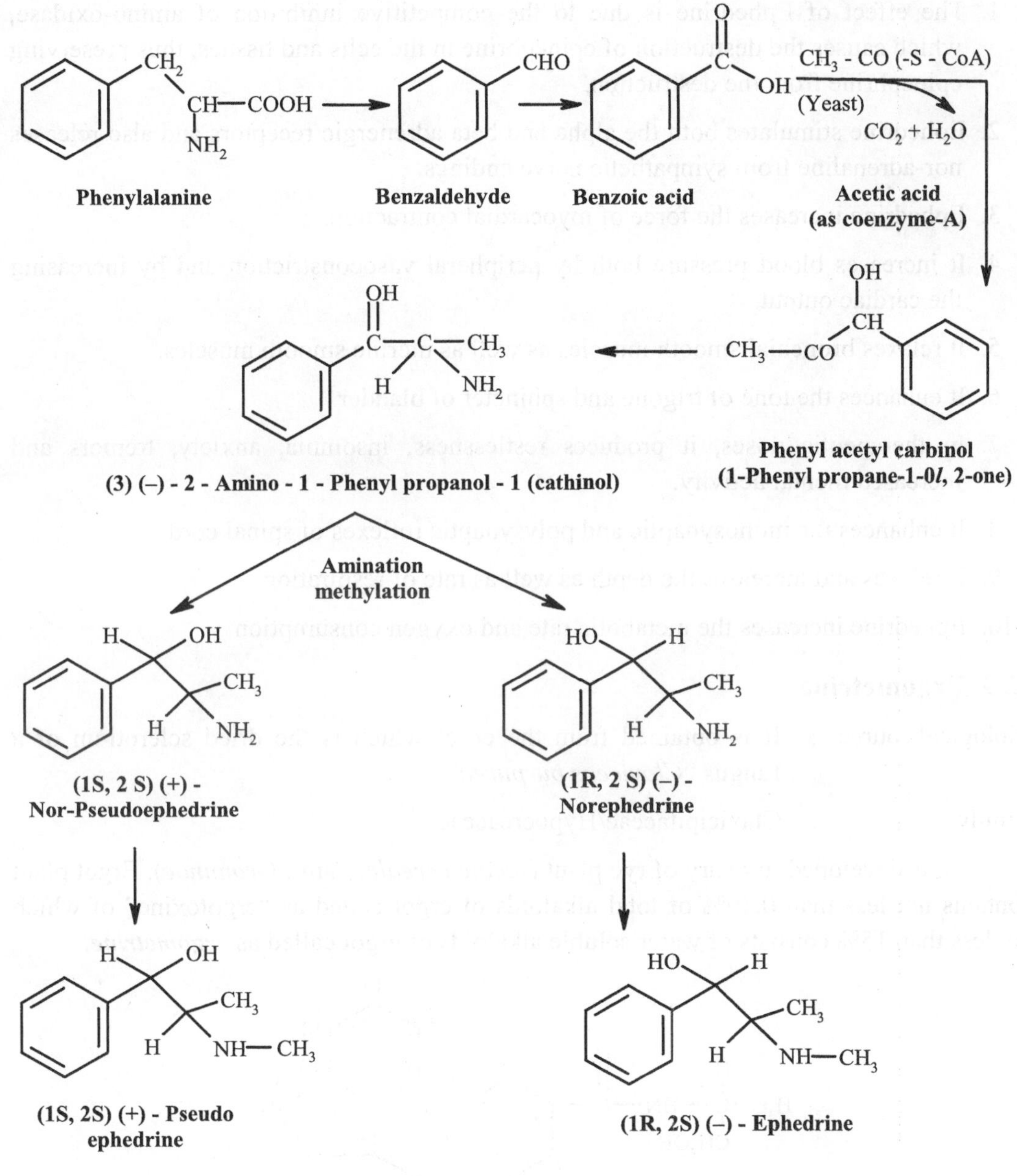

Biogenetic Pathways of Ephedrine

Pharmacological activity

1. The effect of Ephedrine is due to the competitive inhibition of amino-oxidase, which causes the destruction of epinephrine in the cells and tissues, thus preserving epinephrine from the destruction.
2. Ephedrine stimulates both the alpha and beta adrenergic receptors and also releases nor-adrenaline from sympathetic nerve endings.
3. Ephedrine increases the force of myocardial contraction.
4. It increases blood pressure both by peripheral vasoconstriction and by increasing the cardiac output.
5. It relaxes bronchial smooth muscles as well as uterine smooth muscles.
6. It enhances the tone of trigone and sphincter of bladder.
7. In therapeutic doses, it produces restlessness, insomnia, anxiety, tremors and increased mental activity.
8. It enhances the monosynaptic and polysynaptic reflexes of spinal cord.
9. It relaxes and increases the depth as well as rate of respiration.
10. Ephedrine increases the metabolic rate and oxygen consumption.

12.9 Ergometrine

Biological source : It is obtained from the ergot which is the dried sclerotium of a fungus "*Claviceps purpurea*".

Family : Clavicipitaceae/Hypocreaceae

Ergot is developed in ovary of rye plant (*secale cereale*, Fam : *Graminae*). Ergot plant contains not less than 0.19% of total alkaloids of ergot called as "ergotoxine" of which not less than 15% consists of water soluble alkaloids of ergot called as *ergometrine.*

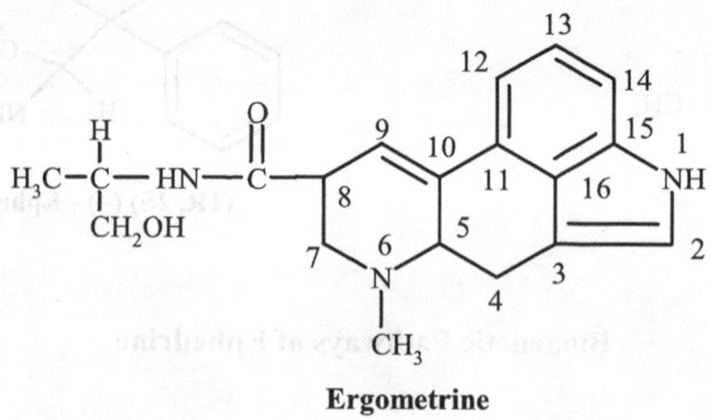

Ergometrine

Chemistry

1. Ergometrine is an amide derivative of (+) – Lysergic acid with 2-amino propanol.
2. Ergometrine (Ergonovine) is generally used in its maleate form.
3. It has two forms: Laevo form → medicinally active
   Dextro form → inert
4. Molecular formula of ergometrine is $C_{19}H_{23}O_2N_3$.
5. Some semi-synthetic derivatives of ergometrine are:
   - Methylergometrine = an amide of lysergic acid with 2-amino butanol.
   - Methysergide = produced by methylation of indole nitrogen of methylergometrine.

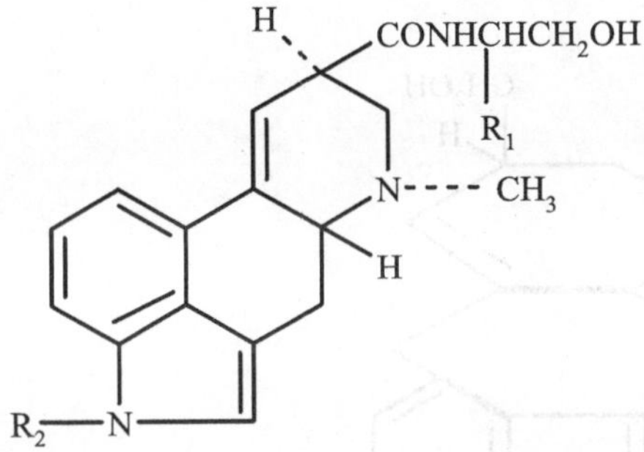

(Used as oxytocic agent).

		R_1	R_2
Methyl ergometrine	⇒	$-CH_2CH_3$	-H
Methysergide	⇒	$-CH_2CH_3$	CH_3

(used in Migraine treatment)

6. Each active alkaloid occurs with an inactive isomer involving isolysergic acid.
7. Lysergic acid has a fused indole-quinoline ring structure, synthesized by tryptophan (less the carboxyl group) and an isoprene unit derived from mevalonate.
8. Ergometrine gives blue fluorescence in water.

Biogenesis

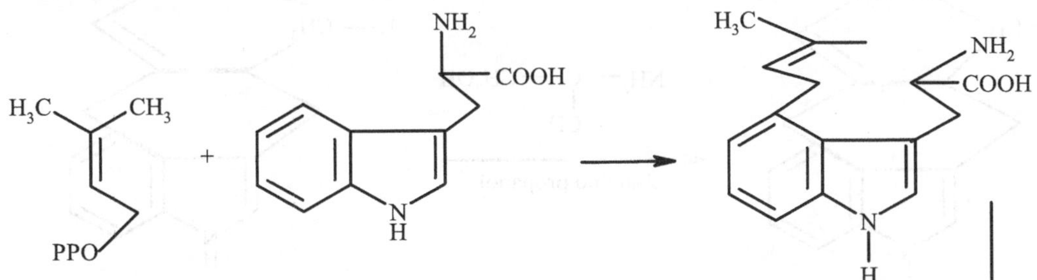

Isopentenyl Pyrophosphate (from Mevalonate)   **Tryptophan**   **Dimethylallyl tryptophan**

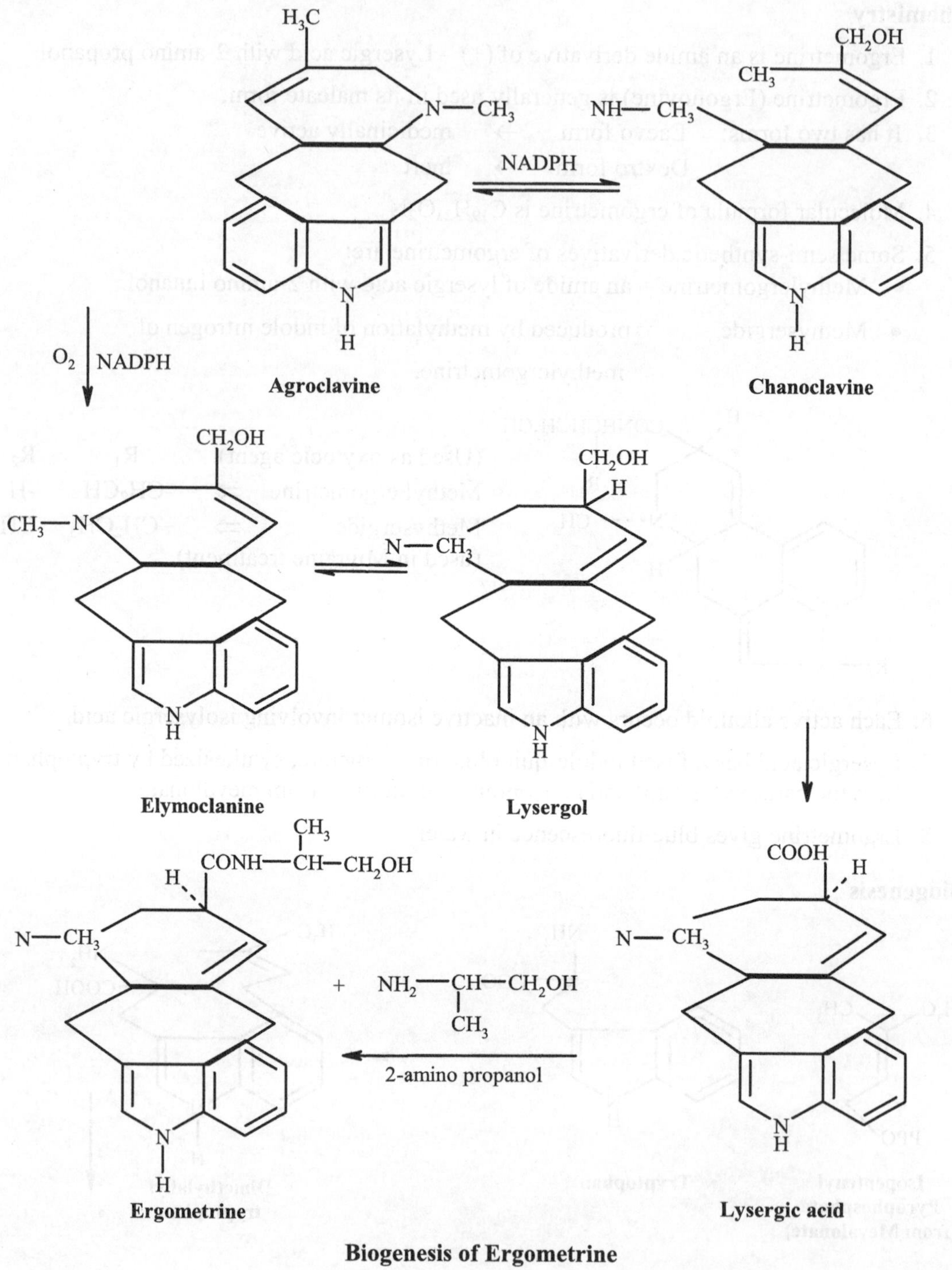

Biogenesis of Ergometrine

Pharmacological Activity

1. Ergometrine causes contraction of uterine smooth muscles (i.e., produces oxytocic action).
2. Sometimes used to enhance the labour pains in delivery cases.
3. Used to prevent and treat post-partum haemorrhage due to uterine atony.
4. A water soluble alkaloid having very high uterine stimulant activity.
5. Produces direct vasoconstrictor effect (in minimal range) to reduce the bleeding.
6. It has no adrenergic blocking activity.
7. Increases the peristaltic activity and potentiates the action of neostigmine on the gut.
8. Ergometrine is a valuable drug after caesarean operations.
9. These drugs may also stimulate 5-HT receptors.

12.10 Sarsasapogenin

Biological source : It is obtained from plant sarsaparilla (*smilax aristolochiaefolia*)

Family : Liliaceae

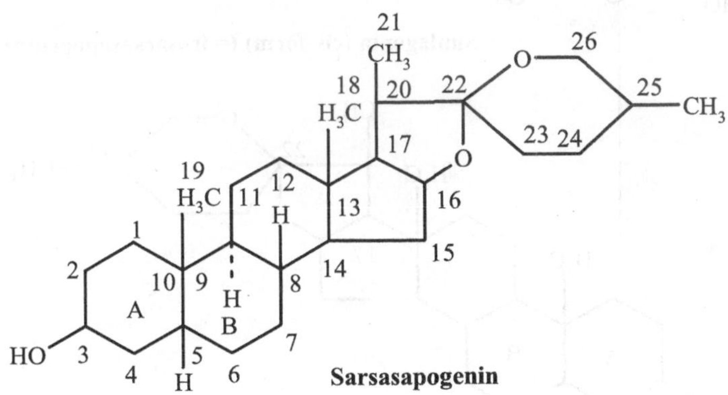

Sarsasapogenin

Chemistry

1. Sarsasapogenin are steroidal saponins (saponins are substances which modify surface tension) in nature.

   Note: Sarsasapogenin is also extracted from the seeds of "*Yucca brevifolia*"

   Family : Agavaceae

2. Sarsasapogenin contain aglycone moiety called as sapogenin which are high molecular weight substances and by acetylation give crystalline forms.
3. Sarsasapogenin contains tetracyclic triterpenoid structural saponins containing glycosidal linkage at C-3 atom.
4. A saponin called as sarsasaponin (Parillin) contains 3-glucose and 1-Rhamnose molecule as a sugar components.
5. In sarsasapogenin, an acetal group or ketone is present in the side chain of molecule.
6. Due to asymmetry of carbon atom at C-22 of acetal ketone, it exists in iso configuration having cis as well as trans form.

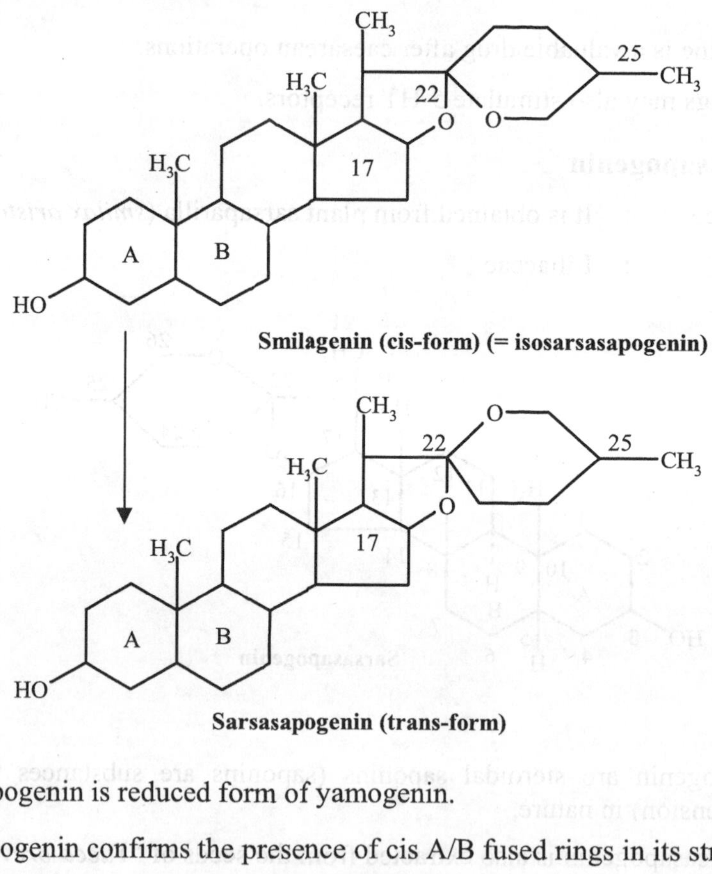

Smilagenin (cis-form) (= isosarsasapogenin)

Sarsasapogenin (trans-form)

7. Sarsasapogenin is reduced form of yamogenin.
8. This sapogenin confirms the presence of cis A/B fused rings in its structure.

Biogenesis

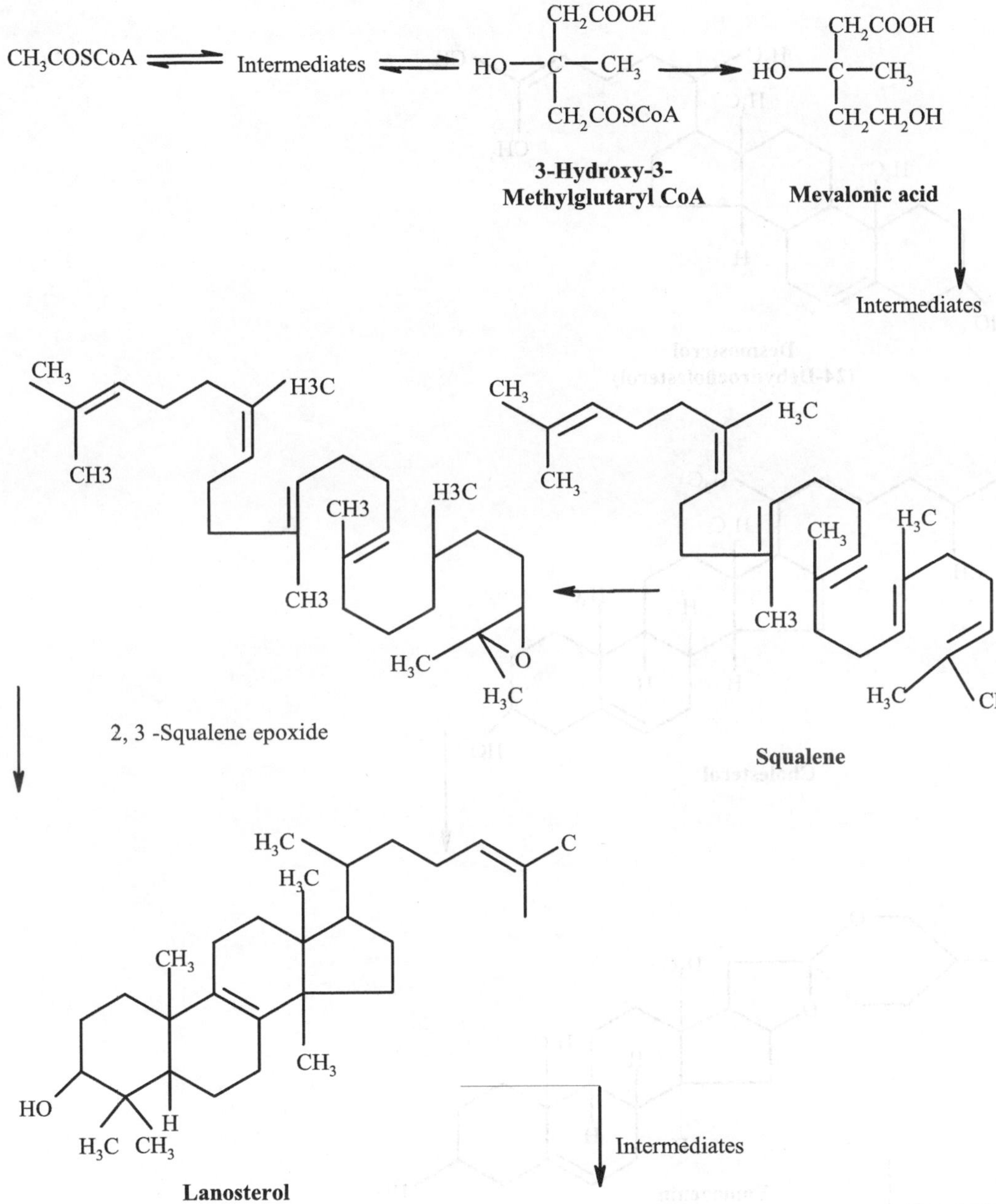

CH3COSCoA
Intermediates
3-Hydroxy-3-Methylglutaryl CoA
Mevalonic acid
Intermediates
Squalene
2, 3 -Squalene epoxide
Lanosterol
Intermediates

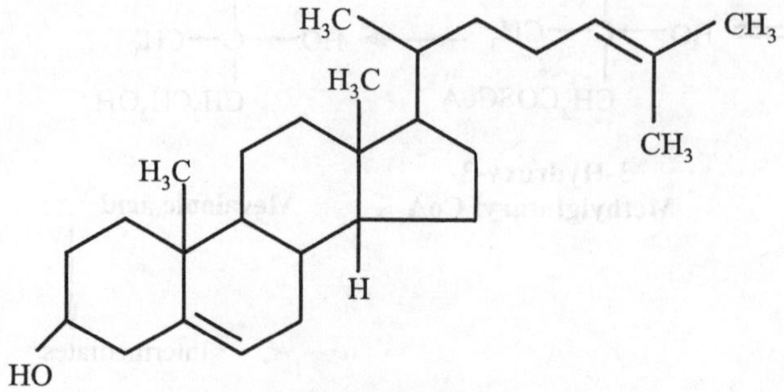

Desmosterol
(24-Dehydrocholesterol)

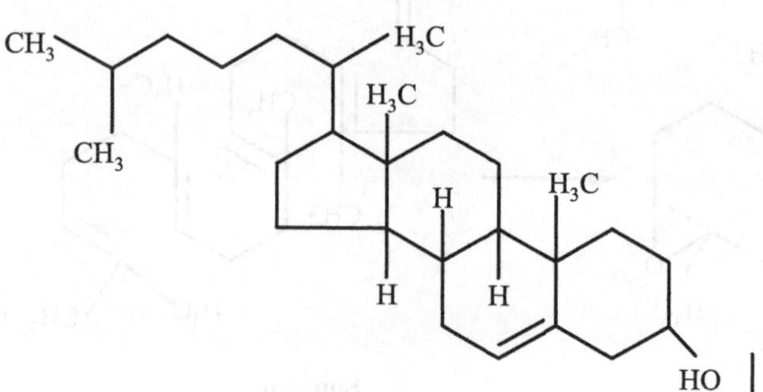

Cholesterol

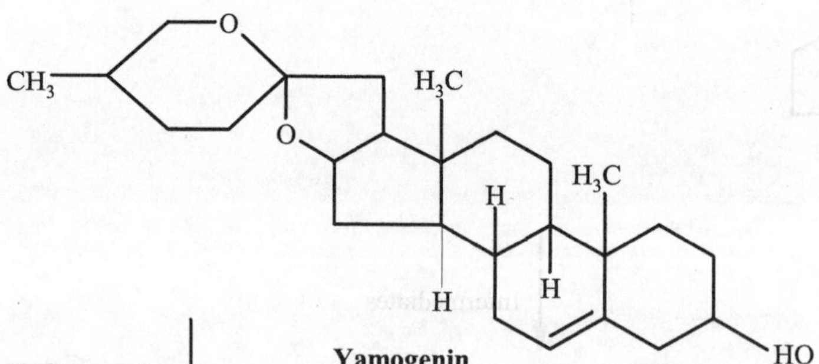

Yamogenin

Hydrogenation

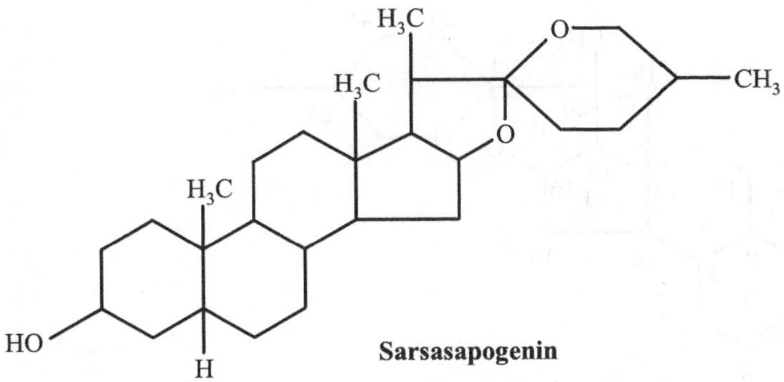

Sarsasapogenin

Biogenetic Pathways of Sarsasapogenin

Pharmacological activity

1. Sarsasapogenin cause haemolysis and hence is toxic to animals, if given parenterally.
2. Very small concentrations of sapogenins paralyze the respiratory functions of gills of fish.
3. The red blood cells carry sterols in their membranes, which upon contact with saponins gets precipitated and their colloidal properties gets altered to give haemoglobin passage to the surrounding medium.
4. These are not absorbed from the intestinal tract.
5. These are irritating to mucosa layer of mouth, stomach and intestines.
6. Bronchial secretion is stimulated by sapogenins.
7. The local irritant effect of sapogenins accounts for their sternutatory property.
8. Sarsasapogenin also increases the absorption of diuretically active substances and stimulate the kidneys to a higher activity, hence, frequently used in rheumatism.

12.11 Diosgenin

Biological Source : It is obtained from dried tubers of plants "*Dioscorea deltoidea*", "*Dioscorea composita*" and other species of dioscorea.

Family : Dioscoreaceae

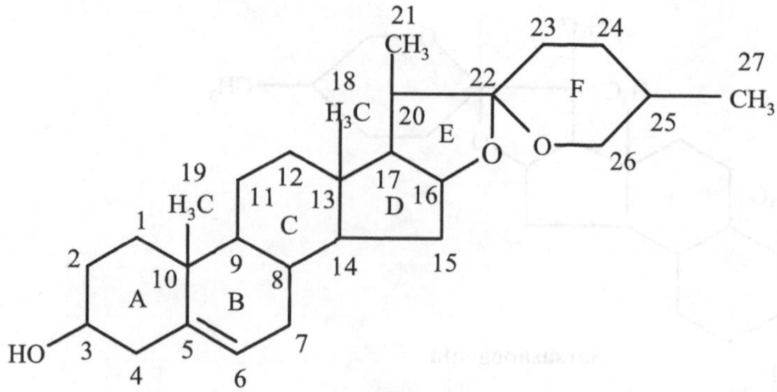

Diosgenin

Chemistry

1. Diosgenin, chemically named as (25 R)- spirost-5-en-3β-ol, the most prominent sapogenins used in industry.

   The structure has two additional rings which are hetero cyclic:

   - Ring E = a five-membered tetrahydrofuran ring
   - Ring F = a six-membered tetrahydropyran ring.

   These two rings are joined at 22-carbon in spiroketal fashion; therefore, parent structure is called as spirostan.

2. Diosgenin is degraded to obtain pregnenolone acetate by acetolysis process.
3. The enzymes saponases occurring in the plants are believed to hydrolyse the saponins into free diosgenin.
4. Diosgenin occurs generally in combined form as glycoside (saponin) and rarely in free state.
5. Diosgenin is present as rhamno-rhamno-glucoside, called as *Dioscin* in the tubers of commercial dioscorea spp.
6. Small amount of diosgenin in the form of its peptide ester with 4-hydroxy isoleucine is present in trigonella spp.

Biogenesis

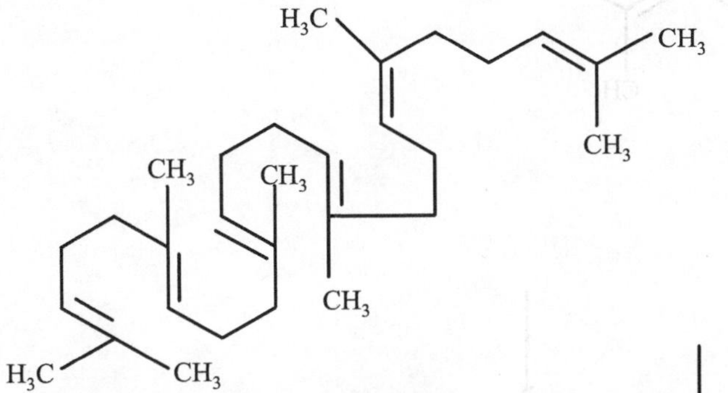

Squalene

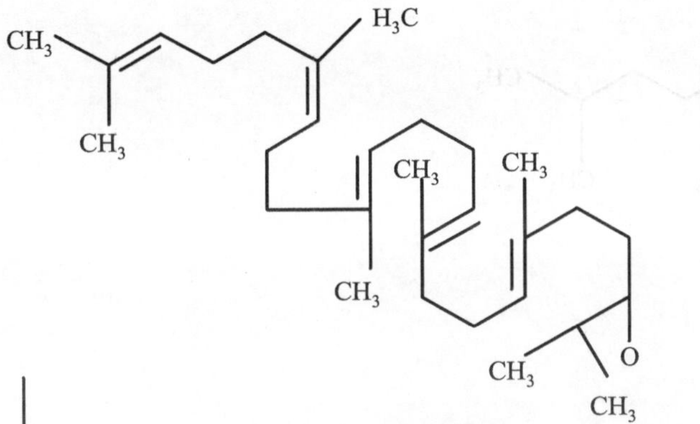

2-3-Squalene Epoxide

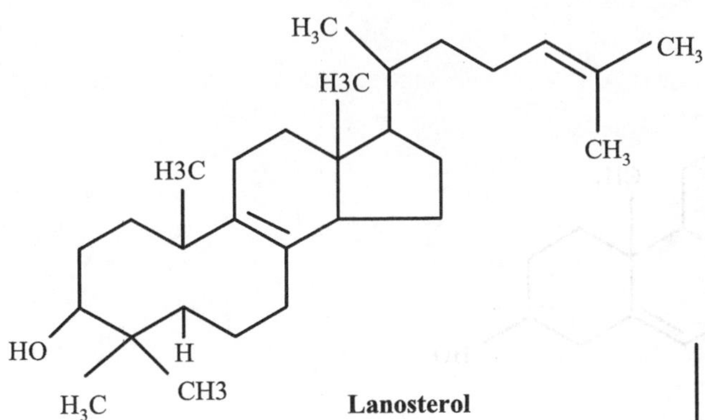

Lanosterol

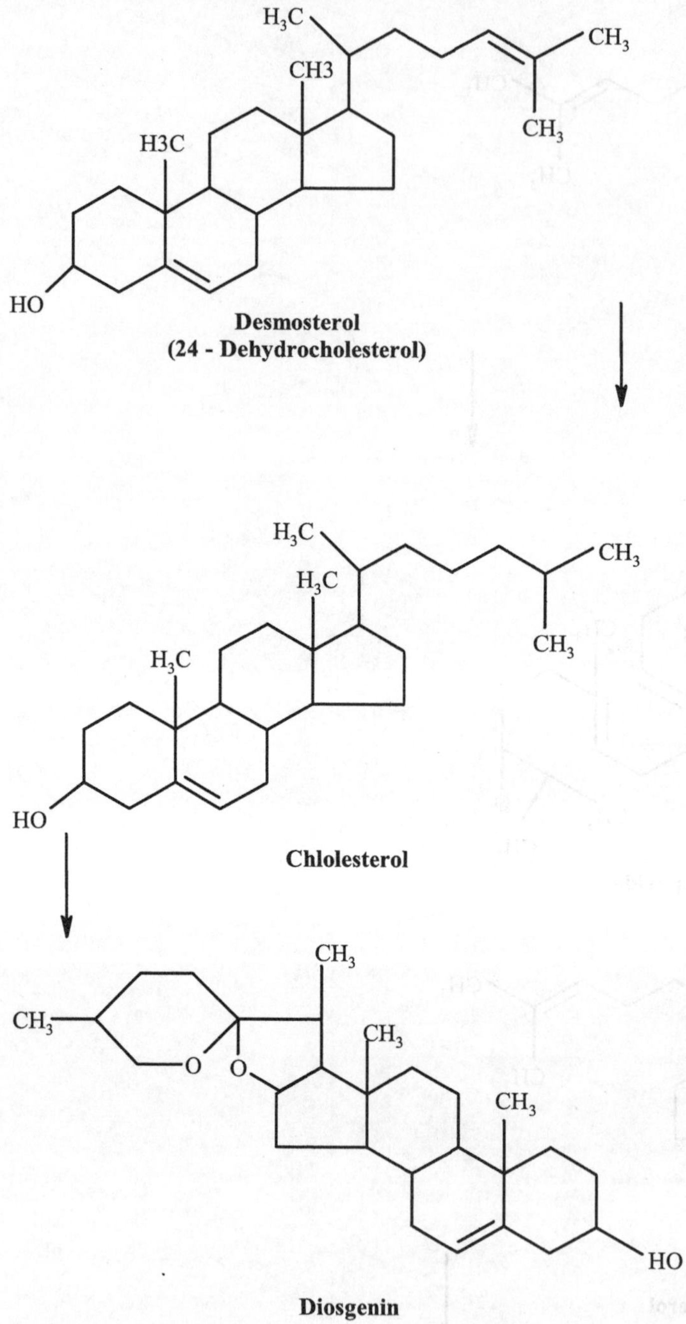

Biogenesis of Diosgenin

Pharmacological activity

1. Diosgenin affects the absorption of pharmacologically active substances.
2. Increases the activity of ciliary epithelium, a process which brings up the expectorate.
3. Used as a main constituent in the treatment of rheumatic arthritis.
4. Diosgenin produces a synergistic effect on the body.
5. Saponins (Diosgenin) stimulate the kidneys to its higher activity.

12.12 Digitoxin

Biological source : It is obtained from dried leaves of "*Digitalis purpurea*" and "*Digitalis lanata*"

Family : Scrophulariaceae

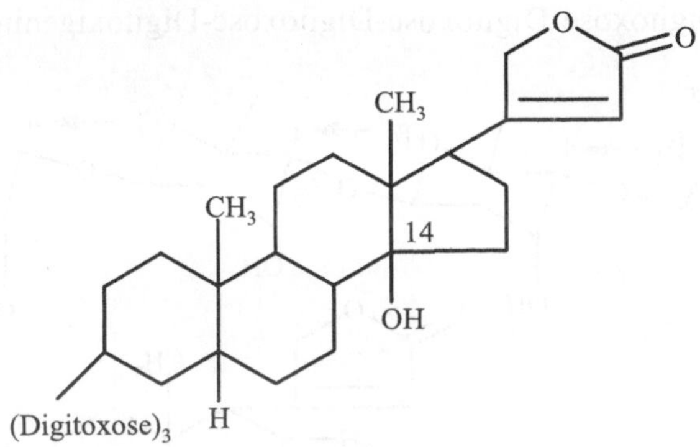

Digitoxin

Chemistry

1. Digitoxin, a glycoside on acid hydrolysis results in separation of aglycone/genin called as degitoxigenin and a sugar, digitoxose.
2. The aglycone moiety is structurally a steroid nucleus with an attached lactone ring.

$$\text{Digitoxin} \xrightarrow[\text{Acid Hydrolysis}]{[H] + 3H_2O} \text{Digitoxigenin} + 3 \text{ Digitoxose}$$

3. Tertiary hydroxyl groups (in position of 14-digitoxigenin) easily splits of as water at elevated temperatures to form anhydrogenins (e.g. anhydrodigitoxigenin).
4. The lactone ring is easily opened in the presence of alkali and salt of aldehydic acid is formed. Thus, the glyosidal form deteriorates.

5. Digitoxin contains basic structure of cardenolides, which contains sugar residues on 3β-hydroxyl group.
6. These have unsaturated lactone ring at c-17 β.
7. The structure contains hydroxyl group at 14 β carbon atom.

Biogenesis

Digitoxin is biosynthesized from purpurea glycoside-A and also from Lanatoside-A.

Method I: Purpurea glycoside-A

(Glucose Digitoxose-Digitoxose-Digitoxose-Digitoxigenin)

↓ –Glucose

Digitoxin

(Digitoxose-Digitoxose-Digitoxose-Digitoxigenin)

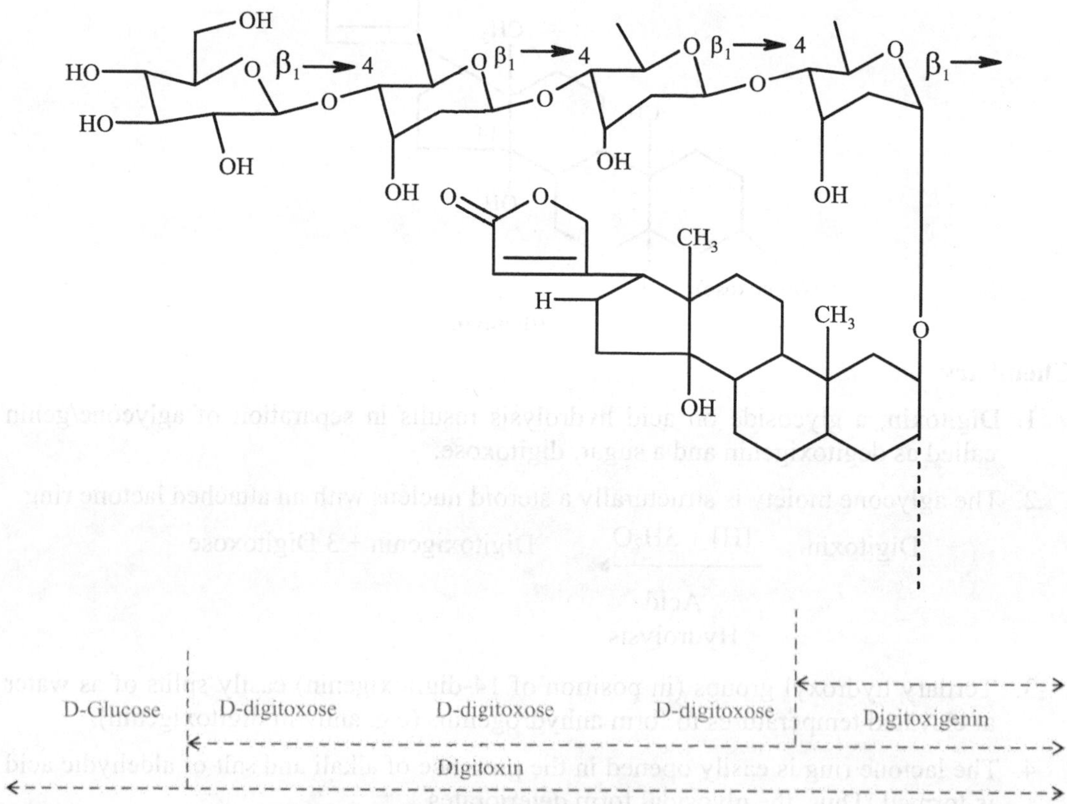

Purpurea Glycoside-A

Method II: Lanatoside-A

(Glucose ¦ Digitoxose-Digitoxose-Digitoxose-Digitoxigenin)

Acetate ↓ –Glucose

Acetyl Digitoxin

(Digitoxose-Digitoxose-Digitoxose-Digitoxigenin)

↓

Acetate

↓ –Acetate

Digitoxin

(Digitoxose-Digitoxose-Digitoxose-Digitoxigenin)

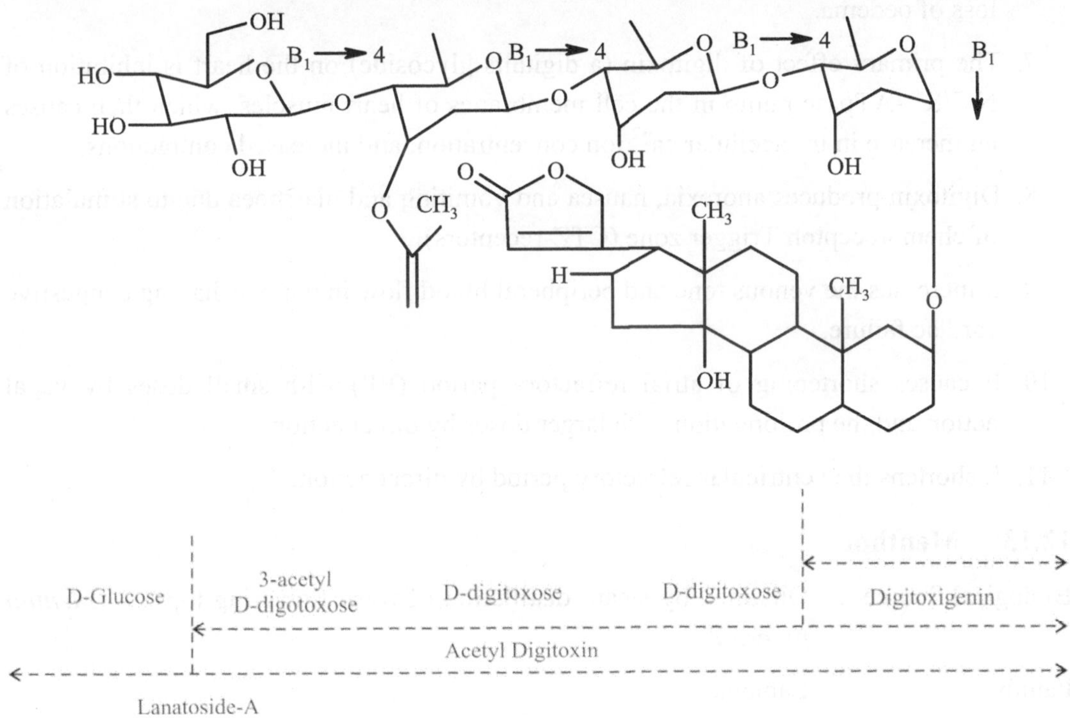

Biosynthetic Pathways of Digitoxin

Pharmacological activity

1. Digitoxin enhances the force of myocardial contractions.
2. In case of heart failure, digitoxin produces inotropic effect thus resulting in a modified cardiac output with regard to more complete emptying of ventricle at systole.
3. Used in treatment of congestive heart failure (CHF).
4. It increases the rapidity and force of systolic contraction of heart muscle, thus increasing cardiac output.
5. Digitoxin increases the ability of purkinje fibres and ventricular muscles to initiate impulses. This leads to development of ventricular extra systoles.
6. On injecting causes increased excretion of sodium and water by the kidney causing loss of oedema.
7. The primary effect of digitoxin (a digitalis glycoside) on the heart is inhibition of Na^{+}/K^{+} -ATpase pump in the cell membranes of heart muscles, which then causes an increase in intracellular ca^{+2} ion concentration, and increased contractions.
8. Digitoxin produces anorexia, nausea and vomiting and diarrhoea due to stimulation of chemorecepton Trigger zone (CTZ-receptors).
9. It increases the venous tone and peripheral blood flow in patients having congestive cardiac failure.
10. It causes shortening of atrial refractory period (RP) with small doses by vagal action and the prolongation with larger doses by direct action.
11. It shortens the ventricular refractory period by direct action.

12.13 Menthol

Biological Source : Obtained by steam distillation of fresh flowering tops of "*Mentha piperita*".

Family : Labiatae

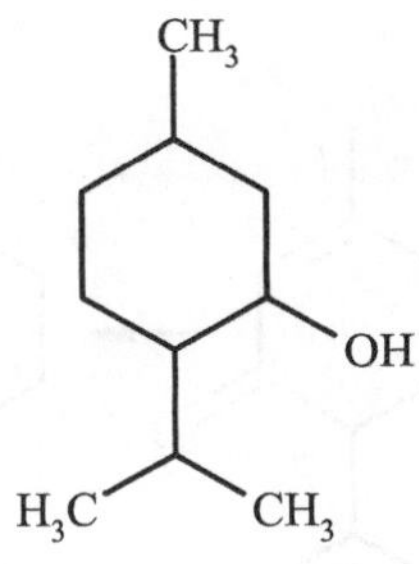

Menthol

Chemistry

1. Menthol is an alcohol (saturated secondary alcohol) obtained from different species of mint oils or prepared synthetically.
2. Natural menthol is laevorotatory, while synthetic menthol is racemic in nature.
3. Menthol is optically active.
4. Menthol contains 3 dissimilar chiral centres at 1, 3 and 4 positions.

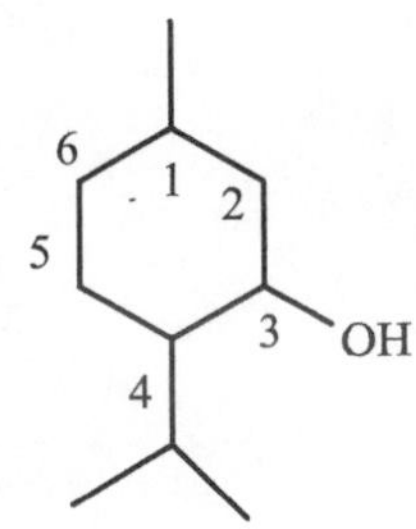

   (Thus eight optically active forms or four racemic modifications are possible called as enantiomorphous pairs). The pairs are:

   - (+) and (–) menthols
   - (+) and (–) isomenthols
   - (+) and (–) neomenthols
   - (+) and (–) neo-isomenthols

5. Synthetic menthol produced by catalytic hydrogenation of menthane, pulegone or thymol.
6. Rates of esterification by isomeric methods:

   Menthol > Isomenthol > Neo-isomenthol > Neo-menthol

Biogenesis

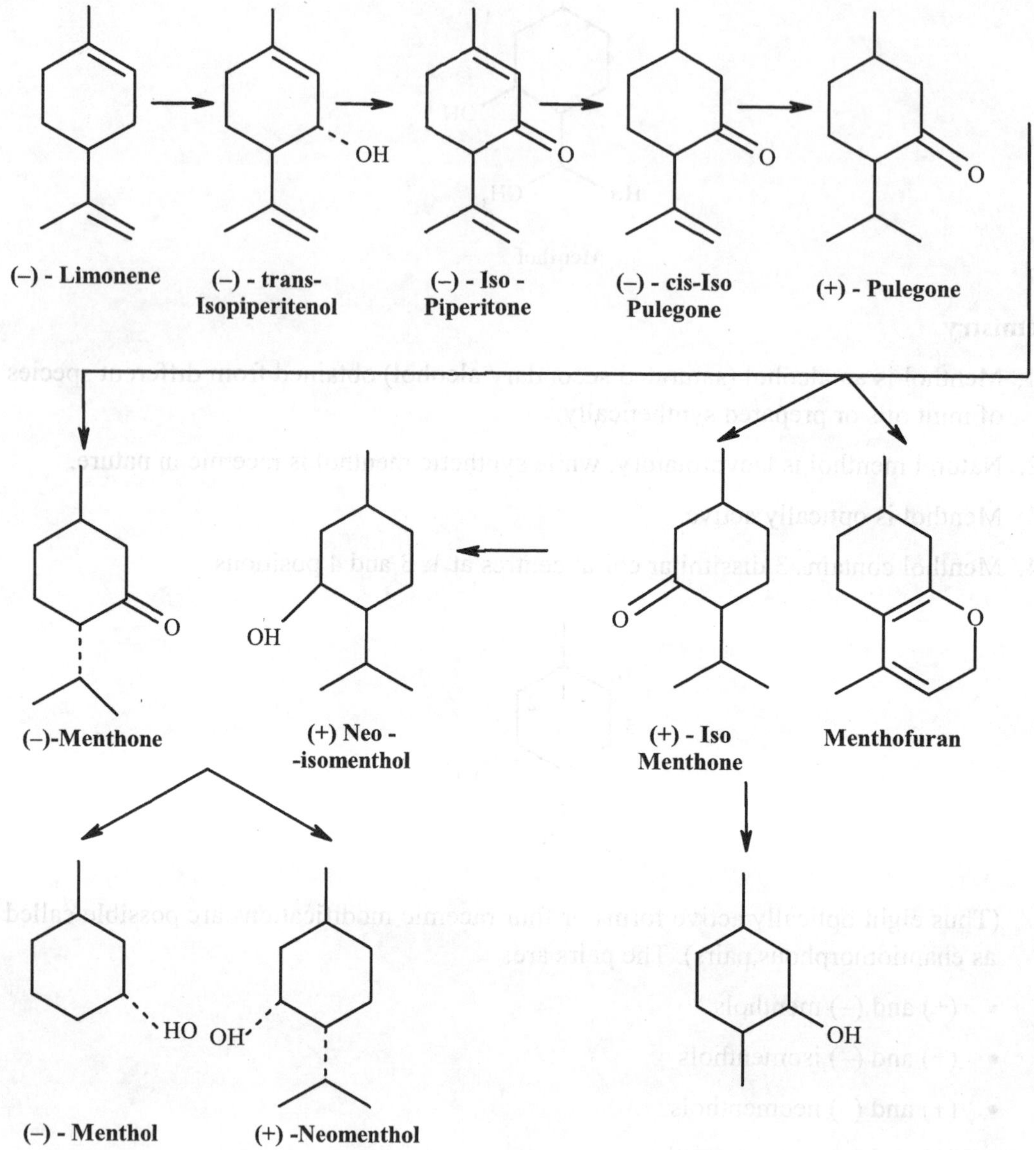

Pharmacological activity

1. Menthol possess calcium channel blocking activity causing spasmolytic and smooth muscle relaxant effects and hence useful in irritable bowel syndrome.

2. They show better pharmacokinetic profile when given by enteric coated capsules for release in large intestine.
3. Muscle relaxant activity of menthol is employed to reduce spasm during endoscopy of colon. For this purpose, emulsified oil is injected through biopsy channel of endoscope.
4. It shows carminative, stimulant and antiseptic property.
5. Generally used for nasal decongestant effect.
6. Produces depressant action on the heart.
7. Topically applied on the skin for itching problems in the form of 0.1% and 2% preparations and is also used in neuralgia (nerve disorder).

12.14 Citral

Biological source : Obtained from steam distillation of leaves and aerial parts of "*cymbopogon flexuousus*", "*cymbopogon citrates*".

Family : Graminae

About 75% citral (in aldehydic form) is present in lemon-grass oil.

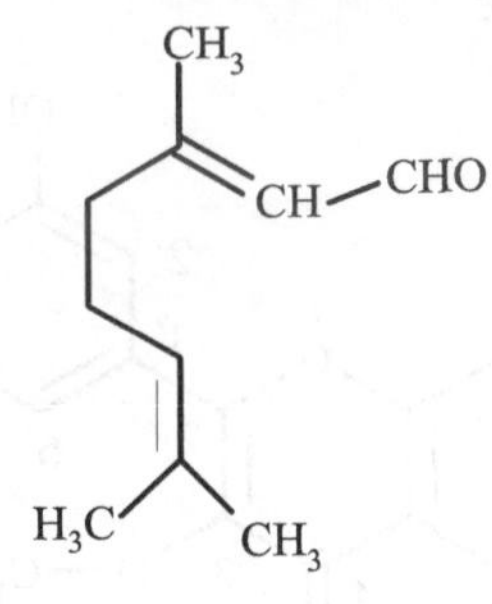

Citral

Chemistry

1. Citral, an aldehydic group containing essential oil component exists both in natural and synthetic forms.
2. Synthetic citral is optically inactive.
3. Natural citral is optically active and possesses two isomeric forms.

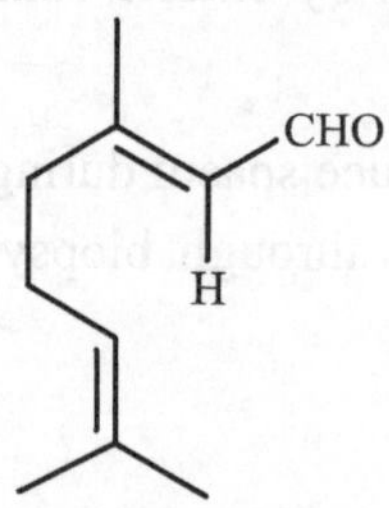

Trans or (E) form (citral-a)
Geranial (b.p = 118 - 119°C)

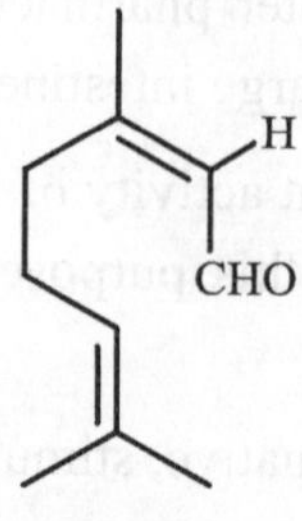

Cis or (z) form (citral-b)
Neral [b.p = 117 - 118°c]

Pharmacological activity

1. Citral, when administered orally or inhaled by the steam, increases the respiratory secretions by direct action.
2. It possesses stimulant and carminative action.

12.15 Rutin

Biological source : Obtained from "*Fagopyrum esculentum*". Also obtained from flower-buds of "*Sophora japonica*" or species of eucalyptus.

Family : Polygonaceae

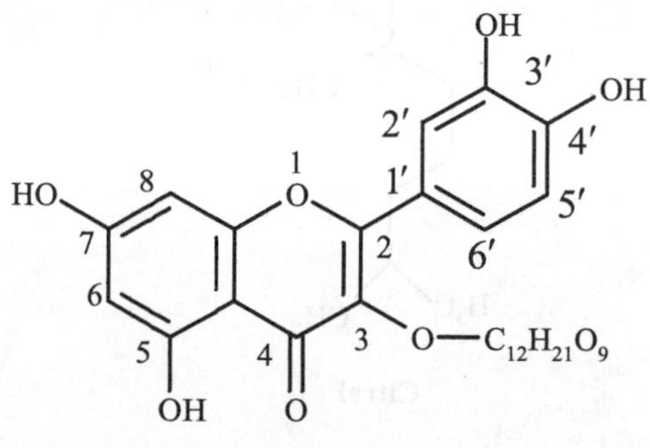

Rutin

Chemistry

1. Rutin is a rhamnoglucoside of quercetin which contains at c-3 position, the sugar rutinase ($C_{12}H_{21}O_9$) composed of glucose + rhamnose.
2. Micro crystalline greenish yellow tasteless powder soluble in CH_3OH, isopropyl alcohol, pyridine and solutions of alkali hydroxides.

3. Rutin on hydrolysis yields quercetin, rhamnose and glucose

$$\text{Rutin} \xrightarrow{\text{(HOH)}} \text{Quercetin} + \text{Rhamnose} + \text{Glucose}$$

Pharmacological activity

1. Rutin employed in veterinary medicine (in the form of ointment).
2. Rutin stops capillary bleeding along with increased capillary fragility.
3. Useful to treat retinal haemorrhages.
4. It is also effective in curing radiation injuries and atomic burns.

CHAPTER 13

CHROMATOGRAPHIC EVALUATION OF HERBAL DRUGS

13.1 Chromatography

Chromatography , (in Greek : Khromatos = colour and graphos = written).

Chromatography may be defined as follows:

1. It is a process which is run in a column of fixed bed.
2. The process consists in separation of substances by filtering their solution through a column of a finely powdered adsorbent filtered in a glass tube, and then washing or developing the column with a solvent.
3. An analytical technique used for purification and separation of organic and inorganic substances which undergo decomposition during fractional crystallization of distillation.

The cromatography process depends on different affinities of solute between two immiscible phases namely:

Stationary phase	:	A fixed bed of large surface area
Mobile phase	:	A fluid or a gas which moves through or over the surface

Advantage

Currently, chromatographic processes are being used as follows:

1. In establishing the identity/non-identity of two substances.
2. In purification of technical products.

3. In separation of mixtures containing stereo isomers or related compounds.
4. In the identification and control of commercial products.
5. In detection and estimation of contaminants in commercial products.
6. In determining concentration of products taking place at greater dilution.
7. In evaluation of herbal and crude drugs.

13.2 Classification

(I) chromatography is divided into two classes:

(i) *Gas chromatography*

- Gas liquid chromatography (GLC
- Gas solid chromatography (GSC)

(ii) *Solution chromatography:*

- Adsorption chromatography
- Column chromatography
- Partition chromatography
- Ion-exchange chromatography
- Reverse-phase chromatography
- Electrophoretic chromatography

(II) Chromatography can also be divided into following types:

(i) *Adsorption chromatography*

(ii) *Exclusion chromatography*:

- Gel permeation technique
- Sieving separation technique

(iii) *Ion-exchange chromatography*

(iv) *Partition chromatography*

- Paper Chromatography
- Column Chromatography
- Thin layer chromatography

Table 13.1 Classification of Multistage fractionation procedures

S.no.	Type of phase	Chromatographic process	Sample (stationary) phase	Second (mobile) phase
1	Liquid-Liquid	Counter current separation	Solution	Immiscible solvent
		Partition	Solution	Immiscible solvent on solid matrix
		Thin layer (TLC)	Solution	Immiscible solvent on fine powder on a glass plate
		Paper	Solution	Immiscible solvent on paper matrix
		Gel	Solution	Solvent held in the interstices of a polymetric solvent
2	Liquid-Gas	Gas liquid	Gas	Solvent held on solid matrix
		Fractional distillation	Gas	Condensed liquid
3	Solid-Liquid	Ion-exchange	Solution	Ion-exchange resins
		Adsorption	Solution	Solid-adsorbent
		Thin layer (TLC)	Solution	Fine powder supported on a glass plate
4	Gas-Solid	Gas solid (GSC)	Gas	Solid adsorbent

1. *Adsorption Chromatography*: A process in which the stationary phase is a solid (e.g. Alumina or silica gel) and mobile phase is either a gas or a liquid. Separation takes place when one component of a two component mixture is more strongly adsorbed than the other by solid stationary phase.

   The distribution coefficient (K) of a substance between two phases of a system is given by:

$$K = \frac{\text{Amount of solute per unit of stationary phase}}{\text{Amount of solute per unit of mobile phase}}$$

2. *Adsorption Column Chromatography*: In this process, mobile phase in the form of liquid passes over stationary phase packed in a column (glass/metallic). Adsorbents used are starch, $CaCO_3$, lime (CaO), Silica gel, alumina (Al_2O_3), charcoal etc. Various mobile phases are used such as petroleum ether, $CHCl_3$, acetone, water, pyridine and organic acids.

Vertical column containing $CaCO_3$ (in powdered form) + petroleum ether extract of chlorophyll (a plant pigment) is passed $\xrightarrow[\text{With alcohol}]{\text{Column irrigated}}$

Develops the colour bands of definite boundaries in a column.

3. *Partition Chromatography*: In this process, the stationary phase is a liquid (H_2O) held on a suitable inert porous solid (cellulose). The mobile phase can be a gas or liquid mixture. Separation between two components of a mixture takes place when one component is strongly retained or adsorbed than the other by stationary phase.

   e.g. Separation of amino acids is carried out using partition columns; employing silica gel column and chloroform as a solvent.

4. *Paper Chromatography*: It is a technique in which the analysis of an unknown substance is carried out mainly by the flow of solvents on specially designed filter paper. An organic solvent partially miscible with water. e.g. Butanol or collidine is generally used.

   Paper chromatography is particularly applicable to water soluble plant constituents namely carbohydrates, amino acids, nucleic acid bases, organic acids and phenolic compounds.

   Two types of paper chromatography:

   (a) *Paper-partition*: Paper is used as an inert support with one solvent as mobile and other as stationary phase for separation.

   (b) *Paper adsorption*: A modified paper (impregnated with an adsorbent such as : silica or alumina) is used as an adsorbent and single solvent (mobile phase) is allowed to flow over unknown components.

5. *Exclusion Chromatography*: In this process, separation of the sample components takes place according to the molecular size.

   Two recently developed exclusion techniques are:

   (a) Gel permeation technique:

   Used in separation of sugars, polypeptides, proteins, lipids, polyethylenes, silicones, polystyrenes etc.

   Separation is effected as per size of solute molecules.

   (b) Sieving separation technique:

   Natural and synthetic zeolites (metal alumino silicates) are used.

A zeolite (molecular sieve) is represented as $M_2/n\ O\ Al_2\ O_3.\ xSiO_2.\ YH_2O$), where

M = Metal cation

n = valency of cation.

6. *Ion Exchange Chromatography*: Ion exchange resins consists of highly polymerized, cross-linked, organic materials containing large number of acidic/basic groups.

Zeolites acts as ion exchangers:

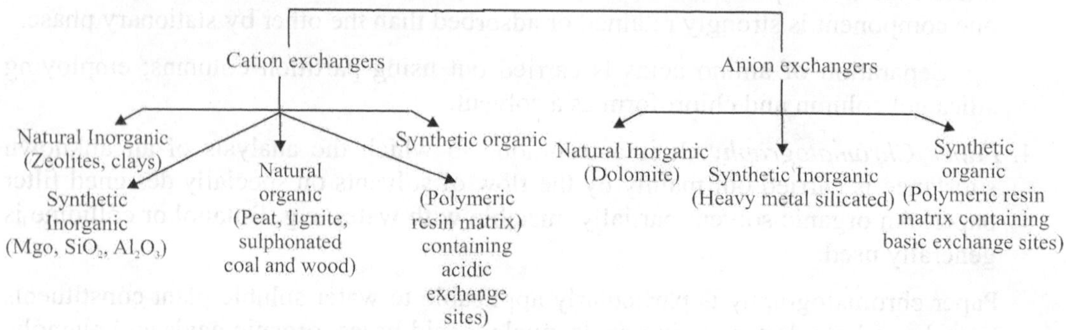

Thus, "Ion-exchange is a reversible process in which ions of like sign are exchanged between a liquid and a solid highly insoluble body in contact with it. The solid is known as an ion exchanger".

An ion-exchange resin is a special type of a poly electrolyte and consists of three dimensional polymeric hydrocarbon network to which are bonded a large number of electrically charged groups, such as sulphonate $\overline{SO_3}$ or quarternary ammonium group (N-$(CH_3)_4^+$).

7. *Reverse Phase Chromatography*: This is the form of partition chromatography in which an organic solvent is held by silica gel or cellulose as the static phase. The impregnation of paper is carried out by materials: alumina, rubber (vulcanized), $CaCO_3$, higher alcohols etc.

- Cortical steroids are separated by using papers dipped in propylene glycol, and excessive solvent removed by pressure.
- Gammexane isomers are separated by using a paper wetted with acetic anhydride and n-hexane/petroleum ether is used as a solvent.
- Br^{32} derivatives of D.D.T are isolated by coating paper through a solution of 3% vaseline in ether, using water, C_2H_5OH and 5% ammonia as a solvent and detected by Geiger counter.

8. *Electrophoresis*: This process involves the migration of colloidal particles through a solution under the influence of an electrical field. The above term is applied both to the migration to individual ions as well as to colloidal aggregates.

   In this process, any charged particle suspended between the poles of an electrical field tends to travel towards the pole that bears the charge opposite to its own.

   The rate of travel of particle depends upon:

   characteristics of the particle;

   properties of electric field;

   nature and temperature of suspending medium.

9. *Gel Chromatography*: It is a process in which fractionation is based on the molecular size and shape of the species in the sample. Also called as:

   gel permeation chromatography,

   size exclusion chromatography, or
   molecular sieve chromatography

   e.g.

   Sephadex gel is used in cross-linking of polysaccharide dextran with epichlorhydrin to obtain a polymer.

   Polyacrylamide cross-linked with methyl bisacrylamide is used as a resin.

   Gels used as stationary phases are either soft-gels /semi-rigid or rigid gels which generally swells in a suitable solvent and the space between polymer chains increases in size.

Some other techniques of chromatography are discussed in further pages. These are discussed with applications in evaluation of herbal drugs. The techniques are:

1. Thin layer chromatography (TLC)
2. High performance liquid chromatography (HPLC)
3. High performance thin layer chromatography (HPTLC)
4. Gas chromatography (GC)

1. *Thin Layer Chromatography (TLC)*: This chromatography involves use of thin layers of an adsorbent held on a glass plate (or other surrounding medium).

   A thin layer plate is prepared by spreading an aqueous slurry of grounded adsorbent over the surface of a glass plate or a microscopic slide and allowed to stand until the layer has set up (It may also be heated in an oven for several hours). Here the chromatogram is developed by ascending elution technique.

   For example: TLC technique is useful in analysis of alkaloids, glycosides, isoprenoids, lipid components, sugars and their derivatives.

Used in analysis of steroids and lipids (detection reagent used is conc. H_2SO_4 sprayed on the glass plates).

Analytical tool for micro analytical separation and determination of natural products.

The R_f values may vary depending upon the purity of solvent, nature of substance to be resolved, composition of solvent, presence of impurities, adsorbent used, and polarity of the solvent.

Adsorbent used in TLC:

- Silica gel widely used
- *Rarely used adsorbents are*: Aluminium oxide, calcium hydroxide, ion exchange resin, magnesium phosphate, polyamide, polyvinyl-pyrrolidone, cellulose and mixture of two or more of the above materials.

Detection:

The prepared TLC plates are sprayed with various suitable reagents for detection of compounds.

- The sensitivity of TLC is such that, separations on less than μg amounts of material can be achieved if necessary.
- The greater speed of TLC is due to more compact nature of adsorbent when spreaded on a plate (advantageous for labile compounds separation).

Table 13.2 Application of TLC in Evaluation of Herbal Drugs

Name of compounds Present in Herbal Drugs	Adsorbents used	Solvent-system used	Rf – value	Detecting Reagents used (by spraying)
Phenolic Compounds				
Resorcinol	Silica gel	$CH_3COOH : CHCl_3$ (1 : 9)	0.17	Vanillin – HCl Reagent used gives → Red colour
Hydroquinone	Silica gel	Ethyl acetate : Benzene (9 : 11)	0.58	None colour
Gallic acid	Cellulose MN-300	$C_6H_6 : CH_3OH : CH_3COOH$ (45 : 8 : 4) and 6.0% aqueous acetic acid	0.05 0.40	Blue colour Blue colour
Salicylic acid	Silica gel	$CH_3COOH : CHCl_3$ (1 : 9)	0.91	Blue after NH_3 fuming

Table 13.2 contd...

Name of compounds Present in Herbal Drugs	Adsorbents used	Solvent-system used	Rf – value	Detecting Reagents used (by spraying)
Chlorogenic acid	Silica gel	Toluene : Ethyl formate : formic acid (2 : 1 : 1)	0.16	UV light → Bright blue and UV + NH_3 → Bright blue
Kaempferol (flavonol)	Polyamide/Silica gel	Forestal → Conc. HCl : CH_3COOH : H_2O (3 : 30 : 10)	0.55	UV light and UV + NH_3 gives → Bright yellow
Apigenin (Flavone)	Polyamide/Silica gel	n-Butyl alcohol : CH_3COOH : H_2O (4 : 1 : 5)	0.89	UV light and UV + NH_3 gives → Bright yellow green
Terpenoids				
Limonene	Silica gel	Benzene : $CHCl_3$ (1 : 1)	-	Conc. H_2SO_4 → Brown
Geraniol	Silica gel	Benzene : $CHCl_3$ (1 : 1)	-	Conc. H_2SO_4 → Purple
Carvone	Silica gel	Benzene : $CHCl_3$ (1 : 1)	-	Conc. H_2SO_4 → Pink
Caraway (Carvone)	Silica gel	Benzene : $CHCl_3$ (1 : 1)	0.43	2, 4 – DNP → orange
Coriander (linalool)	Silica gel	Benzene : $CHCl_3$ (1 : 1)	0.26	Vanillin → mauve
Anise (Anethole, Anisaldehyde)	Silica gel	Benzene : $CHCl_3$ (1 : 1)	Anethole = 0.71 Anisaldehyde = 0.39	2, 4 – DNP → orange
Cumin (Cuminaldehyde)	Silica gel	Benzene : $CHCl_3$ (1 : 1)	0.58	2, 4 – DNP → orange
Fennel (Anethole)	Silica gel	Benzene : $CHCl_3$ (1 : 1)	0.72	2, 4 – DNP → Orange
Diterpenoids	Silica gel	n-hexane : CH_3COOH_3 (17:3)	-	Conc. H_2SO_4
Oleanolic acid	Silica gel	Petroleum : ethyl formate : formic acid (93 : 7 : 0.7)	0.70	$SbCl_3$ in $CHCl_3$
Diosgenin	Silica gel	$CHCl_3$: Acetone (4 : 1)	0.55	$SbCl_3$ in $CHCl_3$ Pink to purple
Gitogenin	Silica gel	$CHCl_3$: CH_3COOCH_3 (1 : 1)	0.21	$SbCl_3$ in $CHCl_3$ → Pink to purple
β-carotene (Carotenoids)	Cellulose	Petroleum : C_6H_6 (49 : 1)	0.84	In day light/UV light

Table 13.2 contd...

Name of compounds Present in Herbal Drugs	Adsorbents used	Solvent-system used	Rf – Value	Detecting Reagents used (by spraying)	
Amino acids and amines					
Glycine	Silica gel G	Phenol : Water (3 : 1)	0.24	Ninhydrin Reagent → Red violet	
Valine	Silica gel G	Phenol : water (3 : 1)	0.40	Ninhydrin → Violet	
Leucine	Silica gel G	n-butanol : acetic acid : H_2O (4 : 1 : 1)	0.44	Ninhydrin → violet	
Aspartic acid	Silica gel G	n-butanol : acetic acid : H_2O (4 : 1 : 1)	0.17	Ninhydrin → Blue-violet	
Phenylalanine	Silica gel G	Phenol : water (3 : 1)	0.55	Ninhydrin →Grey-violet	
Tryptophan	Silica gel G	n-butanol : acetic acid : H_2O (4 : 1 : 1)	0.47	Ninhydrin → Grey-violet	
Methylamine	Cellulose MN-300	n-butanol : acetic acid : H_2O (4 : 1 : 1)	0.24	Ninhydrin → Pink	
Ethanolamine	Silica gel HF-254	n-butanol : acetic acid : H_2O (4 : 1 : 1)	0.50	Ninhydrin → Purple	
Putrescine	Silica gel G	n-butanol : CH_3COOH : H_2O (4 : 1 : 1)	0.06	Ninhydrin → Purple	
Alkaloids				**Behaviour In UV Light**	**Reagents**
Nicotine	Silica gel-G	CH_3OH : NH_4OH (200 : 3)	0.57	Absorbs	Dragendorff
Morphine	Silica gel-G	CH_3OH : NH_4OH (200 : 3)	0.34	absorbs	Iodoplatinate
Solanine	Silica gel-G	CH_3OH : NH_4OH (200 : 3)	0.52	Invisible	Marquis
Codeine	Silica gel-G	CH_3OH : NH_4OH (200 : 3)	0.35	Absorbs	Iodoplatinate
Atropine	Silica gel-G	70% C_2H_5OH : 25% NH_4OH (99 : 1)	0.18	Absorbs	Iodoplatinate
Quinine	Silica gel	CH_3OH : NH_4OH (200 : 3)	0.52	Bright blue	Iodoplatinate

- Dragendorff reagent shows: orange brown spot on a yellow background.
- Iodoplatinate reagent shows: Various range of colour
- Marquis Reagent shows: Yellow to purple spot

2. *Gas or Gas-liquid Chromatography (GLC)*: Gas chromatography is basically a separation technique in which the components of a vapourised sample are separated and fractionated as a consequence of partition between a mobile gaseous phase and a stationary phase held in a column. The partition takes place between a gas and liquid or gas and solid.

   The mobile phase is a gas and stationary phase is a liquid in gas liquid chromatography (GLC). The GLC can be expressed in terms of:

   - Retention volume (R_v): The volume of carrier gas required to elute a component from the column.
   - Retention time (R_t): The time required for elution of the sample.

These parameters are always expressed in terms relative to a standard compound (as RR_v or RR_t) which may be added to the sample extract/ or which could take the form of the solvent used for dissolving that sample.

The main variables in GLC are: Stationary phase of column and temperature of operation.

These are varied according to the polarity and volatility of compounds being separated. Many classes of substances are converted to derivatives (especially to trimethyl silyl ethers) before being subjected to GLC, since this allows their separation at a lower temperature.

GLC provides both quantitative and qualitative data on plant substances, since measurement of area under the peaks is directly proportional to the concentrations of different components in the original mixture. There are two general formulae for measuring these areas:

(i) Peak height × peak width (at half of height) = 94% of peak area

(ii) Peak area is equivalent to that of a triangle produced by drawing tangents.

Applications

(i) GLC find its main applications with volatile compounds, fatty acids, mono and sesquiterpenes, hydrocarbons and sulphur compounds.

(ii) In cosmetics and perfume fields, GLC is helpful in determination of their composition.

(iii) GLC linked to mass spectrometry (MS) and combined GLC-MS apparatus is used for phytochemical analysis.

Applications of GC(GLC) in Evaluation of herbal drugs

1. *GLC Parameters for Phenolic compounds using GLC*:

   Examples: Phenol, o, m, p-cresol, catechol, hydroquinone

Liquid in stationary column: Polyphenyl ether OS124 (PPE)
Trixylenyl phosphate (TXP)
Diethylene Glycol succinate (DEGS)

Temperature: 130-60 $^{\circ}$C/150-80 $^{\circ}$C at 1.5° / min

2. *GLC Parameters for Triterperoids:*

Examples	:	Cholestane, α-amyrin, oleanolic acid methyl ester, primulagenin as trimethyl silyl ether
Liquid in stationary column	:	DEGS (Diethylene glycol succinate), SE-30, ov-1 (methyl siloxane polymer), QF-1. These liquid phases applied to a solid support (chromosorb-w)
Temperature	:	220-250 $^{\circ}$C
Gas flow rate	:	50-100 ml/min

3. *GLC Parameters for Fatty acids and lipids*:

Examples	:	Triglycerides, phospholipids, Glycolipids, stearic acid, Palmitic acid, linoleic acid, phosphatidyl choline, triacyl glycerol.
Liquid in stationary column	:	Poly ethylene glycol (PEG) adipate
Temperature	:	200 $^{\circ}$C

4. *GLC parameters for Amino acids*:

Examples	:	Glycine, Alanine, Tyrosine, Serine, Glutamic acid, Arginine, Histidine, Phenylalanine.
Liquid in stationary column	:	Chromosorb-w (60-80 mesh) coated with 1% polyethylene glycol (carbowax 1546 or 6000)
Temperature	:	125 and 155 $^{\circ}$C
Gas flow rate	:	60 to 240 ml/min

5. *GLC parameters for alkaloids*:

Examples	:	Tobacco	Tropane	Opium
Liquid stationary column	:	5.6% polyethylene glycol	1% Dimethyl Polysiloxane	2-3% silicone SE-30 on Chromo sorb-w
Temperature	:	170-200 $^{\circ}$C	100-300 $^{\circ}$C	204 $^{\circ}$C

6. *GLC Parameters of Cyanogenetic Glycosides*:

Examples	:	Trimethylsilyl ethers, Linamarin, Lotaustralin
Liquidin stationary column	:	10-20% SE-20 on silanized chromosorb W(80-100 mesh)
Temperature	:	210 °C temperature

7. *GLC Parameters of Sugars*:

Examples	:	Natural and synthetic sugars
Liquid in stationary column	:	Silanized chromosorb W column coated with 3% SE-52
Temperature	:	180 °C and inlet pressure of 15 p.s.i

3. *High Performance Liquid Chromatography (HPLC)*:

"HPLC is a method of separation in which the stationary phase is contained in a column, one end of which is attached to a source of pressurized liquid eluent (mobile phase)". By using HPLC, adsorption, partition, ion-exchange and exclusion column separations are successfully possible.

- The stationary phase bonded to a porous polymer is held in a narrow-bore stainless steel column and liquid mobile phase is forced under through a considerable pressure.
- The mobile phase is a miscible solvent mixture, which either remains constant or may be changed in its proportions by including a mixing chamber into the set-up (as in gradient elution technique).
- An increase in temperature shortens the analysis time for most mobile phases. High temperatures are required for highly viscous solvents/samples but a lower pressure is required to pump the mobile phase or to inject the sample.

Applications

HPLC is mainly used for those classes of compounds which are non-volatile in nature, e.g. higher terpenoids, phenolics, alkaloids, lipids and sugars. It works best for the compounds which can be detected in UV or visible regions of spectrum.

***Applications of HPLC in Evaluation of Herbal Drugs*:**

1. *HPLC Parameters for Anthocyanins:*

Examples	:	Mono, Di-, Tri-glyosides, Acylated diglucoside
Column used	:	µ-Bondapak c_{18} or Lichrosorb RP-18
Solvent system	:	water : Acetic acid : CH_3OH (71 : 10 : 19)

2. *HPLC Parameters for Andrographolides*:

Columns used	:	5 μm spherical silica (3.00 mm × 15 cm)
Solvent system	:	$CHCl_3 : CH_3OH$ (9 : 1)
Flow rate	:	0.7 ml/min
Detector	:	UV at 254 nm

3. *HPLC Parameters for Diterpenoids*

Example	:	Methanol extract
Columns used	:	Zorbax ODS C_{18} column (25 × 0.46 cm)
Solvent system	:	$CH_3OH : H_2O$ (9 : 11)

4. *HPLC Parameters for Sterols*:

Examples	:	22-dehydro campesterol
Columns used	:	Lichrosorb RP-18
Solvent system	:	$CH_3OH : H_2O$ (98 : 2)

5. *HPLC Parameters for Carotenoids*:

Examples	:	Lycopene, α-carotene, β-carotene
Columns used	:	Partisil-5 ODS C_{18}
Solvent system	:	Chloroform : Acetonitrile (2 : 25)

6. *HPLC Parameters for Carbohydrates*:

Examples	:	Un-derivatized sugars
Columns used	:	Waters Bondapak, Partisil-10 PAC or Spheri sorb S $5NH_2$
Solvent system	:	Acetonitrile : water (89 : 11)

Table 13.3 HPLC Parameters for Alkaloids

Alkaloids	**Columns used**	**Solvent system**	**Wave length of UV Detection**
Quinazolidine (cytosine)	Lichrosorb SI-100 (50 × 0.3 cm)	15% CH_3OH in C_2H_5-O-C_2H_5 : 2.5% NH_4OH (50 : 1)	220 nm 310 nm
Morphine	5 μm-porous silica gel (30 × 0.39 cm)	Hexane : $CHCl_3$: C_2H_5OH : $C_2H_5NHC_2H_5$ (60 : 6 : 8 : 0.1)	285 nm

Table 13.3 contd….

Alkaloids	Columns used	Solvent system	Wave length of UV Detection
Indole	7 m Merck RP-8 (25 ×0.2 cm)	CH_3OH : H_2O : HCOOH (166 : 34 : 1)	330 nm
Emetine	Merckosorb SI-60 (20 × 0.2 cm)	$CHCl_3$: CH_3OH (17 : 3)	254 nm
Steroidal (solanidine)	Zorbax SIL (50 × 0.46 cm)	Hexane : CH_3OH : CH_3COCH_3 (18 : 1 : 1)	213 nm

4. High Performance Thin Layer Chromatography (HPTLC)

"High Performance Thin Layer chromatography (synonym : planar chromatography), is a modern and powerful analytical technique with separation power, performance, and reproducibility superior to classic TLC."

- Based on the use of high performance TLC plates with small particle sizes and precise instruments for each step of chromatographic processes. (such as sample application, chromatogram development, chromatogram evaluation).
- HPTLC provides the means not only for flexible screening procedures and qualitative analysis but also for demanding quantitative determinations.
- Instruments are easily validated and are fully compliant with GMP.
- HPTLC features highly sensitive scanning densitometry and video technology for rapid chromatogram evaluation and documentation.
- Nowadays, HPTLC instruments are computer controlled and thus improved analytical results are obtained.
- In HPTLC, silica gel (stationary phase) is used as a sorbent.
- Sample preparation in HPTLC needs a very high concentrated solution and the size of sample spot must not exceed 1 mm in diameter.
- Different techniques for spotting samples are:
  (a) Self-loading capillaries: Small volume of samples is applied to HPTLC plate surface using platinum-iridium tubing fused into the end of a length of glass tubing contact spotting.
  (b) Linear development technique: Plate is placed vertically in solvent system in a container. The solvent is usually fed by capillary action.

Applications

- HPTLC used in studying biochemistry of natural products.
- HPTLC technique is used to develop analytical profiles for cardenolides, tropane alkaloids, flavonoids, steroidal compounds, anthracene aglycones, lipids etc.

- HPTLC is applied to obtain "Finger-Print" patterns of herbal formulations; quantification of active ingredients and detection of adulteration.

	Drugs		Solvent system
(i)	Saponins	=	$CH_3OH : CHCl_3$: water (4 : 7 : 1)
(ii)	Cardiac glycosides	=	Dichloromethane : $CH_3OH : HCONH_2$ (8 : 2 : 1)
(iii)	Alkaloids and amino acids	=	n-butanol : CH_3COOH : water (4 : 5 : 1)
(iv)	Terpenes, essential oils and sterols	=	Hexane : Acetone (9 : 1)

Applications of HPTLC in Evaluation of Herbal Drugs

1. Panaxadiol and Panaxatriol (Ginseng):
   - Sorbent used : Silica
   - Solvent system : Chloroform : ether (1 : 1)
   - Reagents used : Spraying with 10% H_2SO_4 acid in CH_3OH, heating at 105 °C for 10 min
   - Quantification : UV absorbance (in densitometry) = 544 nm and 52 nm
2. Aloin (Aloevera spp):
   - Sorbent used : Silica gel
   - Solvent system : Ethyl acetate : HCOOH : water (17 : 2 : 3)
   - Quantification : UV absorbance (in densitometry) = 350 nm
3. Flavonol Glycosides (*Gingko biloba*):
   - Sorbent used : Silica gel
   - Solvent system : $CHCl_3 : C_6H_6 : C_2H_5OH : H_2O$: acetic acid (11 : 4 : 2 : 2 : 1)
   - Reagents used : Spraying with 8% $AlCl_3$ in C_2H_5OH
   - Quantification : UV absorbance (in densitometry) = 370 nm
4. 18 β- Glycyrrhetinic acid (Liquorice):
   - Sorbent used : Silica gel
   - Solvent system : Ethyl acetate : $CH_3OH : NH_3$ (10 : 3 : 1)
   - Quantification : UV absorbance (in densitometry) = 260 nm
5. Carvone (*Cuminum cyminum*):
   - Sorbent used : Silica gel
   - Solvent system : $CHCl_3$: Acetone (100 : 2)

Reagent used : By dipping in anisaldehyde sulphuric acid reagent, heating at 80 °C temperature for about 10 minutes

Quantification : UV absorbance (in densitometry) = 410 nm

6. Cholesterol (from Bear gall bladder powder):

Sorbent used : Silica gel

Solvent system : Ethyl acetate : acetone : petroleum ether (2 : 1 : 11)

Reagents used : Spraying with 10% H_2SO_4 acid in alcohol, heating at 100 °C temperature for 5 minutes.

Quantification : UV absorbance (in densitometry) = 400 nm

Comparison of TLC and HPTLC in evaluation of Herbal Drugs

Similarities

1. TLC and HPTLC are simple to learn and perform for evaluation.
2. Precoated plates are usually employed.
3. The whole chromatogram is easily inspected.
4. Not necessary to elute the individual components.
5. Both the methods are carried out economically because solvent consumption is small.
6. The method of detection does not place any restrictions on the choice of mobile phase.
7. Acidic, basic or purely aqueous eluents can be used.

Dissimilarities

Comparision of Plate Material

Characteristics	TLC	HPTLC
1. Particle size distribution (mm)	2-40	2-10
2. Average Particle size (mm)	10-15	5
3. Layer thickness (mm)	250	100, 200
4. Separation Distance (mm)	100-150	30-70
5. Optimal separation distance (mm)	120	60
6. Running time for optimum distance (min)	30-60	7-20
7. Solvent consumption (Twin through chamber)	25-50 (20 × 20 cm)	10-20 (20 × 10cm)
8. Detection limit, absorbance (ng)	100-1000	10-100
9. Detection limit, Fluorescence (ng)	1-100	0.1-10
10. Separation power	TLC have less separation	HPTLC layers are more

	power than HPTLC	homogenous, have a smoother surface and a higher separation power than conventional TLC plates.

Finger Printing Methods

HPTLC fingerprinting methods serve as a stability indicating method, even when the chromatogram is not differentiated. Finger-printing method can be best understood by studying following example:

1. *HPTLC identification of Vlerian by finger printing method:*

Sample Solution	:	Shake 0.2 gm freshly powdered valerian with 5 ml of CH_2Cl_2 for one minute, allowed to stand for five minutes and then filtered it. Washed the filter with 2 ml of CH_2Cl_2 and evaporated the filtrate to dryness. Dissolved the residue in 0.2 ml of CH_2Cl_2.
Standard Solution (Optional)	:	1 mg of valerenic acid in 0.5 ml of CH_2Cl_2
Anisaldehyde Reagent	:	Mixed 9 ml 98% H_2SO_4 + 85 ml Methanol + 10 ml acetic acid + 0.5 ml anisaldehyde in a water bath/ice bath.
HCl-Acetic acid Reagent	:	Mixed 20 ml acetic acid + 80 ml HCl acid

Chromatographic Condition:

Stationary phase	:	HPTLC plates (10 × 10 cm) silica gel 60 F 254 (Merck/equivalent)
Mobile phase	:	Hexane : Ethyl acetate : acetic acid (65 : 35 : 0.5)
Sample application	:	With Linomat IV on automatic TLC sampler-III ⇒ 3 ml of test solution and standard solution as 10 mm bands, space 6 mm and 8 mm from lower edge.
Development	:	10 × 10 cm twin through chamber saturated for 10 minutes (filter paper) developing distance 55 cm.
Detection	:	• UV = 254 nm

- HCl-Acetic acid reagent is sprayed, dried in cold air, heated to 110 °C for 5 minutes.
  UV spectra = 366 nm.
- Anisaldehyde reagent is sprayed, dried in cold air and heated to 120 °C for 2 minutes.
  UV spectra = 260 nm

2. *HPTLC Fingerprint Identification of Ginseng Medicine*: HPTLC fingerprints of ginseng preparations revealed the instability of ginsenosides in liquid dosage forms containing royal jelly and honey in admixture with ginseng extract.

CHAPTER 14

SPECTRAL ANALYSIS OF HERBAL DRUGS

14.1 Spectroscopy

"Spectroscopy is the branch of analytical chemistry dealing with the study of interaction of electromagnetic radiation with the matter". The spectrum is divided into a series of regions corresponding to the type of absorption or emission obtained.

e.g. In UV and visible regions, electronic transitions of atoms and molecules are observed while in IR region, molecular vibration is observed.

Ultraviolet and Visible Spectroscopy (UV-V is spectra):

1. The absorption spectra of plant constituents is measured in very dilute solution against a solvent blank using an automatic recording spectrophotometer.
2. For colourless compounds: Range for measurements is 200 to 400 nm

   For coloured compounds: Range for measurements is 200 to 700 nm.
3. The wavelengths of maxima and minima of absorption spectrum so obtained are recorded (in nm).
4. The intensity of absorbance at particular maxima and minima is also recorded.
5. Such type of spectral measurements are used in the identification of various plant constituents, for monitoring the eluates of chromatographic columns during purification of plant products, and for screening crude plant extracts for the presence of polyacetylenes compounds.
6. Solvent widely used for UV spectroscopy is 95% ethanol (C_2H_5OH).

(Commercial absolute alcohol should not be used, as it contains residual benzene which get absorbed in short UV range). Other solvents used are water, CH_3OH, hexane, petroleum and ether.

7. Solvents such as $CHCl_3$ and pyridine are not used as they absorb strongly in 200-600 nm region. (Hence, they are suitable for making measurements in visible regions of spectrum with plant pigments such as carotenoids.
8. The spectral utility is increased by repeating measurements made in neutral solution.

   e.g.

   - When alkali is added to alcoholic solutions of phenolic compounds, the UV-spectra shifts towards longer wavelengths (i.e., bathochronic shift) with increase in absorbance.
   - When alkali is added to neutral solutions of aromatic carboxylic acids, UV-spectra shifts in the opposite direction towards shorter wave-lengths (i.e., hypsochromic shift).
9. If a substance shows a single absorption band between 250-260 nm, the compound is a simple phenol, purine/pyrimidine, an aromatic acid.
10. If it shows, three distinct peaks in 400-500 nm region, the compound is carotenoid.

Table 14.1 Spectral Properties of Different classes of plant pigments (in Herbal Drugs)

Class of Pigments	Ultra Violet range (nm)	Visible spectral range (nm)
Chlorophylls (green)	Intense short UV absorption due to protein attachment	640-660 and 430-470
Phycobilins (red and blue)		615-650 and 540-570
Cytochromes (yellow)		545-605 and 415-440
Anthocyanins (Red)	275	475-550
Betacyanins (mauve)	250-270	530-554
Carotenoids (yellow to orange		400-500
Anthraquinones (yellow)	3-4 intense peaks between 220 and 290	420-460
Yellow Flavonols	250-270	365-390

14.2 Infra-Red Spectroscopy (IR-Spectra)

The region which extends about 8000 Å - 35000 Å wavelength is known as infra red region. Infra-Red radiations are associated with much lower energy than UV-vis radiation.

1. IR-spectra is measured on plant substances in an automatic recording IR-spectrophotometers either in solution (in $CHCl_3$ or CCl_4 as 1-5%) or in solid state (mixed with KBr).
2. The region in IR-spectra above 1200 cm^{-1} shows spectral bands due to the vibrations of individual bonds or functional groups in the molecule under examination.
3. The region below 1200 cm^{-1} shows spectral bands due to the vibrations of whole molecule and because of its complexity is called as finger print region. Thus, in this region multiplicity assures the individual identification of bands, but collectively absorption bands help in identifying the material.
4. IR-spectroscopy is most frequently used in phytochemical studies as a "finger printing device", for comparing a natural with a synthetic sample.
5. IR-spectral analysis is extensively used for identifying known essential oil components.

Characteristic Infra-Red Frequencies of some Natural Products

Natural Products	Approximate Positions of characteristic bands above 1200 cm^{-1}
Alkanes	2940 (S), 2860 (M), 1455 (S), 1380 (M)
Alkenes	3050 (W-M), 1850 (W), 1650 (W-M), 1410 (W)
Aromatics	3050 (W-M), 2100-1700 (W), 1600, 1580, 1500 (W-M)
Alcohols and Phenols	3610 (W-M), 3600-2400 (Broad), 1410 (M)
Aldehydes and ketones	2750 (W), 2680 (W), 1820-1650 (S), 1420 (W-M)
Esters and Lactones	1820-1680(S)
Carboxylic acids	3520 (W), 3400-2500 (Broad), 1760 (S), 1710 (S)

S = Strong, M = Medium, W = weak

14.3 Mass Spectroscopy (MS-Spectra)

"Mass spectroscopy, is an instrumental technique in which the sample is converted into rapidly moving positive ions, which are then separated and characterised." The mass spectrometer is an instrument which produces charged ions consisting of parent ion and ionic fragments of original molecule and sorts these ions according to their mass/charge ratio.

1. MS-spectra technique requires only microgram (μg) amounts of material, because it can provide an accurate molecular weight and yields a complex fragmentation pattern which is often characteristic of that particular compound.
2. MS-spectra degrades trace amounts of an organic compound and records the fragmentation pattern according to mass.

   (The sample vapour diffuses into the low pressure system of mass spectrometer where it is ionized with sufficient energy to cause fragmentation of chemical bonds).
3. MS-spectral analytical technique works successfully with low molecular weight plant constituent and has been used for peptide analysis.
4. Those compounds which are too involatile to vaporize in Ms-instrument, are converted into trimethyl silyl ethers, methyl esters or their derivatives.
5. MS spectra is used in conjunction with GLC and combined operation provides at one go a qualitative and quantitative identification of many structurally complex component. GLC used for separation and isolation of the component where as Mass spectra detect it in GLC-Ms apparatus.
6. *e.g.* Zeatin (first naturally occurring cytokinin) = detached and isolated from higher plants.

   Zeatin = Structure (6-(4-hydroxy methyl) –trans-2-butenylamino) purine

   = Formulae ($C_{10} H_{13} ON_5$)

Ms-spectra confirms that zeatin is an adenine nucleus by the study of various characteristic fragment and its structure was determined. Thus, in phytochemical research, Ms-measurements is of great importance.

14.4 Nuclear Magnetic Resonance Spectroscopy (NMR-spectra)

"This spectroscopy involves the magnetic energy of nuclei when they are placed in a magnetic field and transitions occur in the wave region of the spectrum. Generally, the study of radio frequency radiation by nuclei is called NMR-spectra."

1. Proton NMR-spectra provides a means of determining the structure of an organic compound by measuring magnetic moments of its hydrogen atoms.
2. In most of the compounds, hydrogen atoms are attached to different groups (such as $–CH_2$, CH_3, –CHO, $–NH_2$, –CHOH–) and proton NMR-spectrum provides a record of number of hydrogen atoms in these different situations.
3. In NMR-spectra, sample of a substance is placed in the solution in an inert solvent, between the poles of a powerful magnet and protons undergo different chemical shifts according to their molecular environments within the molecule. These are

measured in NMR apparatus in relation to standard and inert compound named tetramethyl silane (TMS).

4. In NNR-spectroscopy, the sample is recovered unchanged after the operation and is used for other determinations.
5. Proton NMR spectroscopy is used by phytochemist as a finger printing technique.
6. The major use of proton NMR is for structural determination and in combination with other spectral techniques.
7. Due to the interaction between protons attached to adjacent carbon atoms, the spectral signals appears as doublets or triplets instead of as single peaks. This confirms that proton NMR-spectra is quite complex.
8. The phytochemical information of any compound can be obtained without analyzing the spectrum in detail.

e.g.

- Sterulic acid (a fatty acid) contains strained cyclo propene ring in its structure confirmed by NMR-spectra.
- Yellow flavonoid pigment named tambuletin contains a flavonol aglycone structure conformed by NMR spectra lateron.

Characteristics of Different Classes of Plant Products

Proton Nuclear Magnetic Resonance Chemical Shifts

Category/Class	Type of Proton	Range of Shift δ (P.P.m)
Alkanes and Fatty acids	$CH_3—R$	0.85-0.95
	$R—CH_2—R$	1.20-1.35
Alkenes	$CH_3—C{=}C$	1.60-1.69
	$—CH = C$	5.20-5.70
Acetylenes	$HC{\equiv}C$	2.45-2.65
Aromatic compounds	Ar—H	6.60-8.00
	$Ar—CH_3$	2.25-2.50
	Ar—CHO	9.70-10.00
Nitrogen compounds	$N—CH_3$	2.10-3.00
	N—CHO	7.90-8.10
	N—H	variable